Cleft Lip and Palate: Diagnosis and Management

Cleft Lip and Palate: Diagnosis and Management

Editor: Binnie Pattinson

MURPHY & MOORE
www.murphy-moorepublishing.com

www.murphy-moorepublishing.com

MURPHY & MOORE

Cataloging-in-Publication Data

Cleft lip and palate : diagnosis and management / edited by Binnie Pattinson.
p. cm.
Includes bibliographical references and index.
ISBN 978-1-63987-108-7
1. Cleft lip. 2. Cleft palate. 3. Cleft lip--Surgery. 4. Cleft palate--Surgery. I. Pattinson, Binnie.
RD524 .C54 2022
617.522--dc23

Murphy & Moore Publishing,
1 Rockefeller Plaza,
New York City, NY 10020, USA

ISBN 978-1-63987-108-7 (Hardback)

Contents

Preface

This book was inspired by the evolution of our times; to answer the curiosity of inquisitive minds. Many developments have occurred across the globe in the recent past which has transformed the progress in the field.

The openings or splits in the upper lip or the roof of the mouth are known as cleft lip and cleft palate. These are defects which are present at birth. It is caused when the tissues of the mouth and face do not fuse in a proper manner. The reasons behind cleft lip and palate can be either environmental or genetic in nature. There are various complications which can be caused by it such as dental issues, feeding difficulties, difficulty in speaking, ear infections, and other emotional and social problems due to differences in appearance. The management of a cleft lip involves multiple medical specialties. A few of them are pediatrics, orthodontics, nursing, genetic counseling, otorhinolaryngology and speech therapy. Most of the topics introduced in this book cover new techniques in the diagnosis and management of cleft lip and palate. Different approaches, evaluations, methodologies and advanced studies on this medical condition have been included in it. Those in search of information to further their knowledge will be greatly assisted by this book.

This book was developed from a mere concept to drafts to chapters and finally compiled together as a complete text to benefit the readers across all nations. To ensure the quality of the content we instilled two significant steps in our procedure. The first was to appoint an editorial team that would verify the data and statistics provided in the book and also select the most appropriate and valuable contributions from the plentiful contributions we received from authors worldwide. The next step was to appoint an expert of the topic as the Editor-in-Chief, who would head the project and finally make the necessary amendments and modifications to make the text reader-friendly. I was then commissioned to examine all the material to present the topics in the most comprehensible and productive format.

I would like to take this opportunity to thank all the contributing authors who were supportive enough to contribute their time and knowledge to this project. I also wish to convey my regards to my family who have been extremely supportive during the entire project.

Editor

1

Orthodontics in Relation with Alveolar Bone Grafting in CLP Patients

Aslıhan Uzel

Abstract

Alveolar bone grafting is an essential step in the overall management of patients with cleft lip and palate (CLP). The numerous advantages of this procedure have been reported in the literature. Failure to rehabilitate the alveolar cleft may give rise to a variety of problems. Lack of investing alveolar bone often precludes the correction of anterior tooth irregularities and limits orthodontic treatment and/or prosthodontic rehabilitation. The success of the graft is multifactorial. The periodontal health of the surrounding graft tissues, the experience and ability of the surgeon, the timing of surgery, and orthodontic management of the cleft area before and after grafting are shown to be the most important factors in this issue. In this chapter, current orthodontic approaches in relation with alveolar bone grafting (ABG) in cleft patients will be discussed.

Keywords: cleft palate, alveolar bone grafting, orthodontics

1. Introduction

Cleft lip and palate (CLP) are among the most common of all congenital facial deformities which affect approximately 1 in every 600 newborn babies worldwide [1]. Congenital CL/P can arise in isolation or together with other syndromes. Alveolar cleft (osseous defect in the alveolus of upper jaw) affects approximately 75% of cleft lip and palate patients [2, 3].

The rehabilitation of individuals with CL/P requires interdisciplinary care by centralization of treatment [1, 4].

As the facial cleft affects the whole stomatognathic system, orthodontics is a core element of the overall treatment process. The orthodontist should aim to provide a dentition that functions well and is capable of lifetime maintenance by routine oral hygiene and dental care. However, the underlying skeletal deformity that reflects intrinsic variation and the consequences of surgery severely restricts occlusal change [5].

There are two major factors which effect orthodontic treatment in patients with CLP:

1. Facial growth disruption

It is well known that facial growth in patient with CP is disturbed. Besides the intrinsic defect, surgery itself contributes to further disruption [3, 6]. A significant feature of facial growth in repaired CP patients is that the maxilla fails to grow at the same rate as the mandible during the adolescent growth spurt. Progressive midfacial retrusion is usually seen by the mid- to late teens. The results of the facial growth studies revealed the general characteristics of the individuals with UCLP: a short retrusive maxilla and vertical elongation of the anterior face, a retrusive mandible, and a reduction in posterior face height [6–9].

2. Alveolar bone deficiency

Lack of the alveolar bone may give rise to a variety of problems, including oronasal fistula, fluid reflux, speech pathology, impaired tooth eruption, lack of bone support for the anterior teeth, dental crowding, periodontal recession and eventual loss of teeth, and maxillary and facial asymmetry. Alveolar defect also limits orthodontic treatment and/or prosthodontic rehabilitation [10–12].

Thus, orthodontic treatment for children with cleft should aim to achieve an optimal occlusion and dentofacial esthetics within the constraints imposed by the underlying skeletal pattern [5].

The integration of orthodontics into the overall treatment of CLP starts any point between birth and end of the teens and highly related to surgical procedures, including lip repair, alveolar bone grafting, distraction, and orthognathic surgery [5].

This chapter reviews current orthodontic approaches in relation with alveolar bone grafting (ABG) in nonsyndromic cleft patients.

2. Alveolar bone grafting

Alveolar bony defect is the main limiting factor for orthodontic treatment. Elimination of the bony defect is provided by alveolar bone grafting (ABG). Since the introduction of secondary alveolar bone grafting (SABG) in 1972, this technique has become an essential step in the overall management of patients with cleft lip and palate (CLP). Providing bone tissue for cleft has following benefits: [10, 12–21]

1. To permit eruption of the permanent canine in the cleft site into sound bone.
2. To provide bony support for teeth on either side of the cleft site.
3. To permit orthodontic tooth movement.

4. To obviate or minimize the need for prosthetic replacement of teeth in the cleft site.
5. To permit placement of osseointegrated implants into the cleft area when indicated.
6. To stabilize maxillary dental arch.
7. To facilitate fistula closure.
8. To improve the contour of the alar base.

The long-term success of the alveolar graft is crucial for providing and lifetime maintaining optimal occlusion and dentofacial esthetics in patients with CLP.

Postgraft stimulation of maturation through remodeling of the graft is extremely important and is provided primarily by natural tooth eruption. Thus, it is generally agreed that the optimum timing for ABG is in the mixed dentition stage (8–11 years), just before the eruption of the permanent canine in line with the cleft side [10, 13, 16, 19, 22–29]. There is no precise recommended chronological age but, when one-half to two-thirds of the canine root is formed [10]. Canines are mostly the reference teeth because lateral incisors in patient with CLP are frequently absent. However, if lateral incisor is present, earlier bone grafting can be indicated at an age around 7–8 years. It has been found that the success rate is significantly reduced when ABG is performed after eruption of the canine. Resorption of the bone graft is a common situation, and the success of ABG depends on several factors. The periodontal health of the surrounding graft tissues, the experience and ability of the surgeon, and graft material are also shown to be the general factors determining success [13, 19, 20, 23, 30, 31].

The importance of the orthodontist in planning, preparations, and follow-up around ABG procedure is also widely recognized. Successful alveolar bone grafting necessitates a joint orthodontic and surgical involvement pre-, peri-, and postoperatively [10, 32, 33].

Before treatment, orthodontists should be able to explain the predicted outcome of bone grafting to patients and their parents [34].

At that point, diagnostic information is very important for planning pre- and post-orthodontic management.

3. Advantages of CBCT in diagnosing and treatment planning of patients with CLP

A bony bridge with sufficient height and width is important for successful bone grafting in the alveolar cleft and to guide eruption and movement of permanent teeth [15, 35–37]. The outcome of the procedure is considered satisfactory when a sufficient volume of remodeled bone tissue is obtained; otherwise, the surgery has to be repeated. Thus, volumetric measurements of CBCT images have been using to evaluate the success of alveolar graft outcomes in the current literature [38]. CBCT, an alternative approach to conventional CT that provides similar diagnostic information with much less radiation exposure, avoids the problems associated with traditional 2D imaging such as image enlargement and distortion, structure

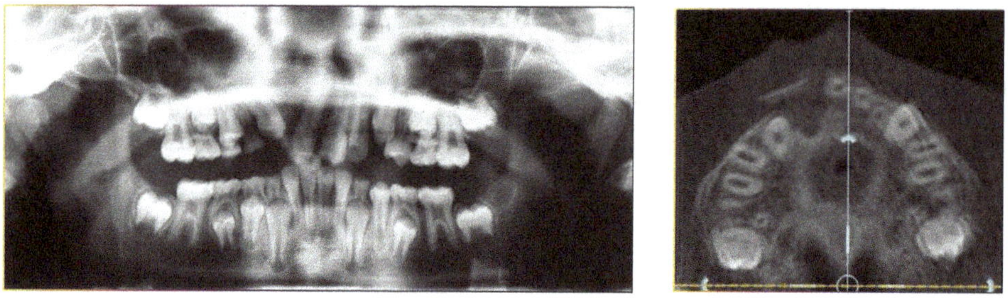

a b

Figure 1. Superimpositions on the 2D imaging might led to misdiagnosis. (a) Grafted area seems to be filled successfully on the pantomograph; (b) axial view of the CBCT image shows that graft is not successful as seen on the panoramic radiograph.

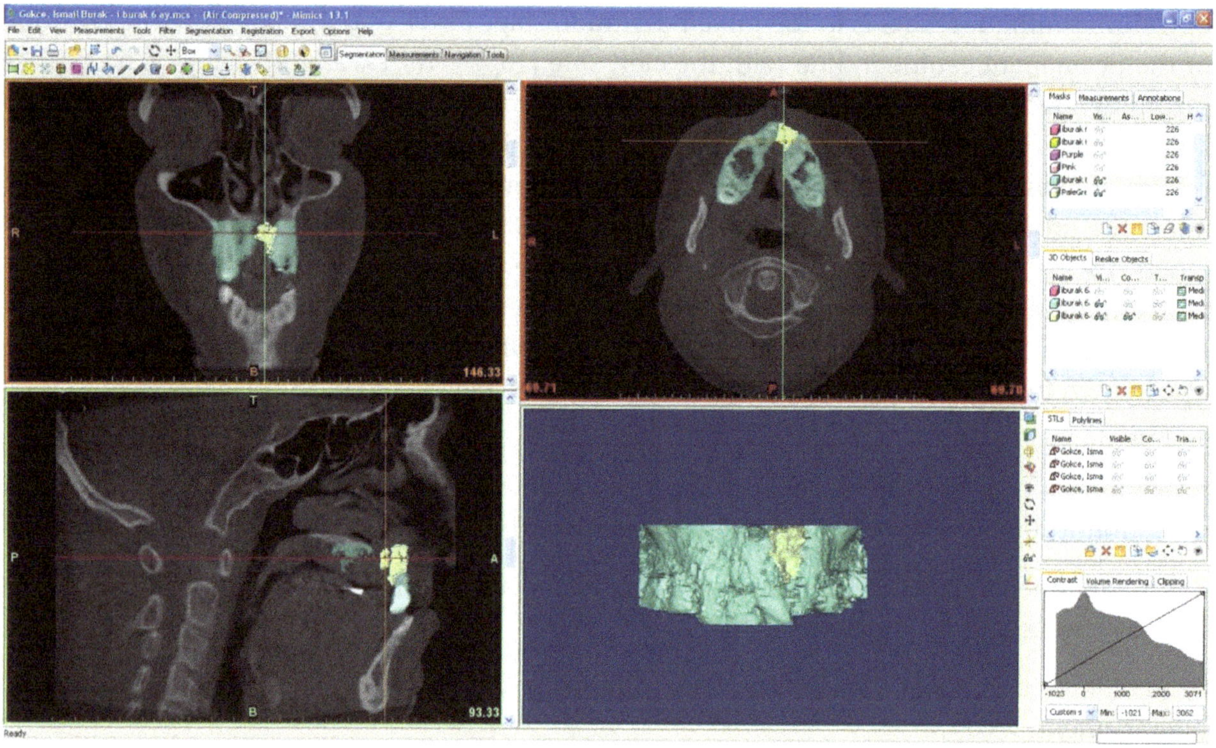

Figure 2. The precise volume and density can be measured by using various software.

overlap, positional problems, and limited number of identifiable landmarks (**Figure 1**). It has been used to quantify the average volume of the graft, location of the bone loss, and periodontal bone support of the cleft-adjacent teeth. CBCT-derived volumetric assessment of alveolar grafts has been reported as a reliable method [24, 29, 37, 39, 40] (**Figure 2**). The success rate of an alveolar graft has been found to be significantly lower with volumetric evaluation than that with conventional radiographic imaging [39, 41, 42].

4. Mixed dentition stage (phase I orthodontic treatment)

Orthodontic treatment of patients with CLP takes much more time (is more extensive) than routine treatment because of the underlying skeletal pattern. There is no need to attempt

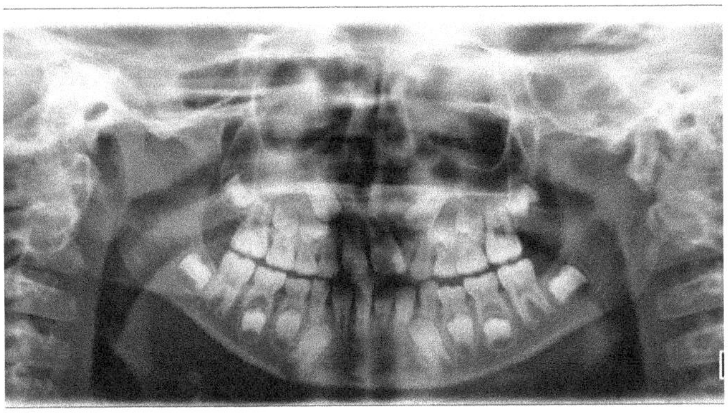

Figure 3. Malpositioned lateral incisor in the cleft area should be extracted 3–4 weeks before ABG.

orthodontic treatment in deciduous dentition stage. This will need much more retention procedures and will impose unnecessary burden of care [5].

Monitoring eruption of the teeth is important by the age 6–7.Radiographic evaluation is needed at the age of 8–9 (after eruption of upper incisors) to detect any possible teeth positioned in the cleft area and to see if lateral incisor is missing or not. If lateral incisor is present, earlier bone grafting can be planned. It is often advisable that any supplemental, deciduous teeth and also malformed and/or malpositioned lateral incisors in the cleft area should be extracted 3–4 weeks before surgery that permits healing of the mucosa (**Figure 3**). Thus, CBCT 6–8 months before ABG is recommended for detailed evaluation of bony support and position of the cleft-related teeth. This time frame will provide enough time to accomplish all necessary pregraft preparations such as tooth extraction and/or orthodontic tooth movement on time and not to delay bone grafting. Sometimes an additional CBCT just before the grafting might be needed to assess the root position of the cleft-related teeth after orthodonticmovement.

4.1. Pre-graft orthodontics

Presurgical orthodontics plays an important role in correcting misaligned incisors or repositioning displaced maxillary alveolar segments. Severe central or canine inclination toward the cleft defect can also interfere with cleft mucoperiosteal dissection. Presurgical orthodontics allows the surgeon better access for placement of the graft and closure of the soft tissue (**Figure 4**). Furthermore, correction of central incisor rotation and inclination prior to SABG enables patients to achieve better oral hygiene and prevents plaque formation. This can therefore prevent chronic, low-grade inflammation activating proteases that degrade grafted bone [5, 32, 33, 38].

One of the presenting problems which occurs early in both unilateral and bilateral clefts is the anteroposterior malpositioning of the incisors. If the anteroposterior malpositioning of the incisors is not corrected, lingual lock of the anterior teeth will further inhibit the development of the maxilla. The proper overjet relationship will allow appropriate growth of the maxilla [19]. By age 7–8, incisor alignment and correction of anterior crossbite can be provided to maximize the forward development of the maxillary dentoalveolar process. However, orthodontic movement of maxillary anterior teeth must be done with great caution because of the closeness of the roots to the bony defect. A very thin bony covering of the central incisor next to the cleft site is a common feature. Often there is just a lamina dura with no cancellous bone.

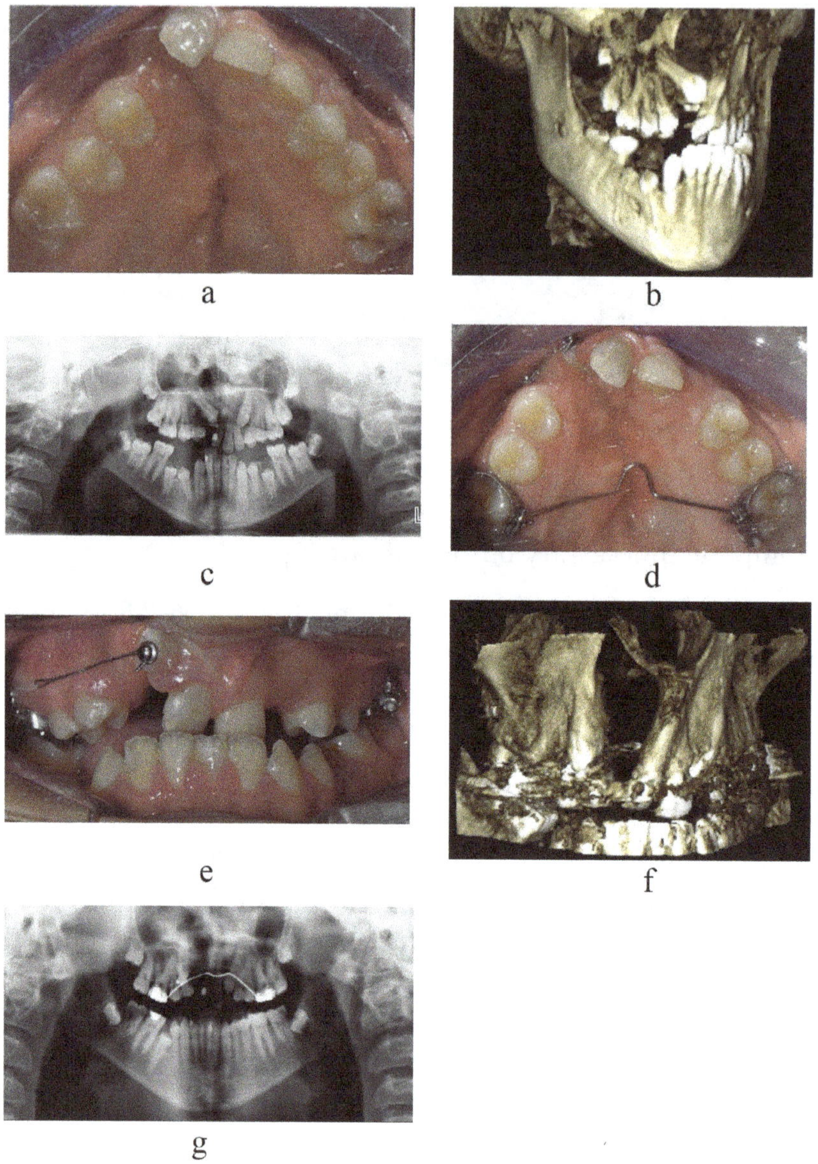

Figure 4. Severe canine inclination toward the cleft defect should be corrected before ABG. (a,b,c) initial views, a. intraoral, b. 3D image c. panoramik radiograph of the patient. (d,e) orthodontic traction of the cleft related canine. (f,g) pregraft 3D image and panoramic radiograph.

The incisor should not be bodily uprighted before successful ABG because of the possibility of bone loss and fenestration of the thin cortical lamina [10, 43].

4.2. Transverse expansion

Constriction of maxillary segments is a very common situation in patients with cleft palate. As the individuals with complete cleft lip and palate do not have midpalatal suture, constriction occurs mostly by the rotation of the lateral segment(s) inward, toward bony defect. Both the absence of the midpalatal bone and the soft tissue traction produced by lip and palate repair promote arch constriction [5, 44, 45].

Significant segmental displacement requires pre-bone graft expansion to rotate the lateral segment(s) outward, facilitate placement of the graft, and provide the surgeon working

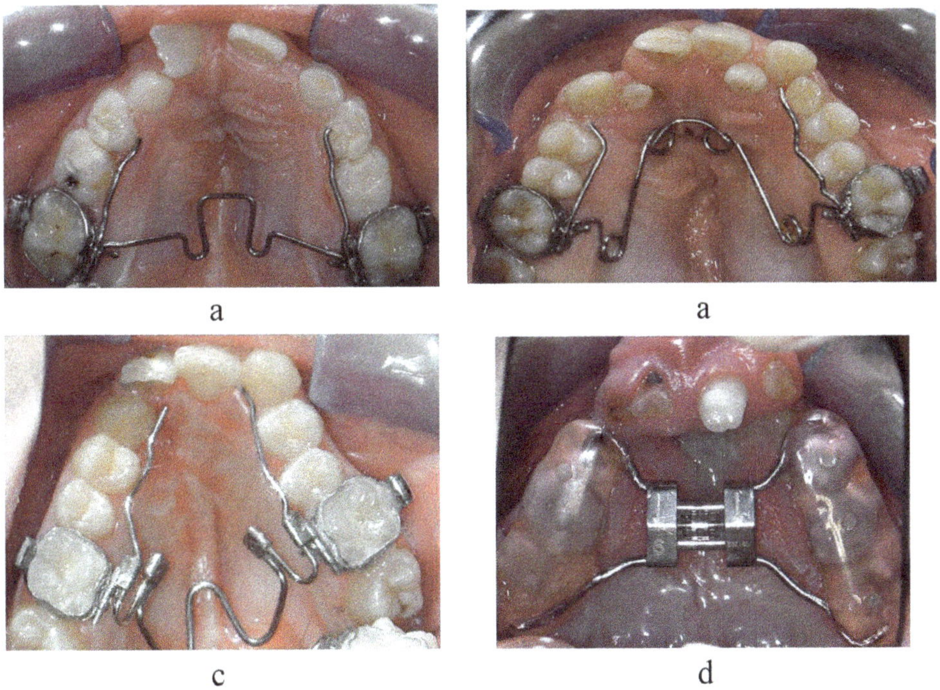

Figure 5. Various types of expanders for maxillary expansion. (a) TPA with lateral expansions, (b) quad helix, (c) NiTi expander, and (d) hyrax.

facility during surgery. If possible, transverse expansion can be combined with the correction of incisor irregularities. In the mixed dentition stage, arch expansion is very important because this process also normalizes the morphology and induces eruption of the canine into the symmetrical maxillary arch [10, 13, 19, 46].

Several types of expanders have been used, and there is no universal protocol for maxillary expansion prior to secondary alveolar bone grafting (**Figure 5**). Both slow maxillary expansion (SME) and rapid maxillary expansion (RME) have been advocated [5, 47, 48].

SME using the quad helix or its variations is frequently used for segmental repositioning as selective expansion anteriorly is required [5]. It has been shown that slow expansion forces are apparently already sufficient to allow a skeletal expansion of the maxilla in complete cleft palate patients [45, 47, 48]. There were *no differences* found between the dentoalveolar effects of SME and RME in patients with BCLP [45, 47].

RME with Haas type or hyrax expanders is also widely used for correcting the maxillary constriction. Asymmetric expansions were found by several authors [46, 48–53]. Isaacson and Murphy reported no correlation between the cleft location and the relative amount of lateral movement of each maxillary segment, emphasizing that RME laterally repositioned the maxillary segments in an unpredictable manner [49]. For greater amount of anterior displacement of the maxilla, fantype or double-hinged RPE expanders have been advocated [54].

According to our clinical experience, there is usually no need for RPE in patients with UCLP. Quad helix or TPA with lateral expansions can solve the problem. However, in some patients with BCLP, significant constriction of the segments necessitates RPE. Thus, patient selection is important in this issue.

5. Postgraft stabilization

The quad helix and/or stabilizing archwire used in BCLP may be removed during the bone grafting procedure for improved surgical access, but these appliances should be replaced before the patient leaves the operating room and left in place for 3 months.

As the bone grafting alone cannot be relied upon to maintain the expansion, a simple palatal arch would be advisable until the permanent dentition has erupted.

Stabilizing a mobile premaxilla with orthodontic arch wire is needed in patients with complete BCLP. Typically the arch wires will be removed during surgery and replaced at the end of the operation to provide retention [5, 10, 19].

6. Postgraft orthodontics

If the graft is done at proper time, before eruption of the cleft-related permanent canine, observation of the permanent dentition is generally all that is necessary. The status of cleft side unerupted teeth does need careful monitoring [5]. Physiologic eruption of the adjacent canine will provide enough stimulation for the alveolar graft. Sometimes orthodontic traction might be needed if the position of the canine is not appropriate for spontaneous eruption. High degrees of canine inclination indicate risk for altered eruption and impaction [5, 32].

If graft is done at age 7–8, correction of incisor irregularities provides also favorable stimulation to the graft.

Orthodontic movement of the cleft-adjacent teeth in the direction of the grafted bone can be instituted at an average of 3 months after the bone grafting, if needed. Combined interceptive bone grafting and orthodontic treatment at an early age avoid more extensive prolonged treatment later in the patient's life [5, 13, 19, 34].

It has been recommended not to delay orthodontic treatment more than 6 months after grafting, in cases in which an a-p crossbite or a residual transverse posterior crossbite exists. One- to two year delay in stimulation of the ABG of the premaxilla (by orthodontic treatment) can lead to serious postoperative problems. Where there is no stimulation of the graft, there tends to be "locking" or lingual collapse of the maxillary central incisors and collapse of the premaxillary arch [19].

6.1. Maxillary space management choice

In patients with CLP, the lateral incisor is missing in about 50% of cases in the permanent dentition. There are two options when maxillary lateral incisors are absent: space closure or space preservation [5].

The success of the bone graft is the determinant factor for this choice. When bone graft is properly done before the eruption of the permanent canine, canine can simultaneously migrate

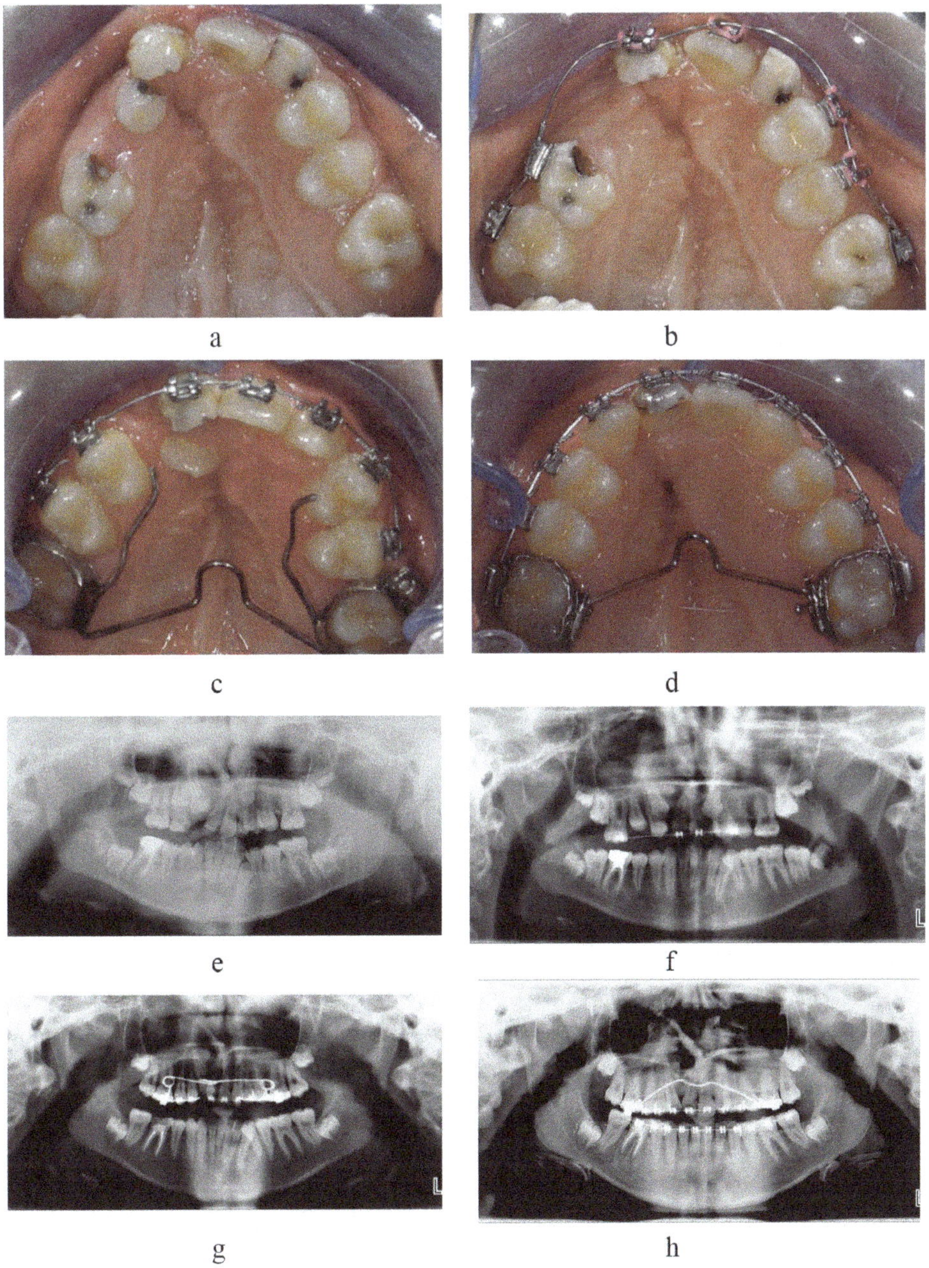

Figure 6. Space closure with canine substitution in patient with successful ABG. (a-d) intraoral occlusal views of the case. a. pre-graft, b. post-graft, c. after eruption of the canine, d. levelling of the upper dentition. (e-h) panoramic radiographs of the case. a. pre-graft, b. post-graft, c. eruption of the canine, h. levelling of the upper arch.

into the newly formed bone and increases its vertical height. Maintaining the alveolar bone height in the cleft area is important to prevent long-term complications, such as gingival retractions and periodontitis [32, 33].

Moreover, the natural dentition has the best prognosis for long-term health of the dentition. Thus, space closure with the canine substitution should be the first treatment choice for patients with CLP [5, 32, 33] (**Figure 6**). The functional stress imposed by orthodontic treatment influences the volume and prevents resorption of the grafted bone. Higher grafting success was found in the case of space closure than in the case of space openings [5, 33].

However, in patients with severely impaired maxillary growth, multiple missing teeth, and/or failure of bone graft, orthodontic space closure may not be feasible, and some form of prosthesis might be needed.

6.2. Extraction choice

Extraction of maxillary teeth may be required in UCLP in non-cleft quadrant, either because of crowding or to allow correction of the dental midline. As the second premolar is frequently malformed, it is the most commonly removed tooth. In some patients removal of the non-cleft lateral incisor allows the rapid restoration of the symmetry. However, this should be considered when compliance with space closure is assured [5].

In the lower arch, the absence of the second premolars is frequent and should be assessed carefully where extractions are necessary to relieve lower incisor crowding.

Extraction of the lower teeth to compensate class III skeletal pattern should be avoided in the early teens.

7. Management of maxillary deficiency in growing cleft patients

Hypoplastic maxilla and progressive midface retrusion are typical characteristics of patients with CLP.

Therefore, maxillary protraction (MP) has been frequently applied in the orthodontic treatment of growing patients with cleft lip and palate to improve the maxillomandibular relationship, occlusion, and facial esthetics. Optimal timing for initiating maxillary protraction for non-cleft children is shown as in the early mixed dentition before age 10. Early mixed dentition is favored over late, because of the closure of the sutures of the nasomaxillary complex [55].

However, SABG is optimally carried out between 9 and 11 years, and there is no consensus on the treatment sequencing of maxillary protraction and SABG in patients with CLP.

Two studies of three-dimensional finite element analysis suggested the advantage of SABG before maxillary protraction [55–57].

In a recent clinical study, short-term results showed that facemask therapy after alveolar bone grafting led to enhance maxillary skeletal advancement and minimize mandibular clockwise rotation more than those in the ungrafted group.

Maeda-lino found that the root lengths of U1 were comparatively short on the cleft side in patients with UCLP treated with MPA before SABG. Thus, they concluded that orthodontic force exerted by the MPA before SABG might result in short dental roots [58].

Moreover, it has been advocated that protraction of severely retruded cleft maxilla, even at an early stage, does not provide lasting skeletal benefit. Its effect in individual cases with CLP is difficult to predict, and many patients require orthognathic surgery after MP treatment [5, 59, 60] (**Figures 7** and **8**). Thus, explanation of the expected effects and associated problems should be given to the patients and parents before MP treatment.

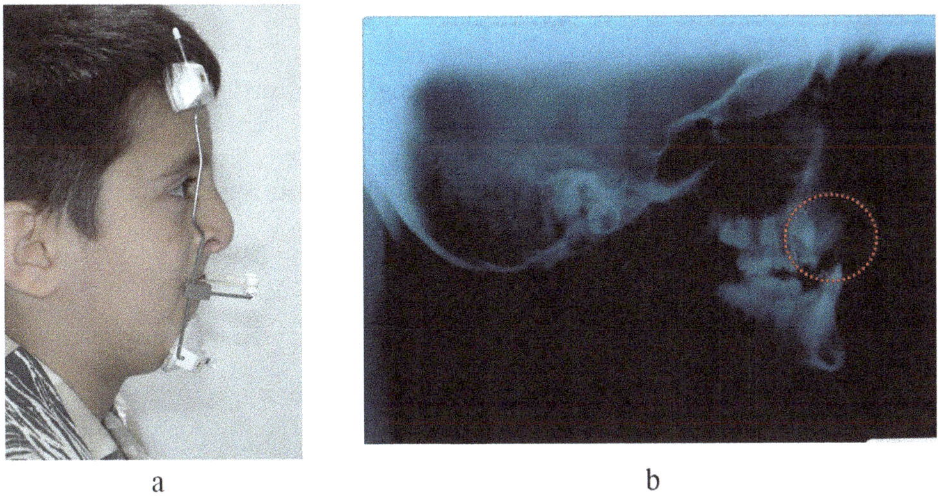

Figure 7. Face mask application using bonded hyrax in patient with BCLP. (a) extraoral view of the patient. (b) initial lateral cephalogram.

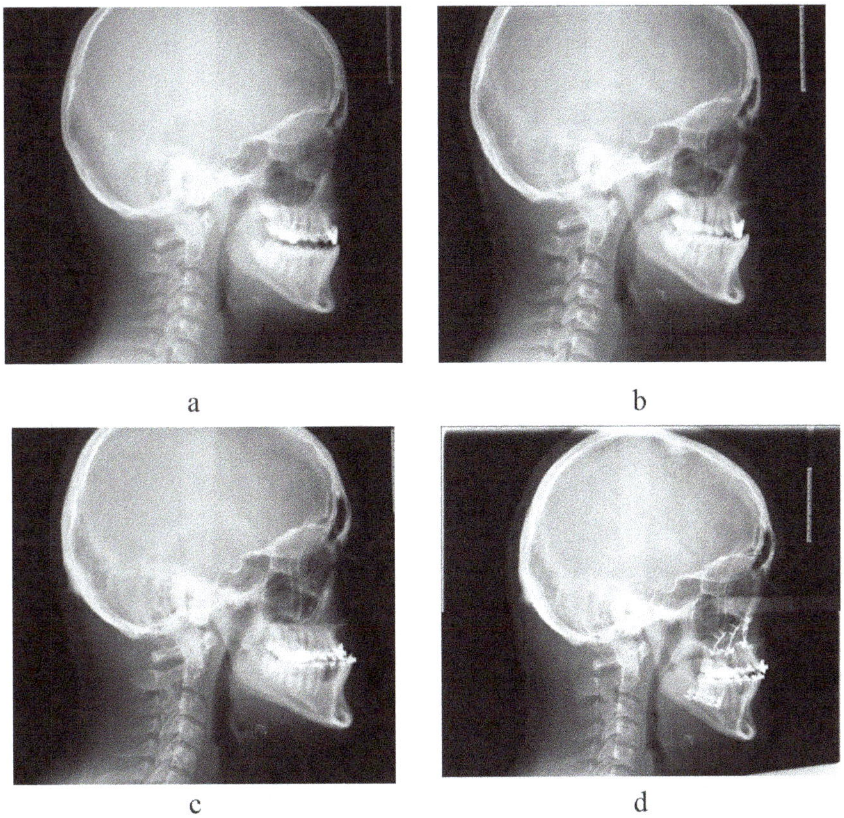

Figure 8. Cephalometric radiographs of the patient after facemask therapy between 10 and 19 years of age and after orthognathic surgery. (a) age 10, after face mask therapy, (b) age 14, follow-up, (c) age 19, ğre-orthogntic surgery, (d) after orthognatic surgery.

7.1. Patients with no to mild skeletal discrepancy

Providing proper overjet relationship at the early mixed dentition by correcting lingual lock of the anterior teeth using either removable or fixed appliances will be sufficient to maximize the forward development of the maxillary dentoalveolar process. Facemask can be a valuable source of anchorage for advancing posterior teeth during space closure after SABG [5, 19].

7.2. Patients with moderate to severe skeletal discrepancy

Early determination of the eventual need for maxillary osteotomy is a very important decision for the orthodontist.

Extracting lower premolar to correct anterior crossbite and trying to camouflage skeletal discrepancy are not appropriate in growing children. In that case, leveling only the upper arch, finishing with crossbite, and monitoring the growth are the best options. Early surgical options can be considered if needed [5].

7.3. Summary of treatment sequencing for mixed dentition stage

Evaluation CBCT–maxillary expansion and/or ortho-tooth movement–fistula closure and alveolar graft–maxillary protraction if needed.

Maxillary protraction protocol: 350–450 gram per side protraction force is adequate 14–15 hours a day for 6–12 months. MP can be started 4–6 weeks after SABG.

Part of this force should be transmitted as intermittent force to the maxillary anterior teeth through oral appliances such as an arch wire and/or lingual arch.

7.4. Unfavorable conditions

If maxillary deficiency accompanies with a wide alveolar cleft and/or fistula, it will be more challenging for both orthodontist and surgeon to treat growing patients [54] (**Figure 9**).

Late bone grafting or prolonged orthodontic treatment prior to bone grafting leads to loss of orthodontic control, marked instability of the premaxilla, and difficulty in maintaining

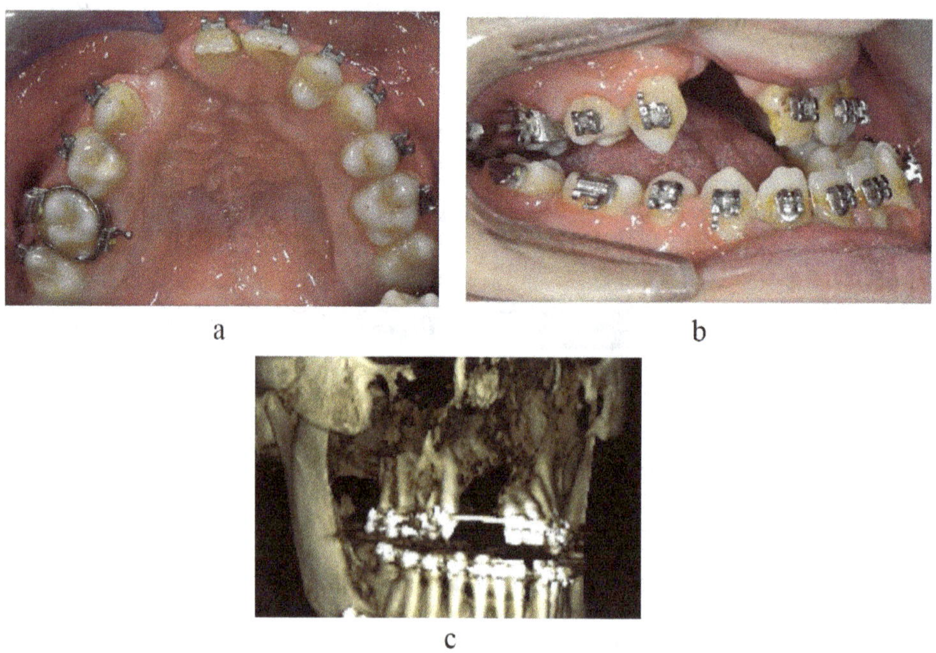

Figure 9. Wide alveolar cleft limits both orthodontic treatment and maxillary osteotomy. (a, b) intraoral views of a wide cleft, (c) 3D image of the case.

anteroposterior growth. In patients with BCLP, the unstable premaxilla with the small amount of maxillary bone attached to the vomer is usually incapable of being maintained with good stability without grafting.

When the premaxilla has been effectively grafted, any need to forward the maxilla at a later date can be accomplished by Le Fort osteotomy with a much diminished possibility of relapse [19].

8. Summary

The success of the orthodontic treatment and SABG is strongly interrelated. Carefully coordinated orthodontic and surgical involvement is critical for the well-being of the patients with CLP.

Author details

Aslıhan Uzel

Address all correspondence to: aslihanuzel@gmail.com

Department of Orthodontics, Faculty of Dentistry, Cukurova University, Adana, Turkey

References

[1] WHO. Global strategies to reduce the health-care burden of craniofacial anomalies. In: Report of WHO Meetings on International Collaborative Research on Craniofacial Anomalies. Geneva, Switzerland: Human genetics programme; 2002

[2] IPDTOC Working Group. Prevalence at birth of cleft lip with or without cleft palate: Data from the international perinatal database of typical oral clefts. The Cleft Palate-Craniofacial Journal. 2011;**48**(1):66-81

[3] ACH W, Sell DA, Grunwel P. Management of Cleft Lip and Palate. London, Philadelphia: Whurr Publishers; 2004

[4] Shaw WC, Semb G. Choosing the best treatment for the child with a cleft. In: ACH W, Sell DA, Grunwel P, editors. Management of Cleft Lip and Palate. London, Philadelphia: Whurr Publishers; 2004. p. 400

[5] Semb G, Shaw WC. Orthodontics. In: Watson ACH, Sell DA, Grunwel P, editors. Management of Cleft Lip and Palate. London, Philadelphia: Whurr Publishers; 2004. p. 299

[6] Kreiborg S, Hermann NV, Darvann TA. Characteristics of facial morphology and growth in infants with clefts. In: Berkowitz S, editor. Cleft Lip and Palate. 2nd ed. Germany: Springer-Verlag Berlin Heidelberg; 2006. pp. 25-235

[7] Semb G. A study of facial growth in patients with unilateral cleft lip and palate treated by the Oslo CLP team. The Cleft Palate Journal. 1991;**28**:1-21

[8] Semb G. A study of facial growth in patients with bilateral cleft lip and palate treated by the Oslo CLP team. The Cleft Palate Journal. 1991;**28**:22-39

[9] Mars M. Facial growth. In: Watson ACH, Sell DA, Grunwel P, editors. Management of Cleft Lip and Palate. London, Philadelphia: Whurr Publishers; 2004. pp. 44-67

[10] Mars M. Alveolar bone grafting. In: Watson ACH, Sell DA, Grunwel P, editors. Management of Cleft Lip and Palate. London, Philadelphia: Whurr Publishers; 2004. pp. 326-337

[11] Semb G. Alveolar bone grafting. Frontiers of Oral Biology. 2012;**16**:124-136

[12] Goudy S, Lott DG, Burton R, Wheeler J, Canady J. Secondary alveolar bone grafting: Outcomes, revisions, and new applications. The Cleft Palate-Craniofacial Journal. 2009; **46**:610-612

[13] Bergland O, Semb G, Abyholm F. Elimination of the residual alveolar cleft by secondary bone grafting and subsequent orthodontic treatment. The Cleft Palate-Craniofacial Journal. 1986;**23**:175-205

[14] Daskalogiannakis J, Ross RB. Effect of alveolar bone grafting in the mixed dentition on maxillary growth in complete unilateral cleft lip and palate patients. The Cleft Palate-Craniofacial Journal. 1997;**34**:455-458

[15] Kindelan JD, Roberts-Harry D. A 5 year post-operative review of secondary alveolar bone grafting in the Yorkshire region. British Journal of Orthodontics. 1999;**26**:211-217

[16] Eppley BL, Sadove AM. Management of alveolar cleft bone grafting-state of art. The Cleft Palate-Craniofacial Journal. 2000;**37**:229-233

[17] Kawakami S, Hura K, Yokozeki M, Takahashi T, Seike T, Nakanishi H, et al. Longitudinal evaluation of secondary bone grafting into the alveolar cleft. The Cleft Palate-Craniofacial Journal. 2003;**40**:569-576

[18] Murthy AS, Lehman JA Jr. Evaluation of alveolar bone grafting: A survey of ACPA teams. The Cleft Palate-Craniofacial Journal. 2005;**42**:99-101

[19] Boyne PJ, Herford AS, Stringer DE. Prevention of relapse following cleftal bone grafting and the future use of BMP cytokines to regenerate osseous clefts without grafting. In: Berkowitz S, editor. Cleft Lip and Palate. 2nd ed. Germany: Springer-Verlag Berlin Heidelberg; 2006. p. 587

[20] Craven C, Cole P, Holier L Jr, Stal S. Ensuring success in alveolar bone grafting: A three-dimensional approach. The Journal of Craniofacial Surgery. 2007;**18**:855-859

[21] Guo J, LI C, Zhang Q, Wu G, Deacon SA, Chen J, et al. Secondary bone grafting for alveolar cleft in children with cleft lip or cleft lip and palate (review). The Cochrane Collaboration issue. 2011;**6**:1-44

[22] Boyne PJ, Sands NR. Secondary bone grafting of residual alveolar and palatal clefts. Journal of Oral Surgery. 1972;**30**:87-92

[23] Boyne PJ, Sands NR. Combined orthodontic-surgical management of residual palato-alveolar cleft defects. American Journal of Orthodontics. 1976;**70**:20-37

[24] Yoshida S, Suga K, Nakano Y, Sakamoto T, Takaki T, Uchiyama T. Postoperative evaluation of grafted bone in alveolar cleft using three-dimensional computed data. The Cleft Palate-Craniofacial Journal. 2013;**50**:671-677

[25] Enemark H, Krantz-Simonsen E, Schramm JE. Secondary bone grafting in unilateral cleft lip palate patients: Indications and treatment procedure. International Journal of Oral Surgery. 1985;**14**:2-10

[26] Feichtinger M, Mossböck R, Karcher H. Assessment of bone resorption after secondary alveolar bone grafting using three-dimensional computed tomography: A three-year study. The Cleft Palate-Craniofacial Journal. 2007;**44**:142-148

[27] Ozawa T, Omura S, Fukuyama E, Matsui Y, Torikai K, Fujita K. Factors influencing secondary alveolar bone grafting in cleft lip and palate patients: Prospective analysis using CT image analyzer. The Cleft Palate-Craniofacial Journal. 2007;**44**:286-291

[28] Sindet-Pedersen S, Enemark H. Comparative study of secondary and late secondary bone-grafting in patients with residual cleft defects. Short-term evaluation. International Journal of Oral Surgery. 1985;**14**:389-398

[29] Tai C-CE, Sutherland IS, McFadden L. Prospective analysis of secondary alveolar bone grafting using computed tomography. Journal of Oral and Maxillofacial Surgery. 2000; **58**:1241-1249

[30] Kalaaji A, Lilja J, Friede H, Elander A. Bone grafting in the mixed and permanent dentition in cleft lip and palate patients: Long-term results and the role of the surgeon's experience. Journal of Cranio-Maxillo-Facial Surgery. 1996;**24**:29-35

[31] Uzel A. Computed tomographic evaluation of secondary alveolar bone grafting in patients with cleft lip and palate. GÜ Diş Hek Fak Derg. 2012;**29**:11-18

[32] Jabbari F, Skoog V, et al. Optimization of dental status improves long-term outcome after alveolar bone grafting in unilateral cleft lip and palate. The Cleft Palate-Craniofacial Journal. 2015;**52**(2):210-218

[33] Liao YF, Huang CS. Presurgical and postsurgical orthodontics are associated with superior secondary alveolar bone grafting outcomes. Journal of Cranio-Maxillo-Facial Surgery. 2015;**43**(5):717-723

[34] Maeda A, Uehara S, Suga M, Nishihara K, Nakamura N, Miyawaki S. Changes in grafted autogenous bone during edgewise treatment in patients with unilateral cleft lip/palate or alveolus. The Cleft Palate-Craniofacial Journal. 2014;**51**(5):525-532

[35] Feichtinger M, Mossböck R, Karcher H. Evaluation of bone volume following bone grafting in patients with unilateral clefts of lip, alveolus and palate using a CT-guided

three-dimensional navigation system. Journal of Cranio-Maxillofacial Surgery. 2006; **34**:144-149

[36] Hamada Y, Kondoh T, Noguchi K, Lino M, Isono H, Ishii H, et al. Application of limited cone beam computed tomography to clinical assessment of alveolar bone grafting: A priliminary report. The Cleft Palate-Craniofacial Journal. 2005;**42**:128-137

[37] Honma K, Kobayashi T, Nakajima T, Hayasi T. Computed tomographic evaluation of bone formation after secondary bone grafting of alveolar clefts. Journal of Oral and Maxillofacial Surgery. 1999;**57**:1209-1213

[38] Chang CS, Wallace CG, Hsiao YC, Chiu YT, et al. Difference in the surgical outcome of unilateral cleft lip and palate patients with and without pre-alveolar bone graft orthodontic treatment. Scientific Reports. 2016;**6**:23597. 1-7

[39] Rosenstein SE, Ross EL Jr, Dado DV, Vinson B, Alder ME. Comparison of 2-D calculations from periapical and occlusal radiographs versus 3-D calculations from CAT scans in determining bone support for cleft-adjacent teeth following early alveolar bone grafts. The Cleft Palate-Craniofacial Journal. 1997;**34**:199-205

[40] Nagashima H, Sakamoto Y, Ogata H, Miyamoto J, Yazawa M, Kishi K. Evaluation of bone volume after secondary bone grafting in unilateral alveolar cleft using computer-aided engineering. The Cleft Palate-Craniofacial Journal. 2014;**51**:665-668

[41] Feichtinger M, Zemanna W, Mossbock R, Kärcher H. Three-dimensional evaluation of secondary alveolar bone grafting using a 3D-navigation system based on computed tomography: A two-year follow-up. The British Journal of Oral & Maxillofacial Surgery. 2008;**46**:278-282

[42] Shirota T, Kurabayashi H, Ogura H, Seki K, Maki K, Shintani S. Analysis of bone volume using computer simulation system for secondary bone graft in alveolar cleft. International Journal of Oral and Maxillofacial Surgery. 2010;**39**:904-908

[43] Long RE Jr, Semb G, Shaw WC, et al. Cleft Palate-Craniofacial Journal. 2000;**37**(6):533-546

[44] Garib DG, Lauris RCMC, Calil LR, Medeiros Alves AC, Janson G, Almeida AM, et al. Dentoskeletal outcomes of a rapid maxillary expander with differential opening in patients with bilateral cleft lip and palate: A prospective clinical trial. American Journal of Orthodontics and Dentofacial Orthopedics. 2016;**150**(4):564-574

[45] de Almeida AM, Ozawa TO, de Medeiros Alves AC, Janson G, Lauris JRP, Ioshida MSY, et al. Slow versus rapid maxillary expansion in bilateral cleft lip and palate: A CBCT randomized clinical trial. Clinical Oral Investigations. 2017;**21**:1789-1799

[46] Ayub PV, Janson G, Gribel BF, Lara TS, Garib DG. Analysis of the maxillary dental arch after rapid maxillary expansion in patients with unilateral complete cleft lip and palate. American Journal of Orthodontics and Dentofacial Orthopedics. 2016;**149**:705-715

[47] de Medeiros Alves AC, Garib DG, Janson G, de Almeida AM. Calil LR analysis of the dentoalveolar effects of slow and rapid maxillary expansion in complete bilateral cleft lip and palate patients: A randomized clinical trial. Clinical Oral Investigations. 2016; **20**:1837-1847

[48] Holberg C, Holberg N, Schwenzer K, Wichelhaus A, Rudzki-Janson I. Biomechanical analysis of maxillary expansion in CLP patients. The Angle Orthodontist. 2007;**77**(2):280-287

[49] Isaacson RJ, Murphy TD. Some effects of rapid maxillary expansion in cleft lip and palate patients. The Angle Orthodontist. 1964;**34**:143-154

[50] Pan X, Qian Y, Yu J, Wang D, Tang Y, Shen G. Biomechanical effects of rapid palatal expansion on the craniofacial skeleton with cleft palate: A three-dimensional finite element analysis. The Cleft Palate-Craniofacial Journal. 2007;**44**:149-154

[51] Wang D, Cheng L, Wang C, Qian Y, Pan X. Biomechanical analysis of rapid maxillary expansion in the UCLP patient. Medical Engineering & Physics. 2009;**31**:409-417

[52] Gautam P, Zhao L, Patel P. Biomechanical response of the maxillofacial skeleton to transpalatal orthopedic force in a unilateral palatal cleft. The Angle Orthodontist. 2011; **81**:503-509

[53] Façanha AJ, Lara TS, Garib DG, da Silva Filho OG. Transverse effect of Haas and hyrax appliances on the upper dental arch in patients with unilateral complete cleft lip and palate: A comparative study. Dental Press Journal of Orthodontics. 2014;**19**:39-45

[54] Liou EJW, Chen PKT. Management of maxillary deformities in growing cleft patients. In: Berkowitz S, editor. Cleft Lip and Palate. 2nd ed. Germany: Springer-Verlag Berlin Heidelberg; 2006. pp. 535-554

[55] Zhang Y, Jia H, Fu Z, Huang Y, Wang Z, Guo R, et al. Dentoskeletal effects of facemask therapy in skeletal class III cleft patients with or without bone graft. American Journal of Orthodontics and Dentofacial Orthopedics. 2018;**153**:542-549

[56] Yang IH, Chang YI, Kim TW, Ahn SJ, Lim WH, Lee NK, et al. Effects of cleft type, facemak anchorage method, and alveolar bone graft on maxillary protraction: A three-dimensional finite element analysis. The Cleft Palate-Craniofacial Journal. 2012;**49**:221-229

[57] Chen Z, Pan X, Shao Q, Chen Z. Biomechanical effects on maxillary protraction of the craniofacial skeleton with cleft lip and palate after alveolar bone graft. The Journal of Craniofacial Surgery. 2013;**24**:446-453

[58] Maeda-Iino A, Marutani K, Furukawa M, Nakagawa S, Kwon S, Kibe T, et al. Evaluation of maxillary central incisors on the noncleft and cleft sides in patients with unilateral cleft lip and palate—Part 1: Relationship between root length and orthodontic tooth movement. The Angle Orthodontist. 2017;**87**:855-862

[59] Kuijpers-Jagtman AM, Long RE Jr. The influence of surgery and orthodontic treatment on maxillofacial growth and maxillary arch development in patients treated for orofacial clefts. The Cleft Palate-Craniofacial Journal. 2000;**37**:1-12

[60] Susami T, Okayasu M, Inokuchi T, Ohkubo K, Uchino N, Uwatoko K, et al. Maxillary protraction in patients with cleft lip and palate in mixed dentition: Cephalometric evaluation after completion of growth. The Cleft Palate-Craniofacial Journal. 2014;**51**(5):514-524

2

A Review of Orofacial Clefting and Current Genetic Mouse Models

Aram J. Keteyian and Yuji Mishina

Abstract

The prevalence of orofacial clefts (OFCs) is nearly 10.2 per 10,000 births in the United States and 9.9 per 10,000 births worldwide. OFCs occur as a result of a break (nonfusion) of orofacial structures during development. This can occur due to a variety of reasons;prenatal exposure to many drugs and environmental factors as well as genetic factors which are implicated in the development of OFCs. While approximately 15 types of clefts have been identified, there are at least four distinct classifications of OFCs. These include complete cleft palate with cleft lip; cleft of the anterior palate, which may/may not involve cleft lip; cleft of the posterior palate; and submucosal cleft. A number of candidate genes have been identified, including transforming growth factor beta (TGFβ) and homeobox genes (e.g., *MSX1*), among many others. What follows is a review of mouse models currently used in research and the classification of their overall contribution to known OFCs.

Keywords: orofacial, cleft lip, cleft palate, genomic, genetics, TGFβ, MSX1, knockout mice, craniofacial, molecular, palatogenesis

1. Introduction

The focus of this chapter is to review a comprehensive list of the genes with known involvement in generating cleft lip with (or without) cleft palate (CL/P) or cleft palate (CP) in mice. Additionally, the associated knockout (KO) and conditional knockout (cKO) models are discussed. Most of the research models currently in use focus on complete CP, and thus not as much is known of the other CP phenotypes. In particular, identifying specific risk genes for CL/P is made simpler when genomic sequencing is done, and clefting associated with syndromes (syndromic) has identified single genetic loci that are involved with abnormalities in palatogenesis. Current mouse models involve a somewhat surprisingly vast array of genes, however, including *Wnt*, *Msx1/2*, *Tbx*, *Pax9*, *Irf6*, *Tgfb*, and *Fgf*. Further elucidation and categorization of these gene families and their associated defects—whether syndromic or non-syndromic—can aid us in further clarifying the molecular mechanisms underlying orofacial clefting and potentially lead us to targeted, more efficient treatments.

We currently utilize four distinct classifications for OFCs: complete cleft palate with cleft lip; cleft of the anterior palate, which may/may not involve cleft lip; cleft of the posterior palate; and submucosal cleft. Subdivided among these four classifications of OFCs are six categories of developmental defects that have been shown to result in cleft palate in KO or cKO mice. The numerous variants of CL/P can generally be found to fit within one of the following categories: [1]

1. Palatal shelf formation failure
2. Abnormal fusion of palatal shelves
3. Delayed/failed elevation of the palatal shelves
4. Failure of palatal shelf development post-elevation
5. Persistence of medial-edge epithelial cells
6. Secondary defect

Each of the known KO/cKO mice mentioned is bred such that the gene missing is one already known to play a role in the development of CL/P. Implicit within these categories are the KO genes known to lead to each particular type of defect, each of which will be outlined as we move through this chapter.

As we look into the future, OFCs need to be classified with more definitive nomenclature. Currently, we use arbitrary terms to define very broadly into which category these congenital malformations fall, i.e., syndromic versus non-syndromic. As studies are broadened to include a wider array of genetic variants and their regulatory regions, more risk genes for CL/P and CP will surely be identified. As a result, more specific phenotypic classifications will emerge as well. The etiology of OFCs is complex, and the presentation is wide ranging; it is important that we continue to use precise genetic mouse models in order to carefully define a given phenotype before reclassifying human cases. The models mentioned in this chapter and those developed in the future are critical to a more sophisticated understanding of OFC anomalies and etiologic variants. Their development and utilization will ideally lead to a greater breadth and depth of treatment intervention options for patients.

2. Current mouse models utilized for elucidation of molecular mechanisms involved in orofacial clefting

As alluded to previously, a great breadth of genes plays critical roles in palatogenesis. Upon further analysis, a subset of gene families and signaling pathways have emerged as containing the most significant molecules related to normal development of the palate. Of note are the following: transforming growth factor beta (TGFβ), hedgehog, Wnt, fibroblast growth factor (FGF), and the mitogen-activated protein kinase (MAPK) signaling pathway. Each signaling pathway has an expansive list of genes with known involvement in palatogenesis (**Table 1**).

Gene	Syndromic/non-syndromic	Orofacial phenotype
Acvr1/Alk2	Submucosal cleft/fibrodysplasia ossificans progressiva	Und
Acvr2a	Und	Und
Akap8/Akap95	Und	Und
Alx1	Frontonasal dysplasia 3	CL/P
Alx3	Frontonasal dysplasia 1	CL/P
Alx4	Frontonasal dysplasia 2, parietal foramina 2, craniosynostosis 5	Cleft alae nasi
Anp32b	Und	Und
Apaf1	Und	Und
Arid5	Und	Und
Asxl1	Bohring-Opitz syndrome; myelodysplastic syndrome, somatic	CL/P
B9d1	Meckel syndrome 9	Und
Barx1	Und	Und
Bmp4	Microphthalmia, syndromic 6	CL/P
Bmp7	Und	Und
Bmpr1a/Alk3	Juvenile polyposis syndrome	CP
Cask	FG syndrome 4, mental retardation, and microcephaly with pontine and cerebellar hypoplasia	CL/P
Cdc42	Und	CL/P
Cdkn1c/p57kip2	Beckwith-Wiedemann syndrome, IMAGe syndrome	CL/P
Ceacam1	Und	Und
Chd7	CHARGE syndrome	CL/P
Chrd	Und	CL
Chuk/Ikk1/Tcf16	Cocoon syndrome	Und
Cited2	Atrial septal defect 8, ventricular septal defect 2	Und
Col2a1	Achondrogenesis, type II; Stickler syndrome, type I; Kniest dysplasia	CL/P
Crebbp/Cbp	Rubinstein-Taybi syndrome	Und
Crk	Und	Und
Ctgf	Und	Und
Ctnnb1	Mental retardation, autosomal dominant 19	Und
Cyp26B1	Craniosynostosis with radiohumeral fusions and other skeletal and craniofacial anomalies	Und
Cyp51	Und	Und
Dhcr7	Smith-Lemli-Opitz syndrome	CL/P

Gene	Syndromic/non-syndromic	Orofacial phenotype
Dhrs3	Und	Und
Dicer1	Rhabdomyosarcoma, embryonal, 2; goiter, multinodular 1; pleuropulmonary blastoma	Und
Dlg1/Dlgh/Sap97	Und	Und
Dlx1	Und	Und
Dlx2	Und	Und
Dlx5	Split-hand/foot malformation 1 with sensorineural hearing loss	CL/P
Dph1/Ovca1	Und	Und
Edn1	Auriculocondylar syndrome 3	CL/P
Efna5	Und	Und
Efnb1	Craniofrontonasal dysplasia	CL/P
Efnb2	Und	Und
Egfr	Und	Und
Eya1	Branchiootic syndrome 1; branchiootorenal syndrome 1, with or without cataracts; anterior segment anomalies with or without cataract	CL/P
Fgf10	Aplasia of lachrymal and salivary glands	Und
Fgf18	Und	Und
Fgf9	Und	Und
Fgfr1	Non-syndromic cleft lip/palate, Hartsfield syndrome, hypogonadotropic hypogonadism 2, Pfeiffer syndrome	CL/P
Fgfr2	Apert Syndrome	CL/P
Foxc2/Mfh1	Lymphedema-distichiasis syndrome	CL/P
Foxd3	Und	Und
Foxe1/Titf2/Fkhl15	Bamforth-Lazarus syndrome	CL/P
Foxf2	Und	Und
Fst	Und	Und
Fuz	Neural tube defects	Und
Fzd2	Und	Und
Gab1	Und	Und
Gabrb3	Epilepsy, childhood absence, susceptibility to, 5	CL/P
Gad/Gad67	Cerebral palsy, spastic quadriplegic, 1	CL/P
Gbr2	Und	Und
Gbx2	Und	Und
Gdf11/Bmp11	Und	Und

Gene	Syndromic/non-syndromic	Orofacial phenotype
Glce	Und	Und
Glg1	Und	Und
Gli2	Culler-Jones syndrome, holoprosencephaly-9	CL/P
Gli3	Greig cephalopolysyndactyly	CL/P
Gpr124	Und	Und
Grb2	Und	Und
Gsc	Short stature, auditory canal atresia, mandibular hypoplasia, skeletal abnormalities	Und
Gsk3b	Und	Und
Hand2/dHand	Und	Und
Hic1	Und	Und
Hoxa2	Microtia with or without hearing impairment	Und
Hs2st1	Und	Und
Hspb11/Ift25	Und	Und
Hspg2	Dyssegmental dysplasia, Schwartz-Jampel syndrome, type 1	Und
Ilk	Und	Und
Impad1/Jaws	Chondrodysplasia with joint dislocations, GRAPP type	CL/P
Inhba	Und	Und
Inpp5e	Mental retardation, truncal obesity, retinal dystrophy, and micropenis	Und
Irf6	Van der Woude syndrome, orofacial cleft 6, popliteal pterygium syndrome 1	CL/P
Itgb1	Und	Und
Itgb8	Und	Und
Jag1	Alagille syndrome	Und
Jag2	Und	Und
Jmjd6/Ptdsr	Und	Und
Kat6a/Moz/Myst3	Und	Und
Kcnj2	Andersen syndrome, atrial fibrillation, familial, 9; short QT syndrome 3	CL/P
Kif3a	Und	Und
Lhx7	Und	Und
Lhx8	Und	Und
Lrp6	Und	Und

Gene	Syndromic/non-syndromic	Orofacial phenotype
Luzp1	Und	Und
Map3k7/Tak1	Und	Und
Mef2c	Chromosome 5q14.3 deletion syndrome, mental retardation, stereotypic movements, epilepsy, and/or cerebral malformations	Und
Meox2	Und	Und
Mn1	Meningioma	Und
Mnt	Und	Und
Msx1	Ectodermal dysplasia 3, Witkop-type Orofacial cleft 5	CL/P
Msx2	Craniosynostosis, type 2; parietal foramina 1, parietal foramina with cleidocranial dysplasia	CL/P
Nabp2/Obfc2b/hSSB1	Und	Und
Nprl3	Und	Und
Ofd1	Joubert syndrome 10, oral-facial-digital syndrome I, Simpson-Golabi-Behmel syndrome, type 2	CL/P
Osr2	Und	CL/P
Pak1ip1	Und	Und
Pax9	Tooth agenesis, selective, 3	Und
Pbx1	Leukemia, acute pre-B-cell	Und
Pdgfc	Und	CL/P
Pdgfra	Gastrointestinal stromal tumor, somatic	CL/P
Pds5a	Und	Und
Pdss2	Coenzyme Q10 deficiency, primary, 3	Und
Phc1/Rae28	Und	Und
Piga	Multiple congenital anomalies-hypotonia-seizures syndrome 2; paroxysmal nocturnal hemoglobinuria, somatic	Und
Pitx1	Clubfoot, congenital, with or without deficiency of long bones and/or mirror-image polydactyly, Liebenberg syndrome	CL/P
Pitx2	Axenfeld-Rieger syndrome, type 1; iridogoniodysgenesis, type 2; Peters anomaly	Und
Pkdcc/Vlk	Und	Und
Pnn	Und	Und
Prdm16	Cardiomyopathy, dilated, 1LL; left ventricular noncompaction 8	
Prickle1	Epilepsy, progressive myoclonic	Und
Prrx1/Prx1/Mhox	Agnathia-otocephaly complex	CL/P
Ptch1/Ptc1	Basal cell nevus syndrome (Gorlin syndrome)	CL/P

Gene	Syndromic/non-syndromic	Orofacial phenotype
Pygo2	Und	Und
Rad23b	Und	Und
Rax	Microphthalmia, isolated 3	Und
Recql4	Baller-Gerold syndrome, RAPADILINO syndrome, Rothmund-Thomson syndrome	CL/P
Ror2	Robinow syndrome, autosomal recessive	CL/P
Rspo2	Und	Und
Runx2	Cleidocranial dysplasia	CL/P
Ryk	Und	Und
Ryr1	Central core disease, King-Denborough syndrome, minicore myopathy with external ophthalmoplegia	Und
Sall3	Und	Und
Satb2	Glass syndrome	CL/P
Sc5d/Sc5dl	Und	Und
Schip1	Und	Und
Sdccag8	Bardet-Biedl syndrome 16, Senior-Loken syndrome 7	Und
Serpinh/Hsp47	Osteogenesis imperfecta, type X	Und
Shh	Holoprosencephaly-3	CL/P
Shox2	Und	Und
Sim2	Und	Und
Slc32a1/Viaat	Und	Und
Smad4	Juvenile polyposis/hereditary hemorrhagic telangiectasia syndrome	Und
Smad7	Und	Und
Smo/Smoh	Basal cell carcinoma, somatic	Und
Smoc	Microphthalmia with limb abnormalities	CL/P
Snai2	Piebaldism	Und
Sox11	Mental retardation, autosomal dominant, 27	Und
Sox5	Und	Und
Sox9	Acampomelic campomelic dysplasia	CL/P
Sp8	Und	Und
Spry1	Und	Und
Spry2	Und	Und
Sumo1	Orofacial cleft 10	CL/P
Tbx1	DiGeorge syndrome	CL/P

Gene	Syndromic/non-syndromic	Orofacial phenotype
Tbx2	Und	Und
Tbx22	Cleft palate with ankyloglossia	CL/P
Tcof1	Treacher-Collins syndrome	CL/P
Tctn2	Meckel syndrome 8	CL/P
Tgfb2	Loeys-Dietz syndrome, type 4	CL/P
Tgfb3	Arrhythmogenic right ventricular dysplasia 1	CL/P
Tgfbr1/Alk5	Loeys-Dietz syndrome, type 1	CL/P
Tgfbr2	Loeys-Dietz syndrome, type 2	CL/P
Trp63/Tp63	Ectrodactyly, ectodermal dysplasia, and cleft lip/palate syndrome 3; orofacial cleft 8, Hay-Wells syndrome, limb-mammary syndrome	CL/P
Tshz1	Aural atresia, congenital	Und
Ugdh	Und	Und
Vax1	Microphthalmia, syndromic 11	CL/P
Vegfa	Und	Und
Wdpcp	Und	Und
Whsc1	Und	Und
Wls/Gpr177	Und	Und
Wnt5a	Robinow syndrome, autosomal dominant	CL/P
Wnt9b	Und	Und
Zeb1	Corneal dystrophy	Und
Zic3	Congenital heart defects, non-syndromic; heterotaxy, visceral, 1; VACTERL association	CL/P
Zpf640/Mzf6d	Und	Und

Genes highlighted here are specifically mentioned in the pathways discussed in this chapter and listed separately in **Tables 2–7**. Phenotypes included are derived from the Online Mendelian Inheritance in Man (OMIM).

Table 1. Summary of genes with known involvement in the etiology of orofacial abnormalities in mice.

Upon cross-referencing the KO mice available through the Jackson Laboratory (http://www.informatics.jax.org/diseasePortal) and performing a literature search on PubMed, Web of Science, and similar scholarly databases, we can provide an accurate account of all currently available mouse models with phenotypes concurrent with our understanding of CL/P. Furthermore, physicians and researchers alike are searching for a coalescence of treatment strategies, including gene therapy, to replace our current therapeutic approaches that consist mainly of a lifetime persistence of surgeries with less than consistent results due, in part, to non-standardization of procedures. What follows is an in-depth look, in order of current dominance in the landscape of research, at the mouse models currently being used to study the etiologic determinants of orofacial clefting.

2.1. TGF beta (TGFβ) signaling pathway

A number of genes from the TGF beta (TGFβ) signaling pathway that play a role in palatogenesis in mice are many (**Table 2**). Members of this "superfamily" play an important role in the development of Meckel's cartilage and the mandible— thus, alteration or inactivation of particular members can lead to cleft palate [2]. TGFβ receptors are dimeric and consist of two types—type I and type II—of receptors with serine/threonine kinase activation. Once activated, these receptors function in such a way that SMAD transcription factors are phosphorylated, and through a cascade, eventually these SMADs make it into the nucleus where they function to modulate the transcription of particular subsets of genes [3]. The SMADs can either activate or repress the gene to which they bind. As such, a combination of dimeric receptors and ligands can result in any number of outcomes for a cell. In particular, TGFβ is

Gene	Syndromic/non-syndromic	Orofacial phenotype
Acvr1/Alk2	Submucosal cleft/fibrodysplasia ossificans progressiva	Und
Acvr2a	Und	Und
Bmp4	Microphthalmia, syndromic 6	CL/P
Bmpr1a/Alk3	Juvenile polyposis syndrome,	CP
Chrd	Und	CL
Cited2	Atrial septal defect 8, ventricular septal defect 2	Und
Foxc2/Mfh1	Lymphedema-distichiasis syndrome	CL/P
Foxd3	Und	Und
Foxe1/Titf2/Fkhl15	Bamforth-Lazarus syndrome	CL/P
Foxf2	Und	Und
Fst	Und	Und
Gdf11/Bmp11	Und	Und
Inhba	Und	Und
Map3k7/ Tak1	Und	Und
Smad4	Juvenile polyposis/hereditary hemorrhagic telangiectasia syndrome	Und
Smad7	Und	Und
Tgfb2	Loeys-Dietz syndrome, type 4	CL/P
Tgfb3	Arrhythmogenic right ventricular dysplasia 1	CL/P
Tgfbr1/Alk5	Loeys-Dietz syndrome, type 1	CL/P
Tgfbr2	Loeys-Dietz syndrome, type 2	CL/P

Table 2. TGF beta/BMP signaling pathway.

involved in several critical functions that take place during embryogenesis, including proliferation, apoptosis, and cell differentiation.

Also, critical to normal development of the palate is the temporal and spatial distribution of the members of the TGFβ signaling pathway. The importance of this timing aspect may be that these structures, similar to morphogens, inducing specific tissue formation at identifiable time points in development [4]. This information can be used in the development of novel treatment strategies in humans with known gene mutations or deficiencies.

Typically, TGFβ receptor activation recruits and phosphorylates SMAD2 and SMAD3 at the carboxyl terminus via TGFβ receptor I. This method of signaling is generally what is meant by the term SMAD-dependent TGFβ signaling. However, TGFβ signaling can occur in lieu of SMAD activation via phosphorylation—pathways known to be activated in this manner include MAPK pathways (i.e., ERK, NJK, and p38) [5]. Inherently, this creates a purported "balance" between the levels of SMAD-dependent and SMAD-independent TGFβ signaling that exists through the development of normal palatogenesis. When we discuss the SMAD-independent pathways, it has been proposed that these are the result of posttranslational modifications which occur to either of the two types of TGFβ receptors. These mechanisms and their subsequent cascades are under current investigation and not yet entirely known [5].

Distinct members of the TGFβ superfamily, utilizing a separate series of SMAD proteins (SMAD1/5/9), are the bone morphogenetic proteins (BMPs). There are a number of BMP ligands known and two distinct receptor types—type I and type II. As mentioned, there appears to be a temporal and spatial distribution of this family, which is critical for the function of BMPs, which are very well researched with regard to palatogenesis. In particular, *Bmp4* cKO mice show clefting of the lip, both uni- and bilaterally [6]. Understandably, BMP receptors play a role in orofacial clefting as well; in addition, there is a distinct involvement in tooth morphogenesis for BMP receptors, notably *Bmpr1a* [7]. This molecule and its related receptors have an essentially unparalleled significance in the etiologic pathogenesis of CL/P. *Bmpr1a* cKO embryos, while also showing tooth morphology defects, die from orofacial clefting [6, 7].

2.2. Hedgehog signaling pathway

When one first thinks of SHH, it is likely that we recall the molecule's importance in left-right patterning of the embryo, dorsal-ventral establishment of the neural tube, and brain development, among other functions. Intrinsic properties of these morphogenic functions include signaling for cell proliferation and survival. The alteration of these properties can lead SHH receptors and/or ligands to function abnormally, thus, in some cases, altering the patterning of cranial neural crest cells during embryonic development. Modulation of the molecules involved in hedgehog signaling has been shown to present with CL/P phenotype in mice.

The full breadth of hedgehog signaling molecules with known involvement in orofacial clefting in mice spans several other pathways (**Table 3**). A notable characteristic of the mechanism of action for *Shh* can be observed in nasal epithelium of mice where *Shh* is reported absent. These mice develop cleft palate, while mice with overexpressed *Shh* are shown to express failure of growth of the maxillary processes and thus no fusion; this leads to cleft palate and several missing bones within the nasal process [8].

Gene	Syndromic/non-syndromic	Phenotypes
Gli2	Culler-Jones syndrome, holoprosencephaly-9	CL/P
Gli3	Greig cephalopolysyndactyly	CL/P
Ptch1/Ptc1	Basal cell nevus syndrome (Gorlin syndrome)	CL/P
Shh	Holoprosencephaly-3	CL/P
Smo/Smoh	Basal cell carcinoma, somatic	Und

Table 3. Hedgehog signaling pathway.

Another notable molecule involved in the hedgehog signaling pathway is *Ptch1*, a transcriptional target of *Shh* as well, which displays a gradient mimicking that of *Shh* in the palatal shelves during early palatogenesis, at E13.5 [8]. Similarly, the palatal mesenchyme adjacent to the medial-edge epithelium (MEE) present in the nasal epithelium expressed *Smo* in significant amounts [9]. In each case with the hedgehog signaling molecules, there is expression in the palatal mesenchyme, with the highest level of expression for most molecules adjacent to the palatal oral epithelium [9]. The awareness of this spatial and temporal expression provides a niche for the insertion or potential innervation of gene products given therapeutically. The effects of an abnormal amount of SHH signaling are palpable. Restoration of the proper balance of SHH signaling throughout development may play a role in treatment options in the near future, and delivery methods are currently underway to target particular areas of known involvement in CL/P.

2.3. Wnt signaling pathway

The Wnt signaling pathway plays another exceptional role in craniofacial morphogenesis in mice (**Table 4**). There are 19 known Wnt proteins found in humans, with combinations of differing ligands and receptors allowing for a mixture of modulatory effects from similar molecules. Between the receptors available, there exist three distinct pathways: the β-catenin-dependent (canonical), β-catenin-independent planar cell polarity (PCP), and β-catenin-independent Ca^{2+} pathways. β-Catenin is a transcription factor that, when Wnt ligands are present, will persist and

Gene	Syndromic/non-syndromic	Phenotypes
Ctnnb1	Mental retardation, autosomal dominant 19	Und
Edn1	Auriculocondylar syndrome 3	CL/P
Fzd2	Und	Und
Gsk3b	Und	Und
Lrp6	Und	Und
Prickle1	Epilepsy, progressive myoclonic	Und
Wnt5a	Robinow syndrome, autosomal dominant	CL/P
Wnt9b	Und	Und

Table 4. Wnt signaling pathway.

translocate into the nucleus; the factor is otherwise degraded [7]. The Wnt pathway is involved in a variety of embryogenic and developmental events, similar to the SHH pathway. In terms of craniofacial development, we see a critical role for the Wnt signaling pathway when we observe the generation, migration, proliferation, and survival of cranial neural crest cells [10].

A notable Wnt ligand involved in canonical signaling is *Wnt9b*. Expressed between the facial processes, alterations in signaling of this molecule have shown to express clefting in mice. Additionally, *Wnt9b* null mice have a distinctly shorter nasal process and shortened maxillary processes, a direct link to bilateral CLP [11]. This expression is apparent with FGF molecules, one of the many molecules involved with and expressively determined by Wnt signaling. A deletion of either the epithelium in which *Wnt9b* is found or a KO of the ligand (gene product) itself results in a similar cleft lip phenotype [11].

While the plethora of numerous other Wnt signaling targets and mediators exist, a receptor of particular interest and importance currently is *Lrp6*. This receptor functions in the canonical Wnt pathway as well and contains members of the Frizzled family as well as a co-receptor, which can be low-density lipoprotein receptor-related protein 6 (LRP6). Research has shown that *Lrp6* null mice demonstrate bilateral clefting of the lip as well and cleft palate and midline clefting of the mandible [12]. These mice also express defects in the neural tube, eye, and brain among others. The orofacial clefting defects were observed at E13.5 in these *Lrp6* null mice, with full penetrance of CLP and mandibular defects [12]. Again, we see a pattern that current research has established wherein a spatial and temporal time table has been created. This knowledge, as it continues to expand with further genomic testing and mouse model availability, should prove highly useful in the development of novel therapies.

2.4. FGF signaling pathway

While it has already been briefly discussed, one can see that the FGF signaling pathway also expands across several currently known molecular cascades. In humans and in mice, mutations resulting in dysfunction of the FGF signaling pathway are known to result in a variety of craniofacial abnormalities and syndromes—one proponent of which is orofacial clefting. An important role of FGF signaling is seen in the induction of the neural crest while being widely expressed in epithelial-mesenchymal interactions elsewhere. Particularly in the facial primordia, FGF signaling is absolutely critical in the proper development and formation of the palate as it is present in both endochondral (i.e., Meckel's cartilage) and intramembranous bones [13]. When we consider palatogenesis, FGF molecules have been shown to be involved in multiple stages—from palatal shelf elevation to fusion of MEE. KO mice have played a key role in our understanding of the function of various FGFs and their relation to orofacial clefting.

There are 23 distinct FGF ligands known and four receptors to which they bind. Alternative splicing generates several receptor variants which allows for multiple binding combinations and, thus, different functionalities temporally during embryogenesis. Various receptors are located in the epithelium and mesenchyme throughout the embryo, and research has elucidated many roles that these molecules play; for our interest, much emphasis has been placed on suture fusion (craniosynostosis) and palatogenesis.

Mutations in FGF receptors have been shown to present with a variety of midfacial syndromes in mice as well (**Table 5**). For example, in humans, gain-of-function mutations in *FGFR2* and *FGFR3* have been consistently observed in individuals with Crouzon syndrome—a genetic disorder that includes craniosynostosis in its list of defects associated with the syndrome. More relevant here, however, is that a KO mouse model in which the *Fgfr1* receptors are missing in the cranial neural crest (CNC) cells directly results in CLP due to failures in the proliferation and migration of said cells [14]. Likewise, research has shown that ectopic activation of *Fgf8* results in increased proliferation and a failure of the palatal shelves to elevate properly [15]. This is exceptionally interesting in that it is a rare case in which an increase in cell proliferative activity has resulted in CP; in many cases, CP is the result of an obvious decrease in the amount of cell proliferation. In the case of *Fgf8* activation, the palatal shelves were still unable to elevate in a normal manner, and thus the palatal morphology was altered, and a CP phenotype was observed.

Gene	Syndromic/non-syndromic	Phenotypes
Fgf10	Aplasia of lachrymal and salivary glands	Und
Fgf18	Und	Und
Fgf9	Und	Und
Fgfr1	Non-syndromic cleft lip/palate, Hartsfield syndrome, hypogonadotropic hypogonadism 2, Pfeiffer syndrome	CL/P
Fgfr2	Apert syndrome	CL/P
Gbr2	Und	Und
Spry1	Und	Und
Spry2	Und	Und

Table 5. FGF signaling pathway.

The FGF signaling pathway has been, and is currently being, extensively studied. Spatial expression of the molecules involved in the pathway has been seen widely throughout the developing mouse embryo, while the temporal expression continues to be expounded upon. Investigations are ongoing to further our knowledge of why characteristically opposing molecular processes (i.e., reduction versus activation of cellular proliferation) may result in the same phenotype. In all, what remains important is that future treatment options are expanding all the time. The more we learn about all the plethora of molecular signals that interact during embryogenesis—which is similar enough between mouse and human—the more physicians and surgeons are able to generate new and better therapies.

2.5. MAPK signaling pathway

The mitogen-activated protein kinase (MAPK) signaling pathway—also known as the ERK pathway—plays a role in craniofacial development of mice as early as E10.5 [16]. MAPK is a protein kinase that functions in conjunction with two others, MAPKKK (e.g., RAF) and MAPKK (e.g., MEK1/2). Upon activation, these effector molecules can act in either the cytosol or the nucleus. Growth factors, including TGFβ, BMPs, and fibroblast growth factor (FGF), can modulate this same protein kinase cascade, and each of the molecules listed is also known to be involved with development of the palate [17]. Additionally, analysis of the potential spatial representation of active (phosphorylated) ERK1/ERK2 in the palate has resulted in the discovery this pathway persists in both the epithelium and the mesenchyme associated with the developing palatal shelves [17].

Immunohistochemistry using an antibody against an activated form of ERK has shown ERK signaling in the frontonasal process, brachial arches, and extraembryonic ectoderm, among other craniofacial-associated regions [16]. Research has also shown associations between MAPK signaling and growth factor pathway genes that include *Fgf9/10/18*, *Alk5*, and *Itgb1* among others and vary craniofacial clefting and defects in mice, including mandibular osteogenic and tongue abnormalities [17]. The inclusion of the mandible and tongue is important in that it adds to the overall complexity of the defect, thus making treatment options that much more of a priority. Current investigations are ongoing to pinpoint time points and the distribution of MAPK signaling and its numerous molecular effectors during embryogenesis in mice (**Table 6**).

Gene	Syndromic/non-syndromic	Phenotypes
Chuk/Ikk1/Tcf16	Cocoon syndrome	Und
Egfr	Und	Und
Grb2	Und	Und
Pdgfra	Gastrointestinal stromal tumor, somatic	CL/P
Crk	Und	Und
Itgb1	Und	Und

Table 6. MAPK signaling pathway.

2.6. Homeobox proteins

Homeobox proteins and their respective KO/mutant mouse models are used to represent easily observable phenotypes. Some of the most well-studied homeobox genes in mice include *Msx1/2*, *Pax9*, and *Alx1* [1]. The reason for their grouping and relatively well-known actions has to do with the fact that transcription factors encoded by homeobox genes act in a site-specific manner [18]. These gene products exist, segmentally, throughout the body and are palpable during nearly all stages of development. As such, we know that there are Hox homeogenes which control bone patterning in the limb buds; similarly, there are separate homeogenes that are associated with craniofacial development in mice (**Table 7**).

Specifically, research has shown that a human *MSX1* missense mutation can lead to orofacial clefting as well as selective tooth agenesis [19]. Mutations in this gene, as seen in other homeogenes, can lead to dysfunctional protein products that act via transcriptional repression. In the case of *Msx1*, the homeodomain interacts directly with the TATA-binding protein (TBP) and acts directly at the start of transcription by repressing the gene completely to which it translocates. In some scenarios, heterodimers will form between homeodomain proteins, and a balance must persist in which they are co-regulatory.

Gene	Syndromic/non-syndromic	Phenotypes
Alx1	Frontonasal dysplasia 3	CL/P
Alx3	Frontonasal dysplasia 1	CL/P
Alx4	Frontonasal dysplasia 2, parietal foramina 2, craniosynostosis 5	Cleft alae nasi
Barx1	Und	Und
Dlx1	Und	Und
Dlx2	Und	Und
Dlx5	Split-hand/foot malformation 1 with sensorineural hearing loss	CL/P
Gbx2	Und	Und
Gsc	Short stature, auditory canal atresia, mandibular hypoplasia, skeletal abnormalities	Und
Hoxa2	Microtia with or without hearing impairment	Und
Msx1	Ectodermal dysplasia 3, Witkop-type orofacial cleft 5	CL/P
Msx2	Craniosynostosis, type 2; parietal foramina 1, parietal foramina with cleidocranial dysplasia	CL/P
Pax9	Tooth agenesis, selective, 3	Und
Pitx1	Clubfoot, congenital, with or without deficiency of long bones and/or mirror-image polydactyly, Liebenberg syndrome	CL/P
Pitx2	Axenfeld-Rieger syndrome, type 1; iridogoniodysgenesis, type 2; Peters anomaly	Und
Prrx1/Prx1/Mhox	Agnathia-otocephaly complex	CL/P
Rax	Microphthalmia, isolated 3	Und
Shox2	Und	Und
Vax1	Microphthalmia, syndromic 11	CL/P

Table 7. Homeobox protein signaling pathway.

As a result of these proteins acting within their respective zones (or "sites"), one can assume that there is an overlap with the adjacent homeodomain. Such overlap is observed between *Msx1* and *Msx2* throughout the craniofacial structures during development—including the skull, suture mesenchyme, and teeth [20]. Inherent in their molecular categorization is the idea that we know where, and upon which tissues, these proteins interact. There are a number of homeogenes involved in craniofacial development that modulate palatogenesis and patterning, among a variety of other roles. Due to their known functions during embryogenesis, further research is ongoing regarding the effect of varying homeogene mutations on cell proliferation, survival, and adhesion. The culmination of knowledge that lies within these determinants of normal development will indubitably result in opportunities for the future application of therapeutic modalities.

2.7. Remaining mouse strains exhibiting CL/P phenotype

Here, we have put into one table a list of the genes with a known association, whether syndromic or non-syndromic, to the development of the palate in mouse (**Table 1**). It should be noted that not all genes in this table have shown their identical, cross species phenotype in humans.

2.8. The future of CL/P therapy

A bonafide surgical protocol remains to be standardized for the repair of CL/P. Fortunately, ongoing research concerning therapeutic interventions for this relatively common birth defect has recently begun to delve into new and improved options for repair with, hopefully, more consistent and stable results for patients. The current "golden standard" treatment option for pediatric oral surgeons involves bone grafting, or alveoloplasty, usually from autogenous sites—but this has many complications associated with both the grafting procedure and the agreed-upon effectiveness in reconstructing the palate over time [21]. Postoperative follow-up has shown success rates ranging from 41 to 73%, which is far from standardized, while there also exists the possibility (in 11–23% of patients) of oronasal fistulas, which come with their own brand new set of complications for the patient [22]. In short, the most effective interventions in use today are far from ideal for the patent and result in long-term risk of complications from grafting procedures, disturbance of adjacent craniofacial development, and, over time, a significant financial encumbrance on the patient. Techniques including gene delivery, in vitro engineered tissue transplantation, and regenerative medicine are being probed for efficacy, and some are showing promising results thus far.

An exceptionally exciting modality is the use of stem cells. One method of delivering these cells is via a biocompatible scaffold upon which cells that have been previously harvested were cultured and attached. Materials including collagen, hyaluronic acid, and hydroxyapatite have been utilized in attempts to develop such scaffolds [23–25]. These scaffolds have been engineered as injectable gels, mesh networks, and foams. Ideally, this aids in the procedure being as minimally invasive as possible while also providing maximum benefit and adequate delivery to the area of interest. This therapy can be modified to include signaling molecules and other types of differentiated cells—which preferably have a known clinical outcome and avoid the possibility of rejection and/or disunity with the surrounding host cells—and injected in a similar fashion or applied to previously engineered palates. Currently, autogenous mesenchymal stem cells (MSCs) are regarded as the optimum choice for in vivo osteogenic reconstructions; these can come from umbilical cord blood, Wharton's jelly, and even the patient's own bone marrow [26]. Tissue regenerative-specific repair of CL/P has been demonstrated with some success, and some are now advocating for in depth considering of its potential to replace traditional autogenous grafting procedures [27].

Regarding clinical studies in progress, one group has shown that in vitro differentiated MSCs derived from bone marrow were delivered with platelet-derived growth factor and significant improvement was observed 3 months post-op [28]. Similarly, recombination therapies are being used to induce osteoblastic differentiation with BMPs formed from stem cells, and resulting immunohistological analysis of the bone that formed has shown normal, vital structure [29]. Finally, platelet-rich plasma (PRP) is being studied with regard to its potential for tissue repair in vivo. A wide variety of growth factors are present in a platelet-rich solution and have been shown to promote angiogenesis and extracellular matrix formation [30]. This intervention has some positive results—it has been shown that PRP can enhance bone regeneration and thus may be a useful alternative to traditional procedures for CL/P patients [31].

A number of prospective therapeutic interventions are currently being investigated, many with exciting outcomes thus far. CL/P etiology is not yet completely understood and is extremely complex. In order to properly apply this research to the human subjects, we must further our research to bridge the gap between an understanding of the signaling pathways, the rescue of the animal phenotype, and the translation of this knowledge into human treatment. As research continues on the pathways mentioned in this chapter, further clinical trials should become available, and treatment outcomes for patients can rapidly and significantly improve. Moving forward, more work is needed to establish a new standard of care and a protocol for various differing types of orofacial clefts, but progress has proceeded rapidly in recent years, and the outlook is bright for the future of care for CL/P patients.

In summary, it remains within animal research where the next steps in the elucidation of potential treatments for CL/P must be made. Understanding the biological, molecular signaling pathways and identifying a broad cause for the clefting phenotype are only the first steps in understanding how to treat it. Now, we need to look toward a greater understanding of the critical downstream events that occur as a result of the KO or cKO models being used; what types of tissue-tissue interactions are changing? What is the scope of the molecular activity being altered as a result of changing the capabilities of one gene? Once more of these questions are answered in animal models, the translation of lab research to the rescue of human phenotypes will become more clear. Until then, it is crucial to continue to identify all that we can in order to bridge the gap between KO/cKO mice, the expansive etiology surrounding their conditions, and the rescue of their control phenotypes.

Author details

Aram J. Keteyian* and Yuji Mishina

*Address all correspondence to: aketeyia@umich.edu

Department of Biologic and Materials Science, School of Dentistry, University of Michigan, Ann Arbor, MI, USA

References

[1] Funato N, Nakamura M, Yanagisawa H. Molecular basis of cleft palates in mice. World J Biol Chem [Internet]. 2015 Aug 26 [cited 2016 Apr 30];6(3):121–138. Available from: http://www.pubmedcentral.nih.gov/articlerender.fcgi?artid=4549757&tool=pmcentrez&rendertype=abstract

[2] Lei R, Zhang K, Liu K, Shao X, Ding Z, Wang F, et al. Transferrin receptor facilitates TGF-β and BMP signaling activation to control craniofacial morphogenesis. Cell Death Dis [Internet]. Nature Publishing Group; 2016 Jun 30 [cited 2016 Jul 16];7(6):e2282. Available from: http://www.nature.com/doifinder/10.1038/cddis.2016.170

[3] Iwata J, Parada C, Chai Y. The mechanism of TGF-β signaling during palate development. Oral Dis [Internet]. Blackwell Publishing Ltd; 2011 Nov [cited 2016 Jul 16];17(8):733–744. Available from: http://doi.wiley.com/10.1111/j.1601-0825.2011.01806.x

[4] Dudas M, Kaartinen V. TGF-β superfamily and mouse craniofacial development: interplay of morphogenetic proteins and receptor signaling controls normal formation of the face. Curr Top Dev Biol. 2005;66:65–133.

[5] Kang JS, Liu C, Derynck R. New regulatory mechanisms of TGF-β receptor function. Trends Cell Biol. 2009;19(8):385–394.

[6] Liu W, Sun X, Braut A, Mishina Y, Behringer RR, Mina M, et al. Distinct functions for Bmp signaling in lip and palate fusion in mice. Development [Internet]. The Company of Biologists Ltd; 2005 Mar [cited 2016 Jul 16];132(6):1453–1461. Available from: http://www.ncbi.nlm.nih.gov/pubmed/15716346

[7] Suzuki A, Sangani DR, Ansari A, Iwata J. Molecular mechanisms of midfacial developmental defects. Dev Dyn [Internet]. 2016 Mar [cited 2016 Jul 16];245(3):276–293. Available from: http://doi.wiley.com/10.1002/dvdy.24368

[8] Cobourne MT, Xavier GM, Depew M, Hagan L, Sealby J, Webster Z, et al. Sonic hedgehog signalling inhibits palatogenesis and arrests tooth development in a mouse model of the nevoid basal cell carcinoma syndrome. Dev Biol. 2009;331(1):38–49.

[9] Rice R, Connor E, Rice DPC. Expression patterns of Hedgehog signalling pathway members during mouse palate development. Gene Expr Patterns. 2006Vol. 6.

[10] Mani P, Jarrell A, Myers J, Atit R. Visualizing canonical Wnt signaling during mouse craniofacial development. Dev Dyn [Internet]. 2010 Jan [cited 2016 Jul 16];239(1):354–363. Available from: http://www.ncbi.nlm.nih.gov/pubmed/19718763

[11] Jin YR, Han XH, Taketo MM, Yoon JK, Abu-Issa R, Smyth G, et al. Wnt9b-dependent FGF signaling is crucial for outgrowth of the nasal and maxillary processes during upper jaw and lip development. Development [Internet]. Oxford University Press for The Company of Biologists Limited; 2012 May [cited 2016 Jul 16];139(10):1821–1830. Available from: http://www.ncbi.nlm.nih.gov/pubmed/22461561

[12] Song L, Li Y, Wang K, Wang YZ, Molotkov A, Gao L, et al. Lrp6-mediated canonical Wnt signaling is required for lip formation and fusion. Development [Internet]. The Company of Biologists Ltd; 2009 Sep [cited 2016 Jul 16];136(18):3161–3171. Available from: http://www.ncbi.nlm.nih.gov/pubmed/19700620

[13] Nie X, Luukko K, Kettunen P. FGF signalling in craniofacial development and developmental disorders. Oral Dis [Internet]. Blackwell Publishing Ltd; 2006 Mar [cited 2016 Jul 18];12(2):102–111. Available from: http://doi.wiley.com/10.1111/j.1601-0825.2005.01176.x

[14] Wang C, Chang JYF, Yang C, Huang Y, Liu J, You P, et al. Type 1 fibroblast growth factor receptor in cranial neural crest cell-derived mesenchyme is required for palatogenesis. J Biol Chem [Internet]. American Society for Biochemistry and Molecular Biology; 2013 Jul 26 [cited 2016 Jul 18];288(30):22174–22183. Available from: http://www.jbc.org/cgi/doi/10.1074/jbc.M113.463620

[15] Wu W, Gu S, Sun C, He W, Xie X, Li X, et al. Altered FGF signaling pathways impair cell proliferation and elevation of palate shelves. Zhang X, editor. PLoS One [Internet]. Public Library of Science; 2015 Sep 2 [cited 2016 Jul 18];10(9):e0136951. Available from: http://dx.plos.org/10.1371/journal.pone.0136951

[16] Corson LB, Yamanaka Y, Lai KMV, Rossant J. Spatial and temporal patterns of ERK signaling during mouse embryogenesis. Development [Internet]. The Company of Biologists Ltd; 2003 Oct [cited 2016 Jul 18];130(19):4527–4537. Available from: http://www.ncbi.nlm.nih.gov/pubmed/12925581

[17] Parada C, Han D, Grimaldi A, Sarrión P, Park SS, Pelikan R, et al. Disruption of the ERK/MAPK pathway in neural crest cells as a potential cause of Pierre Robin sequence. Development [Internet]. Oxford University Press for The Company of Biologists Limited; 2015 Nov 1 [cited 2016 Jul 18];142(21):3734–3745. Available from: http://www.ncbi.nlm.nih.gov/pubmed/26395480

[18] Nassif A, Senussi I, Meary F, Loiodice S, Hotton D, Robert B, et al. Msx1 role in craniofacial bone morphogenesis. Bone. 2014;66:96–104.

[19] Vastardis H, Karimbux N, Guthua SW, Seidman JG, Seidman CE. A human MSX1 homeodomain missense mutation causes selective tooth agenesis. Nat Genet [Internet]. Nature Publishing Group; 1996 Aug [cited 2016 Jul 18];13(4):417–421. Available from: http://www.nature.com/doifinder/10.1038/ng0896-417

[20] Alappat S, Zhang ZY, Chen YP. Msx homeobox gene family and craniofacial development. Cell Res [Internet]. Nature Publishing Group; 2003 Dec [cited 2016 Jul 18];13(6):429–442. Available from: http://www.nature.com/doifinder/10.1038/sj.cr.7290185

[21] Arangio P, Marianetti TM, Tedaldi M, Ramieri V, Cascone P. Early secondary alveoloplasty in cleft lip and palate. J Craniofac Surg [Internet]. 2008 Sep [cited 2016 Jul 19];19(5):1364–1369. Available from: http://www.ncbi.nlm.nih.gov/pubmed/18812864

[22] Tavakolinejad S, Ebrahimzadeh Bidskan A, Ashraf H, Hamidi Alamdari D. A glance at methods for cleft palate repair. Iran Red Crescent Med J [Internet]. Kowsar; 2014 Sep [cited 2016 Jul 18];16(9):e15393. Available from: http://www.ncbi.nlm.nih.gov/pubmed/25593724

[23] Kang SW, Kim JS, Park KS, Cha BH, Shim JH, Kim JY, et al. Surface modification with fibrin/hyaluronic acid hydrogel on solid-free form-based scaffolds followed by BMP-2 loading to enhance bone regeneration. Bone [Internet]. Elsevier; 2011 Feb [cited 2016 Jul 19];48(2):298–306. Available from: http://www.ncbi.nlm.nih.gov/pubmed/20870047

[24] Krishnamoorthy G, Sehgal PK, Mandal AB, Sadulla S. Novel collagen scaffolds prepared by using unnatural D-amino acids assisted EDC/NHS crosslinking. J Biomater Sci Polym

Ed [Internet]. 2013 [cited 2016 Jul 19];24(3):344–364. Available from: http://www.ncbi.nlm.nih.gov/pubmed/23565652

[25] Guda T, Walker JA, Pollot BE, Appleford MR, Oh S, Ong JL, et al. In vivo performance of bilayer hydroxyapatite scaffolds for bone tissue regeneration in the rabbit radius. J Mater Sci Mater Med [Internet]. 2011 Mar [cited 2016 Jul 19];22(3):647–656. Available from: http://www.ncbi.nlm.nih.gov/pubmed/21287244

[26] Diao Y, Ma Q, Cui F, Zhong Y. Human umbilical cord mesenchymal stem cells: osteogenesis in vivo as seed cells for bone tissue engineering. J Biomed Mater Res A [Internet]. 2009 Oct [cited 2016 Jul 19];91(1):123–131. Available from: http://www.ncbi.nlm.nih.gov/pubmed/18767055

[27] Pourebrahim N, Hashemibeni B, Shahnaseri S, Torabinia N, Mousavi B, Adibi S, et al. A comparison of tissue-engineered bone from adipose-derived stem cell with autogenous bone repair in maxillary alveolar cleft model in dogs. Int J Oral Maxillofac Surg [Internet]. Elsevier; 2013 May [cited 2016 Jul 19];42(5):562–568. Available from: http://www.ncbi.nlm.nih.gov/pubmed/23219713

[28] Behnia H, Khojasteh A, Soleimani M, Tehranchi A, Atashi A, Behnia H, et al. Repair of alveolar cleft defect with mesenchymal stem cells and platelet derived growth factors: a preliminary report. J Craniomaxillofac Surg [Internet]. Elsevier; 2012 Jan [cited 2016 Jul 19];40(1):2–7. Available from: http://www.ncbi.nlm.nih.gov/pubmed/21420310

[29] Chin M, Ng T, Tom WK, Carstens M. Repair of alveolar clefts with recombinant human bone morphogenetic protein (rhBMP-2) in patients with clefts. J Craniofac Surg [Internet]. 2005 Sep [cited 2016 Jul 19];16(5):778–789. Available from: http://www.ncbi.nlm.nih.gov/pubmed/16192856

[30] Shirvan MK, Alamdari DH, Ghoreifi A, Arrowsmith SD, Ruminjo J, Landry EG, et al. A novel method for iatrogenic vesicovaginal fistula treatment: autologous platelet rich plasma injection and platelet rich fibrin glue interposition. J Urol [Internet]. Elsevier; 2013 Jun [cited 2016 Jul 19];189(6):2125–2129. Available from: http://linkinghub.elsevier.com/retrieve/pii/S0022534712060053

[31] Oyama T, Nishimoto S, Tsugawa T, Shimizu F, Boyne P, Sand N, et al. Efficacy of platelet-rich plasma in alveolar bone grafting. J Oral Maxillofac Surg [Internet]. Elsevier; 2004 May [cited 2016 Jul 19];62(5):555–558. Available from: http://linkinghub.elsevier.com/retrieve/pii/S0278239104000345

3

Cleft Lip and Palate Patients: Assessment and Management

Letizia Perillo, Fabrizia d'Apuzzo, Sara Eslami and Abdolreza Jamilian

Abstract

Cleft lip or palate is one of the most common types of craniomaxillofacial birth anomalies. Midface deficiency is a common feature of cleft lip and palate patients due to scar tissue of the lip and palate closure. Cleft lip and palate patients should be carefully evaluated by the craniofacial team in order to detect potentially serious deformities. Craniofacial team is involved with diagnosis of facial morphology, feeding problems, guidance of the growth and development of the face, occlusion, dentition, hearing and speech problems, and psychosocial issues and jaw discrepancy of the patients with cleft lip and palate or craniofacial syndromes. Treatment for cleft children requires a multidisciplinary approach including facial surgery in the first months of life, preventive and interceptive treatment in primary dentition, speech therapy, orthodontics in the mixed dentition phase, oromaxillofacial surgery, and implant and prosthetics in adults. Treatment plan from orthodontic perspective can be divided into the following stages based on the dentition stages: (1) presurgical orthopedics, (2) primary dentition, (3) mixed dentition, and (4) permanent dentition. The aim of this chapter is to assess a rational team work approach in the management of the patient with cleft lip and/or palate from birth to adulthood.

Keywords: cleft lip, cleft palate, diagnosis, treatment, maxillary deficiency

1. Introduction

Cleft lip or palate is one of the most common types of cranio-maxillofacial birth anomalies. It accounts for 65% of all head and neck deformities [1]. Maxillary deficiency is a common feature of cleft lip and palate patients due to scar tissue of the lip and palate closure. For treatment of maxillary deficiency, various devices, such as facemask [2], protraction headgear [3], orthopedic mask [4], reverse chin cup [5], tongue appliance [6], tongue plate [7], surgically assisted orthopedic protraction, and distraction osteogenesis have been introduced [8]. Treatment of cleft lip and palate in patients should be started after birth and continues to adulthood. Lip closure and palatal closure are performed at 3 months and around 12 months of age, respectively, as well as secondary alveolar bone graft is done between 9 and 12 years of age [9]. However, orthodontic intervention usually begins during the mixed dentition. Orthodontic treatment in patients with cleft lip and palate are focused on maxillary arch expansion, correction of upper incisor misalignments, gross rotations of incisors, and crossbites and correction of Class III skeletal growth pattern. Patients with cleft lip and/or palate should be treated by teamwork. The team conception allows a systematic treatment plan to be developed and allows the team members to work together properly to identify problems. Orthodontic treatment plan can be divided into the following stages based on the dentition stages: (1) presurgical orthopedics, (2) primary dentition, (3) mixed dentition, and (4) permanent dentition.

In the following sections about diagnosis, classification, and treatment options in different period of time are discussed. Therefore, the aim of this chapter is to assess a rational teamwork approach to the management of the patient with cleft lip and/or palate from birth to adulthood.

2. Diagnostic considerations

Ultrasonography serves as a noninvasive diagnostic tool, now regularly recommended as a routine component of prenatal consideration. This noninvasive diagnostic tool helps to determine gestational age, confirm fetal viability, check placental location, establish the growth and their number of fetuses, and examine fetal anatomy to detect any deformities [10].

3. Treatment planning for cleft lip and palate patients

The treatment of cleft lip and palate should be started right after birth. Treatment for cleft children requires a multidisciplinary approach including: facial surgery in the first months of life, preventive and interceptive treatment in primary dentition, speech therapy, orthodontics in the mixed dentition phase, oral and maxillofacial surgery, and implant and prosthetics in adults. So the treatment to achieve a proper occlusion and function often lasts from birth until adulthood. Patients with cleft lip and palate routinely require extensive and prolonged orthodontic treatment. Close cooperation between the orthodontist, surgeon, prosthodontist, and general dentist is required. Cleft lip and palate patients should be carefully evaluated by the craniofacial team in order to detect potentially serious deformities that can be associated with cleft lip and palate. The team conception allows a systematic treatment plan to be developed and allows the team members to work together properly to identify problems. Maxillary deficiency is a common developmental problem in cleft lip and palate patients. The treatment objectives are to correct the deficient maxillary arch, the anterior and posterior cross bites, correct misaligned maxillary incisors, and also obtain satisfactory overjet and overbite. The following general and local factors must be evaluated before planning any treatment.

3.1. General factors

(a) Health of the patient includes physical, mental, and social.

(b) Family background and attitude.

3.2. Local factors

(a) Width of the cleft.

(b) Adequacy of tissue adjacent to the cleft.

(c) Length of soft palate in relation to nasopharynx.

(d) Configuration of nasopharynx.

(e) Functional activity of palate-pharyngeal muscles.

3.3. Interceptive treatment

Interceptive treatment is recommended because it can

- improve facial and dental esthetics,
- help overcome psychological issues,
- improve speech,
- reduce the risk of decay, and
- avoid the need for major surgery in the future.

3.4. Cleft lip repair

The aim of lip repair is to close the cleft to create esthetics of the face and to restore muscular anatomy of the upper lip. This procedure will serve to develop lip normally with minimal scar tissue. Closure of the lip is accomplished by the plastic or maxillofacial surgeon when the patient is approximately 3 months of age and weighs at least 10 pounds.

3.5. Cleft palate repair

The objective of cleft palate surgery is to close the palate to restore normal function to eating and drinking and to enhance the development of normal speech. The palate forms the floor of the nose and the roof of the oral cavity; thus, a cleft causes a free communication between these two cavities. Treatment of cleft lip and palatal patients is complex because of potential problems with middle ear infections, speech, feeding, occlusion, creating maxillary deficiency due to scar tissue from surgical procedure, and jaw abnormalities. Surgical procedure of the cleft palate is best performed before the child reaches 12 months of age. This procedure is called palatoplasty. Additional surgeries are often needed to achieve the best results [9].

3.6. Nursing care

The role of nursing in the care of patients and or families includes family education, case management, access to team care, assistance with infant feeding, consultation, research, and primary care.

3.7. Feeding problems

An infant with a cleft may have difficulty in feeding due to lack of suction. Cleft lip patients do not usually have feeding problems. But when the palate is involved, feeding can be a crucial challenge. Normally, the palate serves as a barrier to prevent food and liquids from entering the nose. A patient with cleft palate swallows a lot of air and regurgitates food into the nose. Cleft palate patients may need a special bottle and nipple to receive milk. Patients with feeding problems should be visited regularly by a specialist to make sure that they are gaining weight well.

3.8. Speech problems

Difficulty in speech is the number one issue for cleft patients after facial and dental esthetics. They have difficulty in speaking correctly, and treatment can help them to achieve a good tongue posture. Difficulty with speech articulation is common in cleft lip and palate patients. Many patients require speech therapy after surgery. Speech therapist will repeatedly evaluate speech development and will arrange for necessitate speech therapy.

3.9. Dental problems

Dental problems have an effect on chewing, facial esthetics, speech thus these patients frequently require orthodontic treatment. Prevalence of dental anomalies such as variations in tooth number, dislocation, missing, supernumerary, tooth shape, and reduced tooth dimensions has always been found to be higher in cleft lip and or palate patients when compared with general population [11]. Akcam et al. [12] reported that a significant amount (96.7%) of children with cleft had at least one dental irregularity. Shapira et al. [13] found that in the cleft area, most developmental dental anomalies are related to the maxillary lateral incisor, both in the primary and in the permanent dentitions. Shape anomalies, such as enamel hypoplasia and peg shaped, have also been frequently seen in cleft lip and/or palate patients [14]. Tooth agenesis, known as hypodontia or congenital absence of teeth, is the most commonly detected developmental abnormality of the human dentition. All types of clefts are often associated with congenitally missing teeth [15]. Jiroutova and Mullerova [16] studied the frequency of hypodontia in cleft lip and or palate patients and found that the maxillary dentition was affected more often in cleft lip and palate, the mandible was involved more frequently in isolated cleft palate. The dental bud of the upper lateral incisor was affected most commonly in cleft lip and in cleft lip and palate, whereas the second lower premolar was most frequently absent in an isolated cleft palate.

Paranaiba et al. studied prevalence of dental abnormalities in patients with nonsyndromic cleft lip and/or palate in Brazilian population and found that agenesis of the premolars and maxillary lateral incisors were significantly more frequent in patients with unilateral complete cleft lip and palate [17]. In various studies, lateral incisors were reported to be the most commonly missing teeth followed by second premolars [12, 18, 19]. While, in a another study Laatikainen and Ranta [20] found that the maxillary second premolar was the most frequently absent tooth, followed in order of frequency by the upper lateral incisor and the mandibular second premolar.

Polder et al. [21] did a meta-analysis of the prevalence of dental agenesis of permanent teeth of Caucasian populations in North America, Australia, and Europe and found that mandibular second premolar was the most affected tooth, followed by the upper lateral incisor and the upper second premolar. Shapira et al. [22] found a total of 47 missing second premolars in the upper arch and 23 missing in the mandible. In literature, Ranta [23] reported that the incidence of hypodontia rises strongly with the severity of cleft. Paranaiba et al. [17] also found that patients with unilateral cleft lip and palate were affected more significantly by dental anomalies than those with bilateral cleft lip and palate. It should be considered that ethnicity also plays an important role in prevalence of cleft and associated anomalies. Polder et al. reported that prevalence of dental agenesis in Europe and Australia was higher than in North America. In addition, they reported that the prevalence of dental agenesis in females is 1.37 times higher than in males for all three continents. Defects of enamel such as hypoplasia and opacities are common in the teeth adjacent to the cleft site. Decay is higher in these patients compared with the non-cleft populations. Therefore there is a higher incidence of caries in teeth with enamel defects, the issues of prevention and brushing are of great importance in cleft children [24].

3.10. Role of psychologist in cleft lip and palate patients

It is clear that attractive children are seen by others as happier, having more positive social behavior. Children with cleft may have a less attractive appearance and speech problems make it worst. Babies may face bullying and teasing because of their appearance. Parents may be more tolerant of misbehavior in their child and are more likely to spoil their child by being overprotective. Moreover, peer interaction also has an important role in maintaining psychosocial problems. Cleft lip and palate patients are at high risk for developing psychosocial problems especially those relating to self-concept, peer relationships, and appearance. Psychological problems affect development of children with cleft lip and palate. Therefore, these patients are treated by the interdisciplinary team to maximize positive outcome of treatment. Missing teeth, feeding difficulties, the infant's appearance, presence of misaligned teeth, and severe malocclusion can lead to social isolation. Moreover, frequent visits to the doctor and surgeries can be quite stressful. The psychologist provides treatment plan for developmental, emotional, learning, and adjustment abnormalities. They focused on the appearance, speech, patient's self-esteem, psychosocial problems, self-confidence, interpersonal relationships, and emotional handicapped problems [25].

3.11. Role of otolaryngologist in cleft lip and palate patients

Patients with cleft lip and palate have a higher incidence of hearing problems. They have more frequent problems with fluid, ear infections, and otitis media, which can be very painful. It is crucial that to have the infant's hearing tested during the first few months and it is also very important that cleft lip and palate patients have regular hearing tests to screen middle ear problems. This could adjust the development of normal hearing as well as speech. As the child gets older, the rate of ear infections seems to reduce. Any abnormality of the upper airway can affect the function of the Eustachian tube and enhance the possibility of persistent fluid in the middle ear, which is a major cause of repeated ear infections. Hearing loss can be a consequence of repeat ear infections and persistent middle ear fluid. Tubes can be inserted in the ear by an otolaryngologist to relieve fluid build-up and repair hearing. Cleft lip and palate patients are suffering from mouth breathing, feeding, hearing, speech problems, and jaw deformities. There are some areas of overlap with plastic surgery, oral and maxillofacial surgery, otolaryngology, and speech-language pathology. Oral and maxillofacial surgeon evaluates the skeletal discrepancies related to cleft and craniofacial abnormalities such as maxillary deficiency and other skeletal malocclusions. Surgeons work with other members of the group to ensure appropriate and harmonious facial form and dental arch.

3.12. Role of pedodontist in cleft lip and palate patients

The role of pediatric dentistry in treatment of cleft lip and palate cleft patients is the comprehensive preventative and therapeutic oral health care of children, counseling and caries control. These treatments include following steps:

(a) Growth and development monitoring.

(b) Caries prevention and oral hygiene guidance.

(c) Behavior modifications.

(d) Routine dental care.

(e) Preventive and interceptive dentistry.

(f) Interceptive orthodontics where appropriate.

(g) Restorative procedures.

(h) Removal of primary dentition in surgical site.

(i) Periodontal considerations.

3.13. Role of orthodontist in cleft lip and palate patients

In the management of cleft lip and palate patients the orthodontist has an important role in the cleft and craniofacial team. They are involved with diagnosis of facial morphology, guidance of the growth and development of the face, occlusion, dentition, and jaw discrepancy of the patients with cleft or craniofacial syndromes. They provide orthodontic and orthopedic treatment and general expertise for consultation with all of the other members of the cleft team. Different phases of active treatment will be necessary from birth to adulthoods. Orthodontist should consider many factors in determining when to initiate orthodontic treatment. These factors include the ability of the patient to cooperate, the severity of the malocclusion, the amount of jaw discrepancy, type of dental anomalies, existence of missing, dental shape anomalies, supernumerary teeth, and the need for future orthodontic treatment in the early mixed or permanent dentitions.

Orthodontic treatment plan can be divided into following stages based on the time of treatment:

(1) Presurgical orthopedics

(2) During primary dentition

(3) During mixed dentition

(4) During permanent dentition

3.13.1. *Presurgical orthopedics*

Presurgical infant orthopedics is sometimes used to relocate the segments of the cleft in maxilla prior to lip repair. A custom-fitted orthodontic appliance is applied to bring the parts of the lips, upper jaw, and nose closer together. This is called Nasoalveolar Molding (NAM). These appliances can make lip closure easier.

Advantages of presurgical orthopedics:

(a) To facilitate feeding

(b) To help establish normal tongue

(c) To provide psychological boost to the patients

(d) To assist surgeon in the initial repair

(e) To stimulate palatal growth and orofacial functional matrix

(f) To help decrease the number of ear infections

(g) Improve esthetics

(h) Repositioning of premaxilla

Although the evidence does not support the neonatal maxillary orthopedics as an essential or desirable routine procedure; Nonetheless, the molding of the segments achieved by these appliances does make definitive lip repair easier for the surgeon, especially for patients with a severely protruding premaxilla caused by a bilateral cleft lip [26].

3.13.2. *During primary dentition*

Midfacial deficiency is a common feature of cleft lip and palate patients due to scar tissue of the lip and palate closure [25]. During deciduous dentition, no orthodontic and orthopedic treatments are given because it has limited advantage. Orthodontic and orthopedic intervention starts in the mixed dentition.

3.13.3. *During mixed dentition*

Early orthopedic treatment in cleft palate children is essential because the maxillary bones and their component parts may be moved and altered in young children with relative ease and thereby creates a more functional dental arch. Orthodontic interventions in patients with cleft palate are focused at correction of Class III skeletal growth pattern, maxillary arch expansion, correction of upper incisor misalignments, gross rotations of incisors, and cross bite of buccal segments. Maxillary deficiency may be a reflection of the underlying skeletal abnormality for which growth modification and redirection may be indicated with a protraction headgear. Treatment approach to improve the midface deficiency was achieved by using the face mask [2, 27], tongue appliance [6], tongue plate [27], protraction head gear [3, 28], suborbital protraction appliances [4], ankylosed teeth [29], endosseous implants [30], and surgically assisted orthopedic protraction and distraction osteogenesis [8]. Jamilian et al. [6] evaluated the effectiveness of tongue appliance on deficient maxilla in growing cleft lip and palate patients. They showed that tongue appliance improved the deficient maxilla.

Tongue appliance has Adams clasp in first maxillary molars and C clasps in the upper incisors and deciduous teeth in order to increase the retention. A screw is mounted in midpalatal area to correct bilateral posterior crossbite. It was activated twice a week by the patient. Four separate tongue cribs were incorporated in the palatal area, behind the upper incisors. These cribs are long enough to cage the tongue and are adjusted in the clinic to avoid traumatizing the floor of the mouth. Tongue appliance is seen in **Figure 1**. **Figure 2** shows the profile of the patient before application of the tongue appliance and **Figure 3** shows the profile of the same patient after using the appliance. Extraoral appliances are not used suitably by the patients, whereas they prefer to apply small-sized and more convenient appliances. Besides to their large size of extraoral appliances, they need high compliance and many clinicians observe lack of cooperation by patients treated by big extraoral appliances. The philosophy of tongue appliance [31–33] is provided in the following two ways:

(1) The force of the tongue during each swallowing might be 5 pounds. Each patient might have 500–1200 times swallowing in 24 hours. The pressure from the tongue is transferred through the tongue appliance to the deficient maxilla.

(2) There is substantial continuous pressure of tongue. Because tongue is caged behind the cribs that is why this force is continuous in the rest position and centric occlusion. This force pushes the nasomaxillary complex into a forward position. In other words, functional activity and physiological position of tongue create these considerable forces that are conducted by tongue through the palatal cribs and finally transmitted to the deficient maxilla and nasomaxillary complex.

The more anterior the tongue, the greater pressure will be. The more posterior the crib, the greater pressure will be. Jamilian et al. [6] reported that the anterior part of maxillary plane moved superiorly (anteinclination) and posterior part of it relocated inferiorly. In other words, the maxillary posterior segment is extruded slightly and that is why the lower jaw rotated in a clockwise direction. These changes led to correction of the overjet and reducing of SNB and increasing of mandibular plane angle. Click wise rotation of the mandible is not favorable in long face patients.

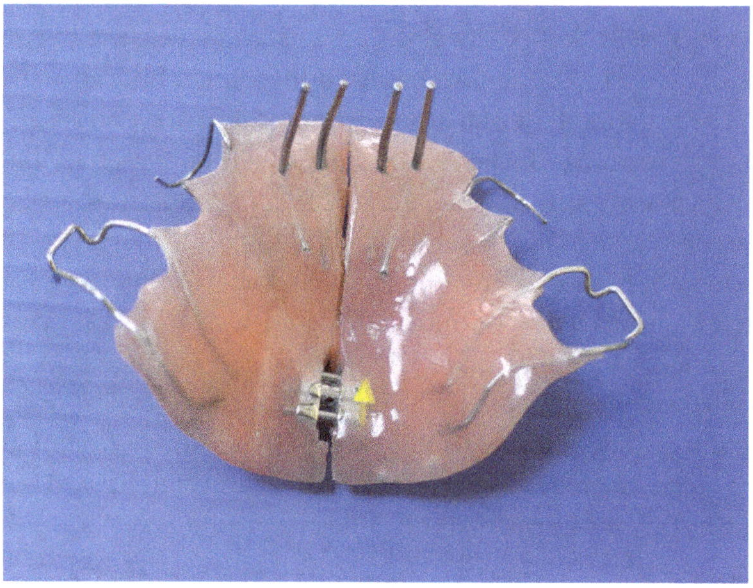

Figure 1. Tongue appliance with expansion screw.

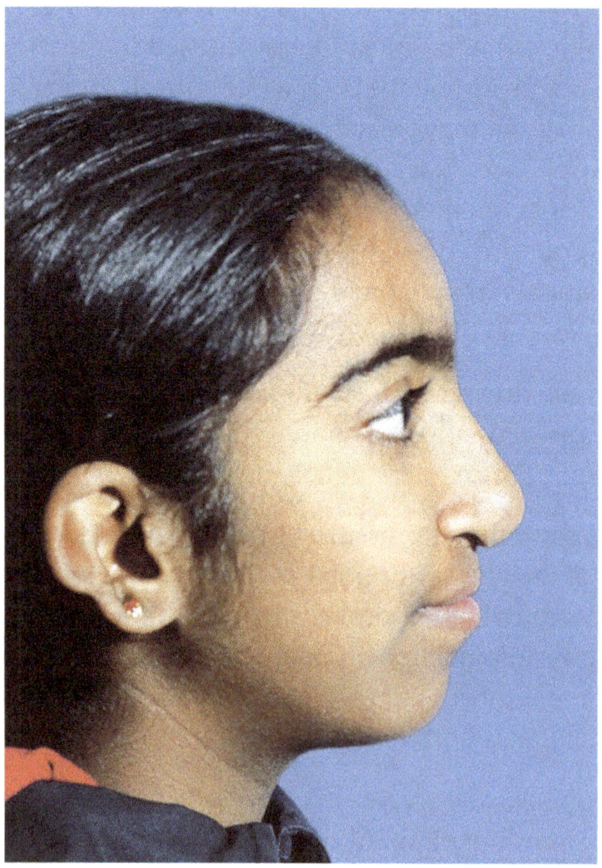

Figure 2. Profile view before treatment.

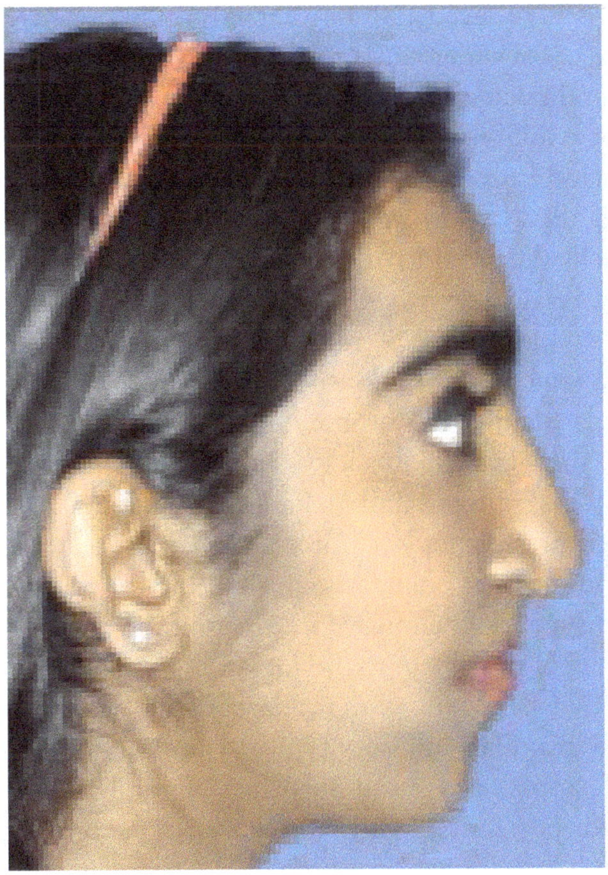

Figure 3. Profile view after treatment.

Tongue plate has been used for correction of maxillary deficiency [27]. Mechanism of tongue plate [7] is very similar to the tongue appliance. The pressure of tongue during rest position and swallowing is transmitted through the tongue plate to the deficient maxilla. The significant pressure of the tongue that is caged behind the acrylic plate transfers the nasomaxillary complex in a forward position. Some patients had some extent of irritation on the tongue from tongue appliance that is why tongue appliance was replaced by tongue plate. This has a smoothed area and these softened edges create it undamaging for the patient. Moreover, it is adjusted in a way to avoid traumatizing the floor of the mouth. Elimination of the cribs in tongue plate might offer a better psychological sense to the patients. Extra oral appliances such as facemask and reverse chin cup [5, 34] improve the deficient nasomaxillary complex but they have an unfavorable effect on the normal mandible. Extra oral appliances rotate the mandible in clockwise rotation and it is unfavorable in normal growth pattern and long face patients. Besides, the cup of facemask can create abrasion particularly in warm climates. Tongue appliance is an intraoral appliance and it is very comfortable and simple. It is constructed easily and it is not expensive. Tongue appliance and tongue plate will be accepted better than extraoral appliances due to less conspicuous of them. Children with cleft lip and palate have suffered from birth; tongue plate and tongue appliance are more comfortable as they create the least stress to patients in comparison with other big extraoral appliances. In spite of many advantages of them, tongue appliance and tongue plate have one disadvantage.

Incisor mandibular angle is reduced due to removal of the pressure of tongue to the lower incisors and acting force of orbicularis oris to them. Tongue appliance and tongue plate have a screw to correct bilateral posterior crossbite. Expansion will lose all maxillary sutures like zygomaxillary, pterygomaxillary, thus, maxilla will transfer more easily in forward direction [35, 36]. On the other hand, upper jaw may be expanded in order to improve dental function, reliving crowding, align upper incisors, eliminate functional shifts, provide access for impacted teeth in the cleft site, provide restorative treatment to carious teeth, improve maxillary deficiency, and nasal airway in mixed dentition [6, 31]. Maxillary skeletal asymmetry in unilateral lip and palate patients may be reflected in a unilateral posterior cross bite, which may be corrected with a removable appliance with a screw or a quad helix type of appliance in the mixed dentition. A bonded or non-bonded hyrax expander are recommended along with extra oral traction, such as facial mask to stimulate maxillary protraction or chin cup to control mandibular growth (**Figures 4** and **5**). Patients with maxillary cleft do not have a midpalatal suture, which requires orthopedic forces to open. Instead there is a midpalatal cleft covered with scarred and repaired palatal tissues limiting the rate and amount of expansion. The slower rate of expansion and the lower force magnitude provided by a quad helix appliance allows the soft tissue of the palate to the increasing maxillary width, avoiding a breakdown of the scar tissue that can result in an oronasal fistula. As the permanent incisors erupt adjacent to the cleft site, maxillary incisors typically are rotated, misplaced, malformed, or hypo plastic. Removable appliance is used to correct upper incisor misalignment. Moreover, incisors may be absent or peg shaped and there may be one or some supernumerary teeth. Maxillary expansion appliances can be anchored on the permanent first molars and extended anteriorly to improve maxillary arch while correcting the cross bite. Usually expansion is followed by maxillary protraction using a traditional Delaire or other protraction appliances. After the expansion and protraction phase, full fixed appliances along with Class III elastics and sometimes extractions, if necessary, are usually needed to correct the malocclusion [33]. **Figures 6** and **7** show the intraoral photograph of a patient before and after orthodontic treatment, respectively. **Figures 8** and **9** show the frontal view of the same patient in pre- and postorthodontic treatment, respectively.

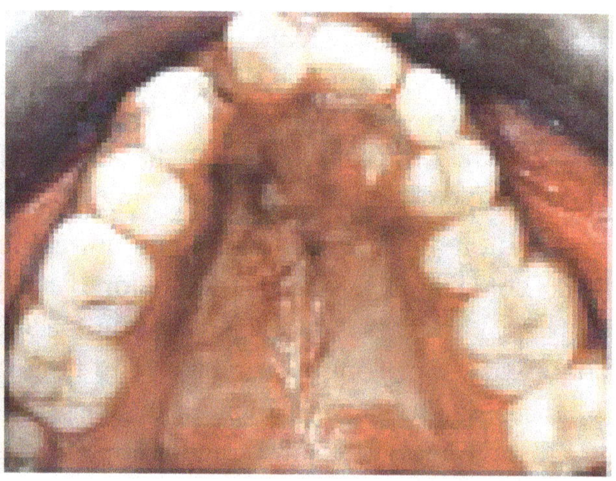

Figure 4. Upper arch before expansion.

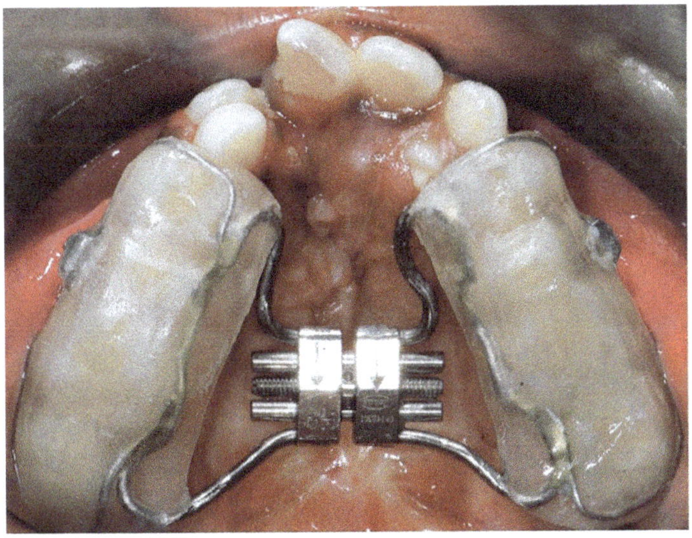

Figure 5. Upper arch during expansion with bonded hyrax.

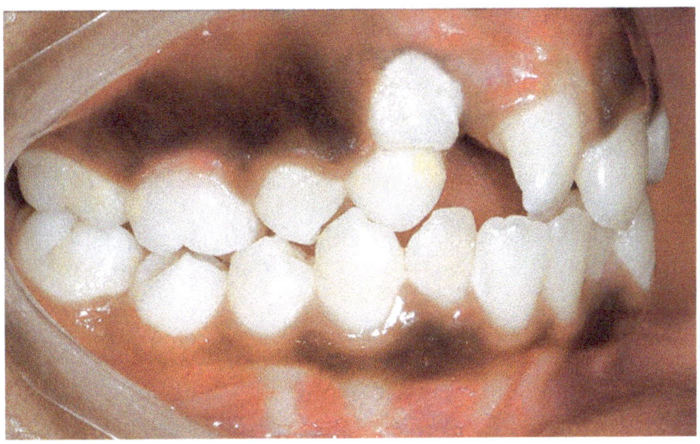

Figure 6. Intraoral view before orthodontic treatment.

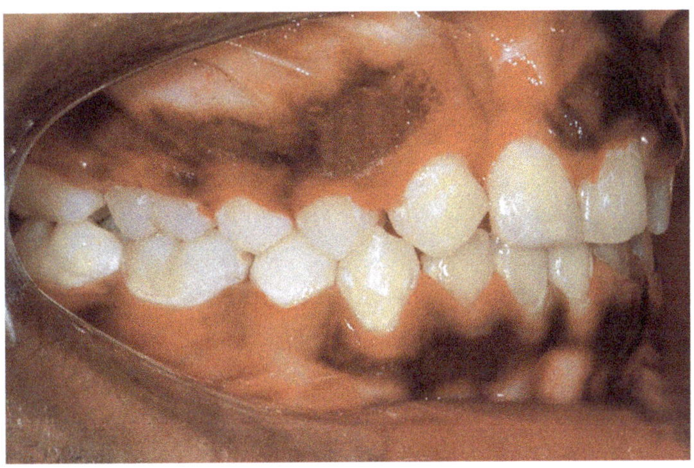

Figure 7. Intraoral view after orthodontic treatment.

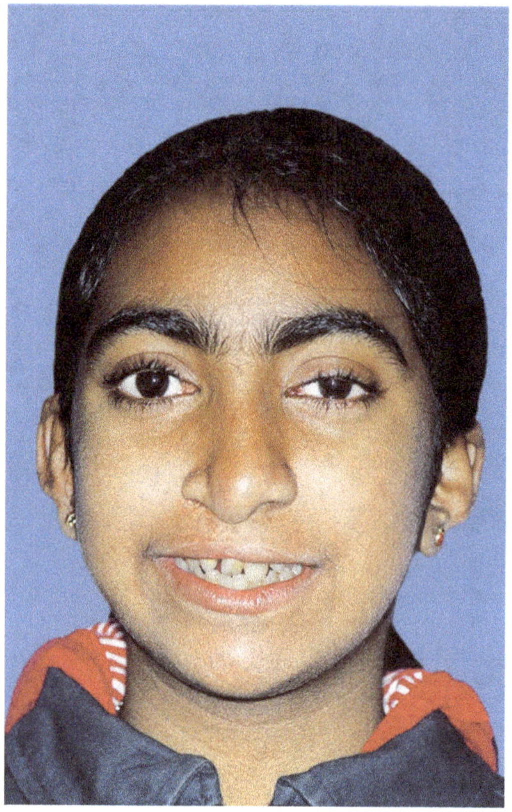

Figure 8. Frontal view before treatment.

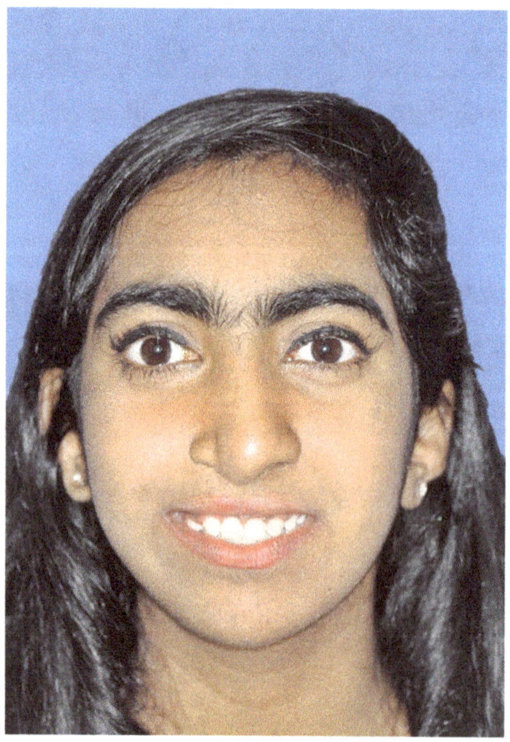

Figure 9. Frontal view after treatment.

3.13.4. Permanent dentition

Comprehensive fixed appliance therapy usually occurs in the permanent dentition with the aim of preparing for alveolar bone graft that can be done by an oral surgeon. This phase usually involves aligning of malposed maxillary incisors. Reverse pull headgear or face mask therapy, expansion of maxillary arch may be continued during this time period. Final alignment of teeth is carried over with or without extraction. Orthodontic management is limited after eruption of permanent dentition. The established malocclusion and discrepancy between the upper and lower arch often require orthognathic surgery.

3.14. Role of oromaxillofacial surgeon in cleft lip and palate patients

Orthognathic procedure may be designated if a malocclusion develops due to abnormal growth of the maxilla. Treatment for adults may involve surgical in severe or camouflage in mild to moderate patients. Orthognathic surgery is performed to patients with deformities of the jaws to improve facial esthetics as well as to correct dental occlusion. Presurgical orthodontics are usually necessary to align the teeth, correct any compensations, decrowding, eliminate any dental midline discrepancy, coordinate arches, and localize space for prosthetic or implant replacement of the teeth. Ideally, the patient is referred to the surgeon after presurgical orthodontics. The postsurgical phase of orthodontics is required for creating perfect occlusion and better interdigitation after surgery.

3.14.1. Pharyngeal flap

Failure to achieve a seal between the posterior pharyngeal wall and soft palate lets leakage of air through the nose and causes cleft palate speech. This has proved not to be a problem in patients with a normal velopharyngeal mechanism. If a patient has speech problems a surgical procedure to create a pharyngeal flap probably will be required. To correct hyper nasality, this procedure contains raising a flap of tissue from the posterior pharyngeal wall and incorporating it into the soft palate. Pharyngeal flap is used when the muscles do not function appropriately or the repaired palate is too short. For adults with speech problems, pharyngeal flap, combined with an intensive schedule of speech therapy, can produce noticeable improvements.

3.14.2. Distraction osteogenesis

Distraction osteogenesis has become a new method for correction of maxillary deficiency [8, 37]. Distraction osteogenesis for maxillary advancement started in 1993 and is now broadly used in cases with skeletal Class III deformity due to maxillary deficiency [38]. Figueroa and Polley [39] reported that distraction osteogenesis was successfully used to advance the maxilla in children with cleft lip and palate. According to them the main advantages of distraction osteogenesis compared with conventional methods of craniofacial reconstruction were reduced time of surgery and cost and the ability to generate new bone. Many advantages and disadvantages of distraction devices have been detailed. For a large advancement in a patient with a cleft lip or palate, distraction osteogenesis may be advantageous. Figueroa and Polley [39] assessed the cephalometric landmarks on 14 patients with cleft palate who were treated with a rigid external distraction technique. Distraction osteogenesis provides less physical and psychological invasion in comparison to conventional LeFort osteotomy: that is, reduced operating time, less blood loss, less postoperative pain, and shorter hospitalization. Also, when intra-arch distraction is applied to lengthen the mandible or maxilla, orthodontic alignment of upper and lower arches are not necessary before the procedure [40]. Intraoral distraction osteogenesis devices are divided into two types namely bone borne or tooth borne. Advantages of these are their smaller size and better patient acceptance; however, the bone attached one has the disadvantage of the need for second intervention to remove the device [41].

Hyrax screw incorporated in an acrylic plate has been applied for treatment of maxillary deficient in cleft lip and palate patients. After creating horizontal cuts similar to LeFort 1 and vertical cuts between the premolars on both sides, a bonded hyrax screw was mounted on an acrylic plate for the slow sagittal expansion of upper arch. The distraction procedure can be initiated after 5 days of latency period.

The expansion is performed by activating the hyrax screw 0.8 mm per day after the latency period (**Figure 10**). Expansion was discontinued after achieving satisfactory overjet and occlusion (**Figure 11**). If open bite occurs during expansion period vertical elastics will be used to correct open bite. Consolidation period lasts 8 weeks and after this period hyrax screw is removed. One of the advantages of anterior maxillary distraction is that velopharyngeal area will be intact. Anterior distraction is used for skeletal deformity and fixed appliance is applied for correction of dental problems [8].

Some researchers suggested that distraction orthogenesis does not seem to have any advantages over surgery. Additionally, the occlusion at the end of distraction is much less defined than what is seen with conventional orthognathic surgery [42].

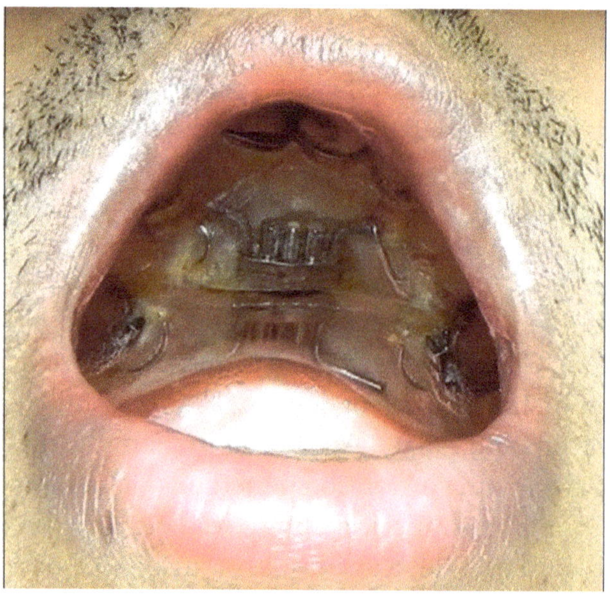

Figure 10. Hyrax screw incorporated in an acrylic plate.

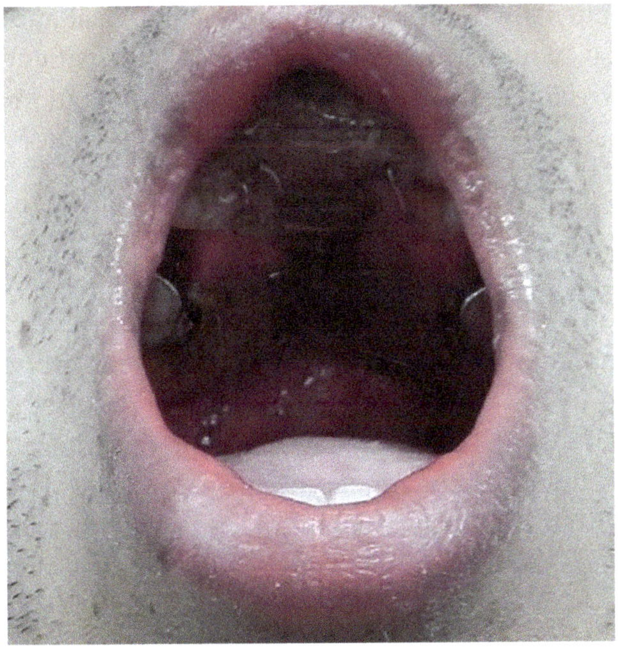

Figure 11. Hyrax screw after activation.

4. Retention

The retention protocol for clefts follows the same principles of orthodontic treatment in Class III malocclusion without clefts. The upper and lower arches should have been coordinated throughout orthodontic and orthopedic intervention. Positive overjet and overbite with adequate intercuspation are necessary for retention. Hawley retainer in the maxillary and mandibular arch is used for retention. Hawley appliance often includes prosthetic teeth that will be displaced later with dental implants or prostheses. Patients are instructed to wear the Hawley appliance for 12 months continuously. After that, if the occlusion is stable, the Hawley retainer is used at night-time for additional six months.

Retention in cleft palate cases is longer than for noncleft patients. The reasons are due to:

(a) lack of bony stability,

(b) contracture of stretched or scar tissues, and

(c) missing teeth.

5. Recommendation

Treatment approach depends on the age and severity of the patients. Growth modification is the best treatment plan when the patient is still growing. We can take advantages of a child's growing years by guiding proper jaw bone formation with small intraoral appliances such as tongue plate and tongue appliance [6, 27]. These small intraoral appliances are recommended in cleft lip and palate patients who suffering from psychological and social problems associated with their malocclusion in early mixed children. Once the patient is an adult, camouflage may be an option for correcting mild deformities and surgery would be proper treatment plan for severe cases.

6. Conclusion

Cleft is the most common craniofacial malformation that an orthodontist may encounter. The orthodontist's role in the cleft lip and palate team requires close relationship with the other team members. Cleft lip and palate patients become more maxillary deficient and mandibular prognathic in their appearance. The most common specialties involved in the care of a child with a cleft are: oromaxillofacial surgeon, plastic surgeon, psychologist, orthodontist, general dentist, otolaryngologist, speech therapist, pediatrician, and prosthodontist.

Treatment plan from orthodontic perspective can be divided into the following stages based on the dentition stages: (1) presurgical orthopedics, (2) primary dentition, (3) mixed dentition, and (4) permanent dentition.

Author details

Letizia Perillo[1], Fabrizia d'Apuzzo[1], Sara Eslami[2] and Abdolreza Jamilian[2*]

*Address all correspondence to: info@jamilian.net

1 Multidisciplinary Department of Medical-Surgical and Dental Specialties, Second University of Naples, Naples, Italy

2 Department of Orthodontics, Cranio Maxillofacial Research Center, Tehran Dental Branch, Islamic Azad University, Tehran, Iran

References

[1] Jamilian, A., F. Nayeri, and A. Babayan, Incidence of cleft lip and palate in Tehran. J Indian Soc Pedod Prev Dent 2007;**25**:174–6.

[2] Buschang, P.H., et al., Face mask therapy of preadolescents with unilateral cleft lip and palate. Angle Orthod 1994;**64**:145–50.

[3] Chen, K.F. and L.L. So, Sagittal skeletal and dental changes of reverse headgear treatment in Chinese boys with complete unilateral cleft lip and palate. Angle Orthod 1996;**66**:363–72.

[4] Delaire, J. and P. Verdon, The use of heavy postero-anterior extraoral forces by an orthopedic mask in the treatment of dentomaxillary sequellae of labiomaxillopalatal clefts. Chir Pediatr 1983;**24**:315–22.

[5] Showkatbakhsh, R. and A. Jamilian, A novel approach in treatment of maxillary deficiency by reverse chin cup. Int J Orthod Milwaukee 2010;**21**:27–31.

[6] Jamilian, A., R. Showkatbakhsh, and M.B. Boushehry, The effect of tongue appliance on the nasomaxillary complex in growing cleft lip and palate patients. J Indian Soc Pedod Prev Dent 2006;**24**:136–9.

[7] Showkatbakhsh, R. and A. Jamilian, A novel method of maxillary deficiency treatment by tongue plate—a case report. Int J Orthod Milwaukee 2011;**22**:31–4.

[8] Srivastava, D., et al., Use of anterior maxillary distraction osteogenesis in two cleft lip and palate patients. Natl J Maxillofac Surg 2015;**6**:80–3.

[9] Rullo, R., et al., Speech outcome in unilateral complete cleft lip and palate patients: a descriptive study. Eur J Paediatr Dent 2014;**15**:293–6.

[10] Grandjean, H., D. Larroque, and S. Levi, The performance of routine ultrasonographic screening of pregnancies in the Eurofetus Study. Am J Obstet Gynecol 1999;**181**:446–54.

[11] Lourenco Ribeiro, L., et al., Dental anomalies of the permanent lateral incisors and prevalence of hypodontia outside the cleft area in complete unilateral cleft lip and palate. Cleft Palate Craniofac J 2003;**40**:172–5.

[12] Akcam, M.O., et al., Dental anomalies in individuals with cleft lip and/or palate. Eur J Orthod 2010;**32**:207–13.

[13] Shapira, Y., E. Lubit, and M.M. Kuftinec, Hypodontia in children with various types of clefts. Angle Orthod 2000;**70**:16–21.

[14] Vichi, M. and L. Franchi, Abnormalities of the maxillary incisors in children with cleft lip and palate. ASDC J Dent Child 1995;**62**:412–7.

[15] Larson, M., R. Hellquist, and O.P. Jakobsson, Dental abnormalities and ectopic eruption in patients with isolated cleft palate. Scand J Plast Reconstr Surg Hand Surg 1998;**32**:203–12.

[16] Jiroutova, O. and Z. Mullerova, The occurrence of hypodontia in patients with cleft lip and/or palate. Acta Chir Plast 1994;**36**:53–6.

[17] Paranaiba, L.M., et al., Prevalence of dental anomalies in patients with nonsyndromic cleft lip and/or palate in a Brazilian population. Cleft Palate Craniofac J 2013;**50**:400–5.

[18] Tortora, C., et al., Prevalence of abnormalities in dental structure, position, and eruption pattern in a population of unilateral and bilateral cleft lip and palate patients. Cleft Palate Craniofac J 2008;**45**:154–62.

[19] Menezes, R. and A.R. Vieira, Dental anomalies as part of the cleft spectrum. Cleft Palate Craniofac J 2008;**45**:414–9.

[20] Laatikainen, T. and R. Ranta, Hypodontia in twins discordant or concordant for cleft lip and/or palate. Scand J Dent Res 1994;**102**:88–91.

[21] Polder, B.J., et al., A meta-analysis of the prevalence of dental agenesis of permanent teeth. Community Dent Oral Epidemiol 2004;**32**:217–26.

[22] Shapira, Y., E. Lubit, and M.M. Kuftinec, Congenitally missing second premolars in cleft lip and cleft palate children. Am J Orthod Dentofacial Orthop 1999;**115**:396–400.

[23] Ranta, R., A review of tooth formation in children with cleft lip/palate. Am J Orthod Dentofacial Orthop 1986;**90**:11–8.

[24] Pope, A.W., Points of risk and opportunity for parents of children with craniofacial conditions. Cleft Palate Craniofac J 1999;**36**:36–9.

[25] Hunt, O., et al., The psychosocial effects of cleft lip and palate: a systematic review. Eur J Orthod 2005;**27**:274–85.

[26] Vig, K.W. and T.A. Turvey, Orthodontic-surgical interaction in the management of cleft lip and palate. Clin Plast Surg 1985;**12**:735–48.

[27] Showkatbakhsh, R., et al., The effects of face mask and tongue plate on maxillary deficiency in growing patients: a randomized clinical trial. J Orthod 2013;**40**:130–6.

[28] Showkatbakhsh, R., et al., The effects of face mask and tongue appliance on maxillary deficiency in growing patients: a randomized clinical trial. Prog Orthod 2012;**13**:266–72.

[29] Omnell, M.L. and B. Sheller, Maxillary protraction to intentionally ankylosed deciduous canines in a patient with cleft palate. Am J Orthod Dentofacial Orthop 1994;**106**:201–5.

[30] Smalley, W.M., et al., Osseointegrated titanium implants for maxillofacial protraction in monkeys. Am J Orthod Dentofacial Orthop 1988;**94**:285–95.

[31] Jamilian, A. and R. Showkatbakhsh, The effect of tongue appliance on the maxilla in Class III malocclusion due to maxillary deficiency. Int J Orthod Milwaukee 2009;**20**:11–4.

[32] Showkatbakhsh, R., et al., Maxillary deficiency treatment by fixed tongue appliance—a case report. Int J Orthod Milwaukee 2013;**24**:31–4.

[33] Showkatbakhsh, R., et al., The short-term effects of face mask and fixed tongue appliance on maxillary deficiency in growing patients—a randomized clinical trial. Int J Orthod Milwaukee 2015;**26**:33–8.

[34] Showkatbakhsh, R., et al., The effects of facemask and reverse chin cup on maxillary deficient patients. J Orthod 2012;**39**:95–101.

[35] Liou, E.J. and W.C. Tsai, A new protocol for maxillary protraction in cleft patients: repetitive weekly protocol of alternate rapid maxillary expansions and constrictions. Cleft Palate Craniofac J 2005;**42**:121–7.

[36] Showkatbakhsh, R., et al., Bone remodeling to correct maxillary deficiency after growth cessation. Natl J Maxillofac Surg 2012;**3**:202–6.

[37] Polley, J.W. and A.A. Figueroa, Rigid external distraction: its application in cleft maxillary deformities. Plast Reconstr Surg 1998;**102**:1360–72; discussion 1373–4.

[38] Kuroda, S., et al., Maxillary distraction osteogenesis to treat maxillary hypoplasia: comparison of an internal and an external system. Am J Orthod Dentofacial Orthop 2005; **127**:493–8.

[39] Figueroa, A.A. and J.W. Polley, Management of severe cleft maxillary deficiency with distraction osteogenesis: procedure and results. Am J Orthod Dentofacial Orthop 1999; **115**:1–12.

[40] Dessner, S., et al., Mandibular lengthening using preprogrammed intraoral tooth-borne distraction devices. J Oral Maxillofac Surg 1999;**57**:1318–22; discussion 1322–3.

[41] Iannetti, G., et al., LeFort III advancement with and without osteogenesis distraction. J Craniofac Surg 2006;**17**:536–43.

[42] Van Sickels, J.E., Distraction osteogenesis versus orthognathic surgery. Am J Orthod Dentofacial Orthop 2000;**118**:482–4.

4

Pediatric Anesthesia for Patients with Cleft Lip and Palate

Alyssa Brzenski, Ofelia Ham-Mancilla,
Silvia Peña-Olvera, Amanda Gosman and
Alicia Sigler

Abstract

Cleft lip and palate are the most common craniofacial deformities in the United States of America and México. Their aesthetic and functional implications influence the lifestyle of the patient: social relationships, school and working performances, self-esteem and health. Surgical repair of the cleft lip is around the third to sixth month of age and the palate repair is when the patient is between six and eighteen months old. There are other surgical repairs during childhood and ideally all of them should be performed by an experienced surgeon teaming up with a pediatric anesthesiologist following the gold standards in cleft care, in a setting where the safety of the patient is paramount.

Keywords: cleft lip, cleft palate, anesthesia

1. Introduction

When anesthetic procedures are performed in cleft patients, there are multiple considerations that have to be taken into account: the actual lip and palate deformities that could lead to a difficult intubation, airway malformations and reactions to the procedure that could lead to laryngospasm or bronchospasm, other malformations or diseases that could alter the prognosis during and after the surgery, the surgical procedure itself that could lead to bleeding or airway obstruction due to swelling, the intubation, the administration of anesthetic medications, the ventilation and use of other medications such as muscle relaxants, pain killers, etcetera, that could alter the homeostasis of the body, and other factors surrounding the anesthetic procedure like the equipment used, the monitoring applied, the site where the surgical act is taking place, the experience of surgeons, anesthesiologists and nurses in charge of cleft care, the availability of a blood bank and an ICU in case of an adverse event. When all of these factors are well controlled and overseen by an experienced team, the risk for an adverse outcome is significantly reduced. This is why there has been an international consensus for guidelines that will lead the cleft team to successful surgical and anesthetic performances. If the team is visiting a foreign country, they must follow the same gold standards of care contained within these guidelines and work within their scope of practice. If the medical setting that they are visiting lacks the equipment, medications and supplies needed for them to perform at their best, then they should bring the equipment, medications and supplies with them.

2. General considerations

Cleft lip (CL) and cleft palate (CP) are one of the most common congenital anomalies found in the United States and the most common craniofacial anomaly seen by plastic surgeons. Nearly one in five hundred live births will result in a child affected by cleft CL and/or CP. The Center for Disease Control estimates that 2650 babies are born with CP and 4440 babies are born with CL with or without a CP annually [1]. In developing countries, such as México, CL and CP is the most common congenital malformation requiring surgical treatment and its incidence is 1:800 to 1000 live births. Of these, 33% have CL. 64% CL and CP. 2% only present a CP and 1%, rare craniofacial clefts. On average, there are 9.6 new cases per day and 3521 cases per year [2].

In the United States, children with CL and CP are primarily cared for in cleft centers with multidisciplinary teams. Teams consisting of otolaryngologists, plastic surgeons, oral surgeons, speech therapists, occupational therapists, dentists and orthodontists work together to ensure optimal timing and care of these patients. Anesthesiologists also integrate into these teams when surgical procedures are required. Studies from the United Kingdom suggest that children who are cared for by these multidisciplinary teams have improved long-term outcomes with improved feeding, speech, and esthetics [3–7]. For many families, the diagnosis of a cleft occurs during the prenatal period. Prenatal counseling may be the first interaction with the cleft team, facilitating a long relationship with multiple specialists to establish expectations regarding the long-term possibilities for children with CP or CL and CP. There are approximately 139,000 Mexicans who have CL and CP. It is a very important public health problem due to the medical, psychological and social impact to the patients and their family. The causes are multifactorial and can be environmental, genetic or a combination [8].

Infants with CL and CP can have difficulty generating oral suction which can make breast feeding and bottle feeding a challenge. Many infants with CL and CP struggle with feeding and may require special bottles, nipples or education to achieve adequate weight gain. Children without access to support services may endure nutritional consequences, which if not taken care of at an early age, can deteriorate or affect growth and development [2, 9].

The goals for surgical repair of CP and CL repair are to reconstruct the affected area, leading to improved feeding, speech, and function of the nasal airway. CL repair in the United States typically occurs first within 2 to 3 months of age with CP repair occurring between 9 and 12 months [10]. The time between birth and this initial repair allows for a thorough work up of other co-morbidities and evaluation of any underlying syndromes. In the majority of children with a cleft there are no other associate syndromes or malformations. However, 20–30% of patients will have some underlying syndrome or systemic abnormalities requiring evaluation and potentially treatment prior to repair of the cleft [11]. Isolated CP has the greatest incidence of associate abnormalities while isolated CL is most likely to be an isolated feature. Thus, a thorough pre-operative evaluation by the cleft team is essential prior to surgical repair.

At least 275 different syndromes [12] have been associated with CL and CP. There are a variety of co-morbidities associated with these syndromes. However, cardiac and airway abnormalities represent the primary concerns of the anesthesia teams prior to repair of cleft abnormalities. Syndromes such as Pierre Robin Sequence, Treacher Collins, Goldenhar Syndrome and 22q deletion, are associated with mandibular hypoplasia, potentially making airway management and repair difficult. Cardiac abnormalities are the most frequent associate co-morbidity in children with clefts [13]. Tetralogy of Fallot, atrial septal defect and ventricular septal defect represent the most common congenital heart disease seen in this patient population. A thorough physical exam and imaging with cardiac echocardiogram should be performed for these children. Cardiac abnormalities should be optimized and potentially repaired prior to repair of the cleft itself. Optimization of other co-morbidities, such as airway anomalies, renal dysfunction, nutrition and additional medical issues, should also be a top priority in the months following birth. Children with CP are prone to middle ear effusions and recurrent otitis media. The dysfunction of the palate muscles impairs regulation of the Eustachian tubes, which may increase the risk of upper respiratory infections.

Patients with CP have an increased risk of gastroesophageal reflux and pulmonary aspiration which may contribute to airway reactivity. Speech impairment also occurs due to the abnormal anatomy of the CP musculature and speech development is further hindered in patients with hypoacusia [12]. In México, the multidisciplinary approach is a must in almost all 53 cleft clinics located throughout the country and the role of the anesthesiologist is vital as well as the pediatrician, cardiologist, geneticist, nutritionist, pneumologist, gastroenterologist and all other specialists that may be involved in the preoperative assessment for the patient. Once the patient has undergone the lip and/or palate surgeries, the multidisciplinary cleft team involving the surgeon, orthodontist, speech therapist, otorhinolaryngologist, audiologist and psychologist become very active in providing their services to improve the physical appearance and the functional activity regarding speech, hearing, feeding, and socialization and self-esteem of the patient [14].

3. Consideration of anesthesia management

During surgical repair, a general anesthetic is required to allow for optimal surgical conditions. Control of ventilation through endotracheal intubation is necessary. Given the abnormalities of the face, concern may exist regarding the difficulty of mask ventilation and endotracheal intubation. Both ease of ventilation and intubation might have significant effects on the management of the induction of anesthesia as well as the equipment that should be present prior to induction of general anesthesia. Unlike the adult population, there are not any objective the normal airway exam. A difficult airway, defined as a difficult laryngoscopy, intubation or mask ventilation, is less common in pediatric patients [15–20]. However, young age (less than 1 year of age) and craniofacial abnormalities increase the risk of a difficult airway [15].

Although there are not set criteria that is useful to identify a child with a CP who will be a difficult laryngoscopy, examination for retrognathia should occur in each child. Viewing the face from the side is an easy way to identify retrognathia. If retrognathia is present, a potentially difficult intubation should be anticipated, and additional precautions should be undertaken. In the United States, a laryngeal mask airway, video laryngoscope and a fiber optic bronchoscope are tools that could be used to aid with a difficult intubation. If providing surgical care in a resource limited location these tools may not be available. An honest, but thorough evaluation of the facility's capabilities should be performed to ensure that the primary goal of doing no harm to the patient is followed.

Pre-operative history should also focus on determining if the infant has an upper respiratory infection (URI). Patients with a URI are at increased risk for perioperative respiratory events such as bronchospasm, laryngospasms, desaturations, breath holding and postintubation croup [21]. Presence of copious sputum and secretions, nasal congestion, recent URI (less than 2 weeks), and history of reactive airway disease increased the risk of perioperative adverse respiratory events [22]. Patients with CL and/or CP with a recent URI are at an increased risk of perioperative respiratory events compared to children without CL and/or CP who have had a recent URI. To minimize the risk of perioperative respiratory events, it is recommended that surgery be postponed for 4–6 weeks after the URI has resolved and that an experienced pediatric anesthesiologist performs the anesthetic [19]. Despite these perioperative events, in the experienced hands of a pediatric anesthesiologist there is not a risk for substantial morbidity or mortality in these patients. Nonetheless, if these symptoms are present it is prudent to postpone surgery for repair of the CL or CP until the child is no longer ill. Gunawardana and Arteau-Gauthier et al. [23, 24] studied risk factors for difficult laryngoscopy in children with CP. These children did not have any identified syndrome. 5–7% of patients in these studies had difficult laryngoscopy, a higher incidence than in other pediatric patients. Large or bilateral clefts, micrognathia and age less than 6 months were associated with increased incidence of difficult laryngoscopy. Large and bilateral clefts can be difficult because the blade of the laryngoscope can fall into the cleft. Should this occur, one can pack the cleft with gauze to improve the laryngoscopy. No patients in these studies were associated with difficult mask ventilation. Since mask ventilation is not difficult in most of these patients, an inhaled induction with volatile anesthetic with control of ventilation is appropriate in most of these patients in experienced hands.

The preanesthetic assessment is very important and should contain the patient's information: age, height and weight and its main goals are:

a) To obtain the medical and surgical background of the patient:

- Family background of anesthetic problems
- Perinatal background such as pregnancy evolution, kind of delivery, complications during delivery, need of special care after birth, prolonged hospitalization [9].

- Non-pathologic background related with nutritional state and development
- Review of systems: pulmonary abnormalities including recent respiratory infections, craniofacial deformities that will make airway and respiratory management more difficult [8], cardiac abnormalities and their treatment and cardiovascular evaluation required latest respiratory infection due to the high incidence of fistula formation or palate wound dehiscence [8], or increasing the incidence of complications of the anesthetic procedure (23%). It has been recommended a period of 4 to 6 weeks between the relief of respiratory infection and the surgical and anesthetic event to avoid such complications [25–26]. Another important issue is allergies to medications, food and toys. Kind of malformations the patient has and other anesthetic procedures in the past and the patient's reactions to them.
- Complete physical examination, including the possibility of difficult venous access and airway.
- Lab work: complete blood count, prothrombin time, partial thrombin time, bleeding and coagulation times, and any other studies for cardiovascular assessment such as EKG, chest X-rays or echocardiogram [25].

b) Evaluate the anesthetic risk and decide on the anesthetic technique to be used.

c) Inform the parents about the anesthetic technique to be used and the possibility of adverse events as well as the amount of time the patient needs to be NPO before the surgery depending on the age of the patient: 2 hours of clear liquids in all ages, to age less than 6 months 4 hours for maternal milk, and 6 hours for non-maternal milk. For patients 6 to 36 months old; 6 hours to solid food and non-maternal milk including formula [26, 14].

d) Preoperative medications: intranasal dexmedetomidine is great for patients older than 6 months because it diminishes secretions that are produced by crying. It must be administered and be continuously monitored in any setting. Midazolam PO is used to treat separation anxiety before taking the children into the operating room.

No matter the setting where the cleft surgery is going to take place, the anesthetic procedure must have the basic monitoring like continuous evaluation of electrocardiography, noninvasive blood pressure, arterial oxygen saturation, temperature, end-tidal carbon dioxide, with capnography. The objective is to obtain a safe management of the patient and to minimize the complications [9, 27]. When the surgical outreach trips for clefts in children occur in a general hospital not a pediatric hospital, it is important to provide that institution with the appropriate monitors and equipment for the adequate management and safety for the patient.

There is no standard anesthetic that has been shown to be superior in the care of children for repair of CL and CP. Typically, CL are repaired at 2–3 months of age to improve feeding and repair the muscular of the mouth. CP is repaired between 9 and 12 months of age. The goal is to optimize speech development. However, earlier repair could increase the likelihood of midface hypoplasia in the future. No premedication is required for children of these ages undergoing CL and CP repair. At this stage in life, separation anxiety is not yet a major concern. Most children present for surgery from home and have no established intravenous access. Most anesthesiologists utilize an inhalational induction with volatile anesthesia. If a difficult airway is anticipated, then this induction may be changed. The induction stage is the one with the most risk of adverse events. The main adverse event reported in the literature at the Instituto Nacional de Pediatría in Mexico City is laryngospasm which was noted in 77% of the cases [28]. Once intravenous access is obtained intubation with a RAE (Ring, Adiar and Elwyn) endotracheal tube is used. The pre-formed bend in this endotracheal tube lies on the chin, optimizing the surgical exposure for the surgeon. For a CP repair a throat pack may be used and a Digman retractor is typically placed to further improve surgical visualization. Care must be taken to ensure that the endotracheal tube is not moved when these devices are placed, as endobronchial intubation or inadvertent extubation can occur. In addition, the Digman retractor can compress the endotracheal tube when initially raised. Communication with the surgeons is important to ensure optimal oxygenation and ventilation continues throughout the surgical repair. Multiple anesthesia techniques can be used for the children undergoing CL or CP repair. In the United States, use of a volatile anesthetic with or without opioids or regional anesthesia [29–31] is commonly used. Anesthesia with propofol-remifentanil can also be used with similar anesthetic results [30].

There is an important incidence of adverse events during this stage such as accidental extubation and occlusion of the endotracheal tube by surgical instruments or malposition of the patient. It's also important to mention the laryngospasm and bronchospasm during the palate repair. Hypothermia in patients of two months to two years of age is directly proportional to the length of the surgery and the temperature of the surgical room [27]. In the Instituto Nacional de Pediatría, hypothermia was a frequent concern and it is critical to keep the surgical room at an adequate temperature to avoid other adverse events that could alter the behavior or stability of the patient during the moment of the extubation. To avoid the adverse events such as laryngospasm and bronchospasm it is important to set criteria for the best moment of extubation.

4. Perioperative and postsurgery analgesia

Pain control during the entire perioperative procedure is especially important in CL and palate surgeries. Multi-modal pain therapy with narcotic, non-narcotic and regional anesthesia can help ensure optimal pain control. In the United States, the surgeon will typically inject local anesthetic and epinephrine prior to the repair of both CL as well as CP. The main goal of this injection is to provide vasoconstriction in surgical field. However, when local anesthetic is utilized the patient will benefit from some additional pain control. The duration of which is dependent on the type of local anesthetic used. Opioids can be used intraoperatively to smooth the hemodynamic response to surgical pain. Some anesthesiologists in the United States are increasingly using the short acting narcotic remifentanil. Remifentanil is potent and quick acting, but is metabolized quickly allowing its effects to dissipate quickly. Remifentanil can also be used to facilitate a smooth emergence and extubation in these patients. However, remifentanil may not be available in all facilities throughout the world, making it difficult to utilize in resource limited locations.

Regional anesthesia can provide excellent analgesia in children undergoing surgical repair of CL. The infraorbital nerve provides sensory innervation to the skin on the unilateral skin and mucous membranes from the upper lip through the check and to the lower eyelid. Sensory innervation for the nasal alae is also provided (**Figure 1**). Blockade of the infraorbital nerve should provide pain relief for most of the tissue affected by a CL repair. A 2016 Cochrane Review of infraorbital nerve blocks during CL repair demonstrated that bilateral infraorbital nerve blocks result in lower opioid consumption during the surgical procedure as well as lower pain scores in the Post-Anesthesia Care Unite (PACU) [32]. The pain relief was superior to fentanyl [33], placebo [34], and local infiltration [35]. Nicodemus et al. [36] demonstrated that pain relief lasted 19 hours when a mixture of bupivacaine with epinephrine was used for the block. Infraorbital nerve blocks can be easily placed via two approaches; intraoral or extra-oral. The intraoral approach directs a 25 g needle in the mouth and until the gingiva-labial fold near the canine toward the infraorbital notch. The infraorbital nerve emerges from the infra-orbital foramen below the eye which is easily palpated in most patients. Care must be taken to avoid advancing the needle past the foramen into the eye in neonates and infants. Given the small size of these patients, the toxic dose of local anesthesia should be calculated when the surgeon also utilizes local anesthetic with epinephrine for vasoconstriction in the surgical field. Typically, only 0.5–1 mL of local anesthetic is utilized.

The sensory innervation of the palate is more complex than the lip, requiring blockade of the greater palatine, lesser palatine and the nasopalatine. Each of these nerves is branches of the maxillary division of the trigeminal nerve. The suprazygomatic approach to maxillary nerve blockade allows a single injection to provide improved pain control for CP repair [37–38]. Overall, pain was better controlled, and fewer narcotics were required for the first 48 hours following

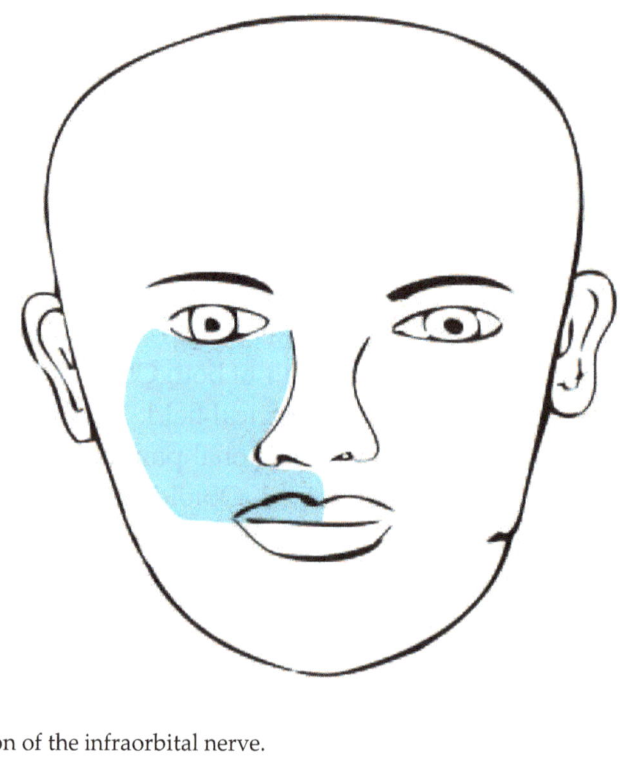

Figure 1. Sensory innervation of the infraorbital nerve.

surgical repair. Unfortunately, suprazygomatic maxillary nerve block is not frequently used due to lack of familiarity by most anesthesiologists in the United States currently. However, unlike infraorbital nerve blocks the nerve block alone is not sufficient to provide adequate analgesia. Typically, narcotics are used in the United States to supplement the residual discomfort.

Multi-modal pain management incorporates the use of non-narcotic medications. Acetaminophen, non-steroidal anti-inflammatory medications and the alpha-2 agonists, like dexmedetomidine, are commonly used in pediatric patients to reduce the total amount of opioids required following surgical procedures, and to reduce the side effects of opioids such as respiratory depression. In infants undergoing primary CP repair acetaminophen is effective in reducing pain scores and overall opioid consumption [39], with intravenous acetaminophen providing the lowest pain scores and lowest opioid consumption compared to placebo and oral administration. Rectal acetaminophen historically has been used given its ease of administration. However, overall opioid consumption is not decreased when rectal acetaminophen is used; suggesting other routes of administration might be preferred [40]. Alpha-2 agonists, such as dexmedetomidine, and ketamine given intraoperatively can also decrease postoperative pain [41].

5. Postoperative care

Postoperatively, there is not a concern for respiratory compromise with CL repair. CP repair differs as obstruction is possible following extubation. The surgical repair itself reduces the size of the airway and excessive sedation from anesthesia and opioids can cause the tongue to lose muscle tone causing obstruction. If the Digman retractor is up for long periods of time, the tongue itself can have some swelling. Obstruction is problematic as blind placement of an oral airway can result in disruption of the fresh surgical repair. Therefore, a plan should be formulated intraoperatively to avoid obstruction in the postoperative period. Dexamethasone is frequently given early during the surgical repair to reduce any swelling. A tongue stich or nasal trumpets can also be placed by the surgeon following CP repair to relieve obstruction should it result. These techniques are not uniformly used by cleft teams in the United States [42] and there is no increase in reintubation rates when tongue stitch is avoided [43], but it is our practice to place a tongue stitch on all our CP patients. The tongue stitch remains in place while the patient is in the PACU, but is removed before transfer to a medical floor for monitoring overnight.

During the postoperative stage, the main care is based on continuous monitoring the supplementary oxygen depending on the needs of the patient. The bleeding assessment is the proper management of pain and the start of oral intake of clear liquids before allowing the patient to be discharged. It is important to establish which patients are candidates for ambulatory management, which ones have a higher risk to present adverse events like bronchospasm, laryngospasm, desaturation and respiratory difficulty. High risk patients with palate repair could end up having to stay in the hospital or intensive care unit longer than expected and this should be a consideration [28]. It's recommended that the stay at the PACU is 1 hour at least [26]. In the Instituto Nacional de Pediatría in Mexico City, the management of pain after surgery is based on paracetamol at 15 mg/kg or an AINE like ketorolac at 1 mg/kg, and other

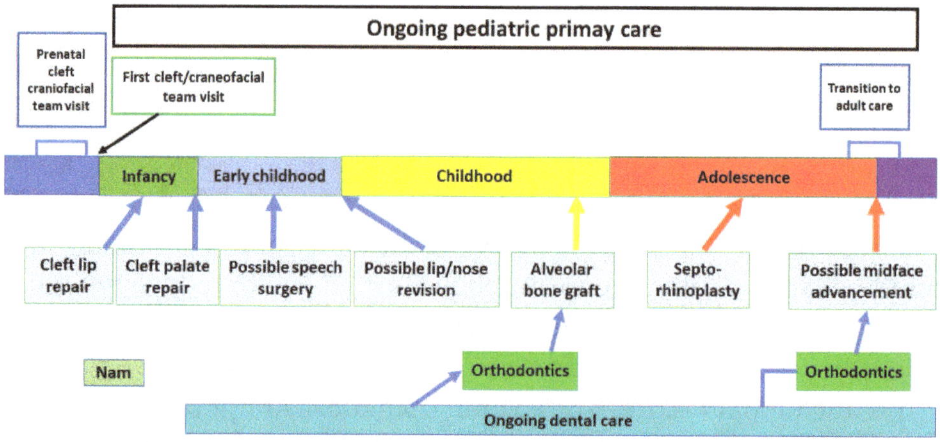

Figure 2. Edited from Lewis CW, Jacob LS, Lehmann CU, AAP SECTION ON ORAL HEALTH. The primary care pediatrician and the care of children with cleft lip and/or cleft palate [44].

options such as a combination of both, or paracetamol with an opioid such as tramadol, or AINE with an opioid. During the surgical outreach trips for clefts, at the surgical setting, there should always be a postanesthetic care unit well equipped to monitor and observe the pediatric patients. The availability of an intensive care unit and a pediatric ventilator should be part of the criteria for any site where one of these trips will take place.

Following the primary repair of CL and CP, children with CP with or without CL have multiple future treatments and potential additional surgical interventions (**Figure 2**).

After multiple surgical procedures, children can be anxious about future procedures. Any past stressful procedure may create lasting difficulty for the future perioperative period. The anesthesiologist should assess for anxiety and create a plan that eases the fears of the patient. In addition, anesthesiologists should be aware of past procedures and what was done. This is especially important following a pharyngoplasty. Nasal intubation following pharyngoplasty can tear or disrupt the past surgical repair. All attempts at nasal intubation should be avoided if possible.

6. The international team of cleft lip and palate

Internationally, there is a need for surgical teams to help aid in surgical repairs of CL and CP. A full discussion of the techniques of establishing sites for these surgical services is beyond the scope of this chapter. However, it is important for the anesthesiologists to recognize differences occur when surgical teams go to other countries. When resources are limited, the choices one makes may differ from the choices made in one's home country. Similarly, a different environment may affect outcomes [45]. Before proceeding with any medical procedures, it is helpful to understand local culture and medical practices. For example, in the United States it is very common that patients receive opioid medications for recovery on the hospital medical floor following surgery. In some countries, the infrastructure and the comfort with postoperative narcotics is not present. Thus, an adapted anesthetic plan should be implemented to ensure that the ultimate goal of adequate pain relief is met with non-narcotic medications. In these countries reliance in nerve blocks and other non-opioid pain medication becomes valuable (**Table 1**).

The most important idea when surgically treating patients in other countries is to remember to *"first do no harm."* The pre-operative evaluation becomes vital to ensuring safety in these kids. It is unlikely that an extensive cardiac evaluation may have been done. A murmur on exam or a history consistent with heart failure warrants further workup before proceeding to surgery. Similarly, a difficult airway should not be underestimated when in a resource limited location. If a potential difficult airway is identified, with known risk factors such as retrognathia, young age and a syndrome associated with a difficult airway, an assessment of resources is important. A plan should be made prior to proceeding in case extubation is not possible following the procedure. Finally, a history and physical should thoroughly inquire about the possibility of a current or recent upper respiratory infection. If risk factors for perioperative respiratory complications from the upper respiratory infection are identified, surgical repairs should be postponed.

In general, once appropriate surgical patients are identified, anesthetic care is similar regardless of the location. The medications available and local customs for postoperative care will help shape the anesthetic designed and the plan for postoperative care.

All reconstructive and craniofacial surgeons that oversee cleft care should treat any patient abroad as if they are at their usual surgical facility at home; always following the quality guidelines for their best performance and safety for the patients. There are different protocols for cleft care all over the world, but the visiting surgeon should adapt to the local multidisciplinary team in charge and ensure that there will be the proper follow up for the patients. A complete documentation should be the rule for the entire team working in the operating room. This will simplify preoperative assessment in the future and enable the team to properly evaluate current and future issues that could lead to any adverse outcome and will help

Syndromes associate with CL and CP	Common features
Pierre Robin Sequence	Micrognathia, glossoptosis
Treacher Collins syndrome	Micrognathia, ear defects, congenital heart disease
Goldenhar's syndrome	Unilateral mandibular hypoplasia, unilateral ear deformity
Down syndrome	Macroglossia, atlantoaxial instability, congenital heart disease
Fetal alcohol syndrome	Congenital heart disease, developmental delay
22q deletion syndrome	Congenital heart disease, hypocalcemia, thymic hypoplasia
Klippel-Feil syndrome	Fusion of the cervical spine, renal disorders
Stickler syndrome	Connective tissue disorder, glaucoma and cataracts, hearing loss, joint hypermobility

Table 1. Shows some syndromes associated with CL and/ or CP and common characteristics.

improve the quality of care provided. All facilities should meet the basic standards to care for all patients, if these standards are not met by the facility, the visiting team is required to bring with them the supplies and equipment necessary to meet these basic standards such as:

1. Electrical power that is dependable and continuous.
2. Working modern anesthesia machines.
3. Dependable oxygen supply.
4. Full-functioning monitoring for each patient in the operating rooms.
5. Working suction should be present at each operating room table and in the recovery area.
6. Basic laboratory and radiology services should be immediately available.
7. Blood banking.

Every team should include a surgeon who is familiar with the planned procedures, preferably a board certified surgeon, a board certified anesthesiologist experienced in the care for children undergoing same or similar procedures, who should be supervising no more than two procedures at any given time, certified nurse anesthetists with experience in the care of children undergoing the same or similar procedures, a board certified pediatrician, operating room, recovery area and ward nurses experienced in the care of children.

The visiting team should always bring the airway equipment including appropriate laryngoscopes and blades, laryngeal mask airways, self-inflating bag-valve-mask in all care areas, emergency cricothyroidotomy kit and fiber-optic bronchoscope. Emergency medications, emergency vascular access kits, defibrillator, portable pulse oximetry, Stat laboratory and portable oxygen supply must be included among the supplies and equipment needed during cleft surgical outreach trip [46].

7. Conclusions

Anesthesia in cleft patients should be performed in a setting with the proper equipment, medications and supplies to provide the safest procedure by experienced anesthesiologists since these patients have high risk for respiratory complications such as difficult intubation, laryngospasm, bronchospasm, or if they have had an upper respiratory infection within the month preceding the surgery, then they may suffer complications like pneumonia or bronchopneumonia. If any other complication may arise from the surgical or anesthetic procedure, the anesthesiologist should be able to diagnose it and manage it and the patient should be transferred to a post anesthetic care unit or intensive care unit, depending on the severity of the complication. Favorable outcomes are directly related to carefully selecting the patient that will undergo cleft surgery, anesthesiologists properly trained to manage this kind of cases and having all the human and material resources to provide the best care during and after the surgical procedure.

Conflict of interest

None of the authors have any conflict of interest.

Author details

Alyssa Brzenski[1], Ofelia Ham-Mancilla[2], Silvia Peña-Olvera[2], Amanda Gosman[3] and Alicia Sigler[4*]

*Address all correspondence to: aliciasiglerplasticsurgeon@gmail.com

1 University of California San Diego, San Diego, CA, USA

2 Instituto Nacional de Pediatría, Ciudad de México

3 UC San Diego School of Medicine, University of California San Diego, San Diego, CA, USA

4 Clínica Ambulatoria Shriners, Tijuana, Baja California, México

References

[1] Parker SE, Mai CT, Canfield MA, Rickard R, Wang Y, Meyer RE, Anderson P, Mason CA, Collins JS, Kirby RS, Correa A. National Birth Defects Prevention Network. Updated national birth prevalence estimates for selected birth defects in the United States, 2004-2006. Birth Defects Research. Part A, Clinical and Molecular Teratology. 2010;**88**(12): 1008-1016. DOI: 10.1002/bdra.20735

[2] Polaiah KP, Madhavi KN, Sivaiah T. A study of airway complications among the patients of cleft lip and cleft palate during intraoperative and postoperative period at government general hospital, Guntur. Journal of Evolution of Medical and Dental Sciences. 2015;**4**(9):1488-1492

[3] Al-Ghatam R, Jones TE, Ireland AJ, Atack NE, Chawla O, et al. Structural outcomes in the cleft care UK study. Part 2: Dento-facial outcomes. Orthodontics & Craniofacial Research. 2015;**18**(Suppl 2):14-24. DOI: 10.1111/ocr.12109

[4] Ness AR, Wills AK, Waylen A, Al-Ghatam R, Jones TE, et al. Centralization of cleft care in the UK. Part 6: A tale of two studies. Orthodontics & Craniofacial Research. 2015; **18**(Suppl 2):56-62. DOI: 10.1111/ocr.12111

[5] Persson M, Sandy JR, Waylen A, Wills AK, Al-Ghatam R, et al. A cross-sectional survey of 5-year-old children with non-syndromic unilateral cleft lip and palate: The cleft care UK study. Part 1: Background and methodology. Orthodontics & Craniofacial Research. 2015;**18**(Suppl 2):1-13. DOI: 10.1111/ocr.12104

[6] Sell D, Mildinhall S, Albery L, Wills AK, Sandy JR, Ness AR. The cleft care UK study. Part 4: Perceptual speech outcomes. Orthodontics & Craniofacial Research. 2015;**18**(Suppl 2): 36-46. DOI: 10.1111/ocr.12112

[7] Smallridge J, Hall AJ, Chorbachi R, Parfect V, Persson M. Functional outcomes in the cleft care UK study--part 3: Oral health and audiology. Orthodontics & Craniofacial Research. 2015;**18**(Suppl 2):25-35. DOI: 10.1111/ocr.12110

[8] Adenekan AT, Faponle AF, Fadekemi Oginni FO. Perioperative adverse airway events in cleft lip and palate repair. Southern African Journal of Anaesthesia and Analgesia. 2011;**17**(6):370-373. DOI: 10.1080/22201173.2011.10872808

[9] Gómez-García R, Lara-Navarro R. Incidencia de labio y paladar hendido en México: 2003-2006. Revista ADM. 2008;**45**(6):309-313

[10] Waylen A, Ness AR, Wills AK, Persson M, Rumsey N, Sandy JR. Cleft care UK study. Part 5: Child psychosocial outcomes and satisfaction with cleft services. Orthodontics & Craniofacial Research. 2015;**18**(Suppl 2):47-55. DOI: 10.1111/ocr.12113

[11] Dixon MJ, Marazita ML, Beaty TH, Murray JC. Cleft lip and palate: Understanding genetic and environmental influences. Nature Reviews. Genetics. 2011;**12**(3):167-178. DOI: 10.1038/nrg2933

[12] Leslie EJ, Marazita ML. Genetics of cleft lip and cleft palate. American Journal of Medical Genetics. Part C, Seminars in Medical Genetics. 2013;**163C**(4):246-258. DOI: 10.1002/ajmg.c.31381

[13] Wyse RK, Mars M, Al-Mahdawi S, Russell-Eggitt IM, Blake KD. Congenital heart anomalies in patients with clefts of the lip and/or palate. The Cleft Palate Journal. 1990; **27**(3):258-264

[14] López-Muñoz AC, Busto-Aguirreurreta N, Braulio T. Guías de ayuno preoperatorio: Actualización. Revista Española de Anestesiología y Reanimación. 2015;**62**(3):145-156. DOI: 10.1016/j.redar.2014.09.006

[15] Heinrich S, Birkholz T, Ihmsen H, Irouschek A, Ackermann A, Schmidt J. Incidence and predictors of difficult laryngoscopy in 11,219 pediatric anesthesia procedures. Paediatric Anaesthesia. 2012;**22**(8):729-736. DOI: 10.1111/j.1460-9592.2012.03813.x

[16] Lee A, Fan LT, Gin T, Karmakar MK, Ngan Kee WD. A systematic review (meta-analysis) of the accuracy of the Mallampati tests to predict the difficult airway. Anesthesia and Analgesia. 2006;**102**(6):1867-1878. DOI: 10.1213/01.ane.0000217211.12232.55

[17] Shiga T, Wajima Z, Inoue T, Sakamoto A. Predicting difficult intubation in apparently normal patients: A meta-analysis of bedside screening test performance. Anesthesiology. 2005;**103**(2):429-437

[18] Alarcón-Almanza JM. Labio y paladar hendido. Rev Mex Anestesiol. 2010;**33**(S1):S76-S78

[19] El-Ganzouri AR, McCarthy RJ, Tuman KJ, Tanck EN, Ivankovich AD. Preoperative airway assessment: Predictive value of a multivariate risk index. Anesthesia and Analgesia. 1996;**82**(6):1197-1204

[20] Parnis SJ, Barker DS, Van der Walt JH. Clinical predictors of anaesthetic complications in children with respiratory tract infections. Paediatric Anaesthesia. 2001;**11**(1):29-40

[21] Tait AR, Knight PR. The effects of general anesthesia on upper respiratory tract infections in children. Anesthesiology. 1987;**67**(6):930-935

[22] Coté CJ. The upper respiratory tract infection (URI) dilemma: Fear of a complication or litigation? Anesthesiology. 2001;**95**(2):283-285

[23] Gunawardana RH. Difficult laryngoscopy in cleft lip and palate surgery. British Journal of Anaesthesia. 1996;**76**(6):757-759

[24] Arteau-Gauthier I, Leclerc JE, Godbout A. Can we predict a difficult intubation in cleft lip/palate patients? Journal of Otolaryngology - Head & Neck Surgery. 2011;**40**(5):413-419

[25] Reséndiz-Álvarez Y. Manejo anestésico para pacientes con labio y paladar hendido. Rev Mex Anestesiol. 2015;**38**(Suppl 1):245-246

[26] Kularni KR, Patil MR, Shirke AM, Jadhav SB. Perioperative respiratory complications in cleft lip and palate repair: An audit of 1000 cases under "smile train project". Indian. Indian Journal of Anaesthesia. 2013;**57**:562-568. DOI: 10.4103/0019-5049.123328

[27] Bolton P. Anaesthesia for cleft lip and palate surgery. Anaesthesia and Intensive Care Medicine. 2006;**5**:157. DOI: 10.1383/anes.2006.7.5.157

[28] Jindal P, Khurana G. A retrospective analysis of anesthetic experience in 2917 patients posted for cleft5 lip and palate repair. Anesthesia, Essays and Researches. 2013;**7**(3):350-354. DOI: 10.4103/0259-1162.123233

[29] Takemura H, Yasumoto K, Toi T, Hosoyamada A. Correlation of cleft type with incidence of perioperative respiratory complications in infants with cleft lip and palate. Paediatric Anaesthesia. 2002;**12**(7):585-588

[30] Steinmetz J, Holm-Knudsen R, Sørensen MK, Eriksen K, Rasmussen LS. Hemodynamic differences between propofol-remifentanil and sevoflurane anesthesia for repair of cleft lip and palate in infants. Paediatric Anaesthesia. 2007;**17**(1):32-37. DOI: 10.1111/j.1460-9592.2006.01999.x

[31] Simion C, Corcoran J, Iyer A, Suresh S. Postoperative pain control for primary cleft lip repair in infants: Is there an advantage in performing peripheral nerve blocks? Paediatric Anaesthesia. 2008;**18**(11):1060-1065. DOI: 10.1111/j.1460-9592.2008.02721.x

[32] Feriani G, Hatanaka E, Torloni MR. Da silva EM: Infraorbital nerve block for postoperative pain following cleft lip repair in children. Cochrane Database of Systematic Reviews. 2016;**4**:CD011131. DOI: 10.1002/14651858.CD011131.pub2

[33] Rajamani A, Kamat V, Rajavel VP, Murthy J, Hussain SA. A comparison of bilateral infraorbital nerve block with intravenous fentanyl for analgesia following cleft lip repair in children. Paediatric Anaesthesia. 2007;**17**:133-139. DOI: 10.1111/j.1460-9592.2006.02032.x

[34] Ahuja S, Datta A, Krishna A, Bhattacharya A. Infra-orbital nerve block for relief of postoperative pain following cleft lip surgery in infants. Anaesthesia. 1994;**49**:441-444

[35] Prabhu KP, Wig J, Grewal S. Bilateral infraorbital nerve block is superior to peri-incisional infiltration for analgesia after repair of cleft lip. Scandinavian Journal of Plastic and Reconstructive Surgery and Hand Surgery. 1999;**33**:83-87

[36] Nicodemus HF, Ferrer MJR, Cristobal VC, aI. Bilateral infraorbital block with 0.5% bupivacaine as postoperative analgesia following cheiloplasty in children. Scandinavian Journal of Plastic and Reconstructive Surgery and Hand Surgery. 1991;**25**:253-257

[37] Mesnil M, Dadure C, Captier G, Raux O, Rochette A, Canaud N, Sauter M, Capdevila X. A new approach for peri-operative analgesia of cleft palate repair in infants: The bilateral suprazygomatic maxillary nerve block. Paediatric Anaesthesia. 2010;**20**:343-349. DOI: 10.1111/j.1460-9592.2010.03262.x

[38] Chiono J, Raux O, Bringuier S, et al. Bilateral suprazygomatic maxillary nerve block for cleft palate repair in children: A prospective, randomized, double-blind study versus placebo. Anesthesiology. 2014;**120**(6):1362-1369. DOI: 10.1097/ALN.0000000000000171

[39] Nour C, Ratsiu J, Singh N. Analgesic effectiveness of acetaminophen for primary cleft palate repair in young children: A randomized placebo controlled trial. Paediatric Anaesthesia. 2014;**24**(6):574-581. DOI: 10.1111/pan.12393

[40] Bremerich DH, Neidhart G, Heimann K, Kessler P, Behne M. Prophylactically-administered rectal acetaminophen does not reduce postoperative opioid requirements in infants and small children undergoing elective cleft palate repair. Anesthesia and Analgesia. 2001; **92**(4):907-912

[41] Kayyal TA, Wolfswinkel EM, Weathers WM, et al. Treatment effects of dexmedetomidine and ketamine on postoperative analgesia after cleft palate repair. Craniomaxillofacial Trauma and Reconstruction. 2014;**7**(2):131-138. DOI: 10.1055/s-0034-1371446

[42] Dorfman DW, Ciminello FS, Wong GB. Tongue suture placement after cleft palate repair. The Journal of Craniofacial Surgery. 2010;**21**(5):1601-1603. DOI: 10.1097/SCS.0b013e3181ebccb1

[43] Gallagher S, Ferrera A, Spera L, et al. Utility of tongue stitch and nasal trumpet in the immediate postoperative outcome of cleft palatoplasty. Plastic and Reconstructive Surgery. 2016;**137**(2):569-573. DOI: 10.1097/01.prs.0000475786.60069.a3

[44] Lewis CW, Jacob LS, Lehmann CU. AAP section on oral health: The primary care pediatrician and the care of children with cleft lip and/or cleft palate. Pediatrics. 2017; **139**(5):e20170628. DOI: 10.1542/peds.2017-1921

[45] Maine RG, Hoffman WY, Palacios-Martínez JH, Corlew DS, Gregory GA. Comparison of fistula rates after palatoplasty for international and local surgeons on surgical missions in Ecuador with rates at a craniofacial center in the United States. Plastic and Reconstructive Surgery. 2012;**129**(2):319e-326e. DOI: 10.1097/PRS.0b013e31823aea7e

[46] Schneider WJ, Politis GD, Gosain AK, Migliori MR, Cullington JR, Corlew DS, Wexler AM, Flick R, Van Beek AL. Volunteers in plastic surgery guidelines for providing surgical care for children in the less developed world. Plastic and Reconstructive Surgery. 2011;**127**(6):2477-2486. DOI: 10.1097/PRS.0b013e3182131d2a

5

Cleft Lip and Palate in the Dog: Medical and Genetic Aspects

Enio Moura and Cláudia Turra Pimpão

Abstract

The same types of cleft lip and/or cleft palate (CL/P) that affects humans also naturally affect dogs. Therefore, the dog has become an important spontaneous animal model for the study of human oral clefts. In order to provide an overview of CL/P in dogs to people with an interest in this area, we present in this chapter the main medical aspects, ranging from the etiology to the prevention, and also the main genetic aspects, including inheritance mechanisms and highlighting the homology between the two species, and the most recent molecular findings.

Keywords: dog, cleft lip, cleft palate, cleft lip and palate, oral clefts, genetics

1. Introduction

In the last 20 years, the domestic dog has become one of the main animal models for the study of genetic disorders and congenital defects due to advances in genetics and genomics. The frequent occurrence of birth defects in dogs, with the cleft lip and palate being among the most common, is a byproduct of breeding practices. Since the mechanisms responsible for the morphogenesis of mammals are highly conserved and the genomic similarity between dogs and humans is high, in addition to sharing the same environment, spontaneous cases of cleft lip and palate in dogs are exceptionally useful for studies on the pathogenesis and genetics of oral clefts and the morphogenesis of the face [1–3].

In this chapter, we present an overview of the medical and genetic aspects of cleft lip and palate in dogs, in the hope that it will be useful to veterinary clinicians, researchers, and other professionals interested in genetics and developmental biology.

2. General considerations

2.1. Considerations on homology

It is easy even for a layperson to see that human anatomy and physiology have their equivalence throughout the zoological scale of vertebrates, especially when it comes to tetrapods. It is also not difficult to deduce that the mechanisms of development are similar or even identical, especially when we compare eutherian mammals. However, when we think of genes, genotypes, and their mechanisms of action, there is a tendency to conclude that everything is quite different. Nevertheless, in reality, "our genome" is not as exclusively ours as we generally imagine. Dogs and mice share over 90% of our genes [4], enabling us to suppose that genetic programs that control embryonic development are similar in the three species. Genes with a common evolutionary origin, maintaining the same function in different species, are known as orthologs (**Figure 1**). They are clear evidence that the homology of structures among species also have a molecular base. For instance, the *ADAMTS20* gene is one of the necessary genes for the normal palatogenesis of mice, to the extent that homozygous individuals for a mutation with loss of function have a palatal cleft [5]. Recently, a recessive mutation in the canine ortholog was identified in dogs with a cleft palate [6].

Knowledge of the developmental biology and genetics of one species helps us to understand those of another. Much has been learned regarding craniofacial morphogenesis by studying chickens and mice [7–9]. The dog, which has contributed so much to the development of

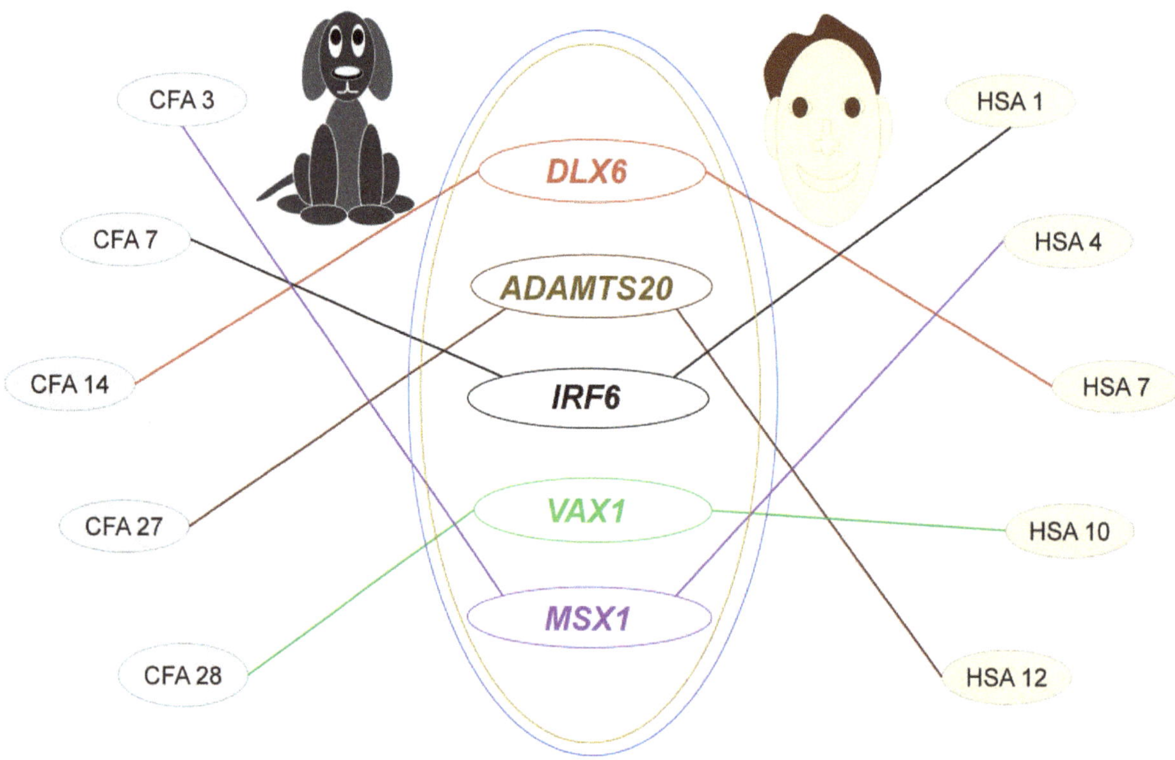

Figure 1. Shared genome. Examples of orthologs with the respective chromosomal assignment in the dog (CFA) and man (HSA). In two of them (*ADAMTS20* and *DLX6*), mutations are known that cause cleft lip and palate in a breed of dogs, while in the other three, mutations are known that have been associated with cleft lip and palate in humans.

surgical techniques used today to correct oral defects, can also help to expand our knowledge of the pathogenesis and genetics of orofacial defects.

2.2. Considerations on the morphogenesis of the lip and palate

Orofacial development is a sequence of events in space and time that involve cellular multiplication, migration and differentiation, tissue fusion, and apoptosis and are dependent on the action of various signaling molecules and transcription factors [10].

The primitive mouth is called the stomodeum. It emerges as a slight depression on the ectodermal surface, delimited by mesenchymal structures where cells from the neural crest proliferate. Although these cells are ectodermal in origin, they settle and integrate with the mesenchyme of the head of the embryo. They are fundamental to the development of the craniofacial structures. Five structures surround the stomodeum: frontonasal prominence, from which the primary palate will originate; right and left maxillary prominences, from which the secondary palate will originate; and right and left mandibular prominences, from which the mandible will originate (**Figure 2**). The maxillary and mandibular prominences are derived from the first branchial arch [10, 11].

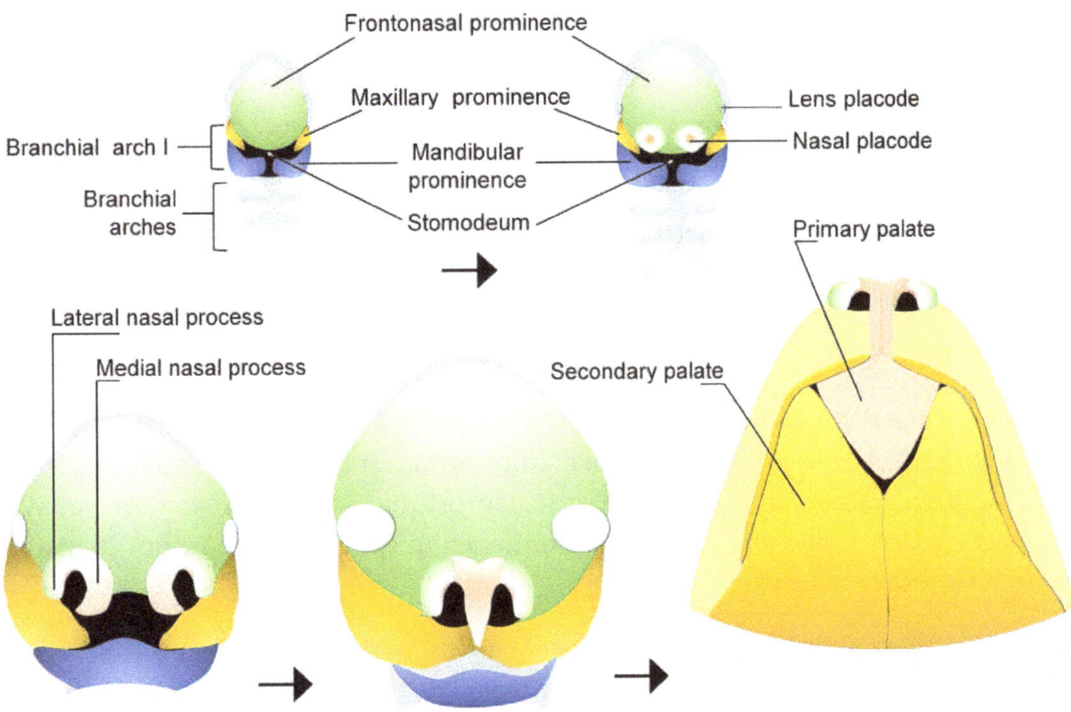

Figure 2. Palatogenesis. Semischematic drawing representing the formation of the primary and secondary palate in dogs.

2.2.1. Formation of the primary palate

The primary palate is the primordium of the hard palate (incisive bone) rostrally located at the incisive fissures (incisive foramen in humans). During development, the frontonasal prominence forms a pair of lateral and medial nasal processes. The fusion of the lateral and medial parts of each process delimits the nasal cavities that are forming. The medial processes are then lengthened and projected between the maxillary prominences, are fused with them, and transformed into the primary palate and medial part of the upper lip [11].

2.2.2. Formation of the secondary palate

The secondary palate is the primordium of the palate caudally located at the incisive fissures (hard palate and soft palate, so-called because its formation is completed after the formation of the primary palate). Initially, the maxillary prominences are projected vertically by the sides of the tongue, and are then raised and projected horizontally on the tongue until they meet. A fusion then occurs between the two in the medial line forming a continuous epithelial seam, which will subsequently disappear. Rostrally, the secondary palate is also fused with the primary palate and, dorsally, with the projection (nasal septum) formed by the united medial nasal processes. The maxillary prominences also form the lateral parts of the upper lip [11].

At approximately 23 days of gestation, in the canine embryo it is possible to see the frontonasal, maxillary, and mandibular prominences. At approximately 28 days, the first ossification of the maxilla and mandible occurs [12].

3. Medical aspects

3.1. Frequency

A cleft lip and/or palate can affect purebred dogs or mongrels. Any canine breed can be affected, especially if we consider cleft lip and palate caused by environmental teratogens. However, the relatively frequent occurrence in some breeds indicates a strong contribution of genetic factors [13].

Indeed, certain breeds of dog are more likely to have cleft lip and palate, especially brachycephalic dogs [14]. At least, this is the clear impression of numerous veterinary practitioners who work with small animals worldwide. Unfortunately, no statistics are yet available that enable definitive statement regarding frequency in different breeds, nor in canine species as a whole.

In boxers, a frequency of 0.6% has been recorded, while in beagles has been 0.11%, and in Pyrenees shepherd dogs, 2.2%. In Portuguese water dogs, cleft palate has been reported in 2.3% of litters [15–18].

In some cases, the high frequency observed at veterinary clinics in certain breeds may be due to the popularity of those breeds at a given time. It is also possible that the frequency is high in certain lines due to constant inbreeding, but not high in the breed as a whole. In a lineage of old Spanish pointer dogs a frequency of 15–20% was found [19].

Table 1 shows the breeds that are considered as having a predisposition to oral clefts or for which cases have been registered.

Affenpinscher	Chihuahua	Nova Scotia duck-tolling retriever
Akita inu	Collie	Old Spanish pointer dog
American cocker spaniel	Dachshund	Papillon
American pit bull terrier	English bulldog	Pekingese
American Staffordshire terrier	English pointer	Poodle
American water spaniel	English toy spaniel	Portuguese water dog
Australian shepherd	Finnish spitz	Puli
Australian terrier	Fox terrier	Pug
Basset hound	French bulldog	Pyrenees shepherd dog
Beagle	German shepherd dog	Rottweiler
Bearded collie	Giant schnauzer	Samoyed
Bernese mountain dog	Golden retriever	Schipperke
Bichon frise	Great Pyrenees	Scottish terrier
Boston Terrier	Irish setter	Shetland Sheepdog
Bouvier des flandres	Italian greyhound	Shih Tzu
Boxer	Labrador retriever	Silky terrier
Brittany spaniel	Maltese	Staffordshire bull terrier
Brussels griffon	Manchester terrier	Swiss sheep dog
Bull terrier	Mastiff	Welsh corgi, cardigan
Bullmastiff	Miniature pinscher	West Highland white terrier
Cairn terrier	Miniature schnauzer	Yorkshire terrier
Cavalier King Charles spaniel	Norwegian elkhound	
Refs. [13, 14, 17–23].		

Table 1. Breeds with records of CL/P.

3.2. Classification

Successful communication between professionals (veterinary practitioners, geneticists, surgeons, dentists, etc.) who treat patients with CL/P depends on an appropriate and correct registration of these abnormalities adhering to common criteria by everyone involved. Thus, the adoption of a classification is highly important. Furthermore, a consistent register based on a classification helps to establish the cause, planned treatment, prognosis, and studies of comparative anatomy [24].

The different classifications used in human medicine can be adapted for use with dogs, as has been done by some researchers based on the first classifications of human oral clefts [24, 25]. Many of the classifications of human clefts are modifications of the classification of Kernahan and Stark [26], which will be adopted here for the purposes of this chapter. It is based on the morphology and pattern of embryonic development of mammals. The clefts are clustered into three groups, each with three subgroups, with all of them considering the degree of impairment of the structures as total or partial (**Figures 3** and **4**):

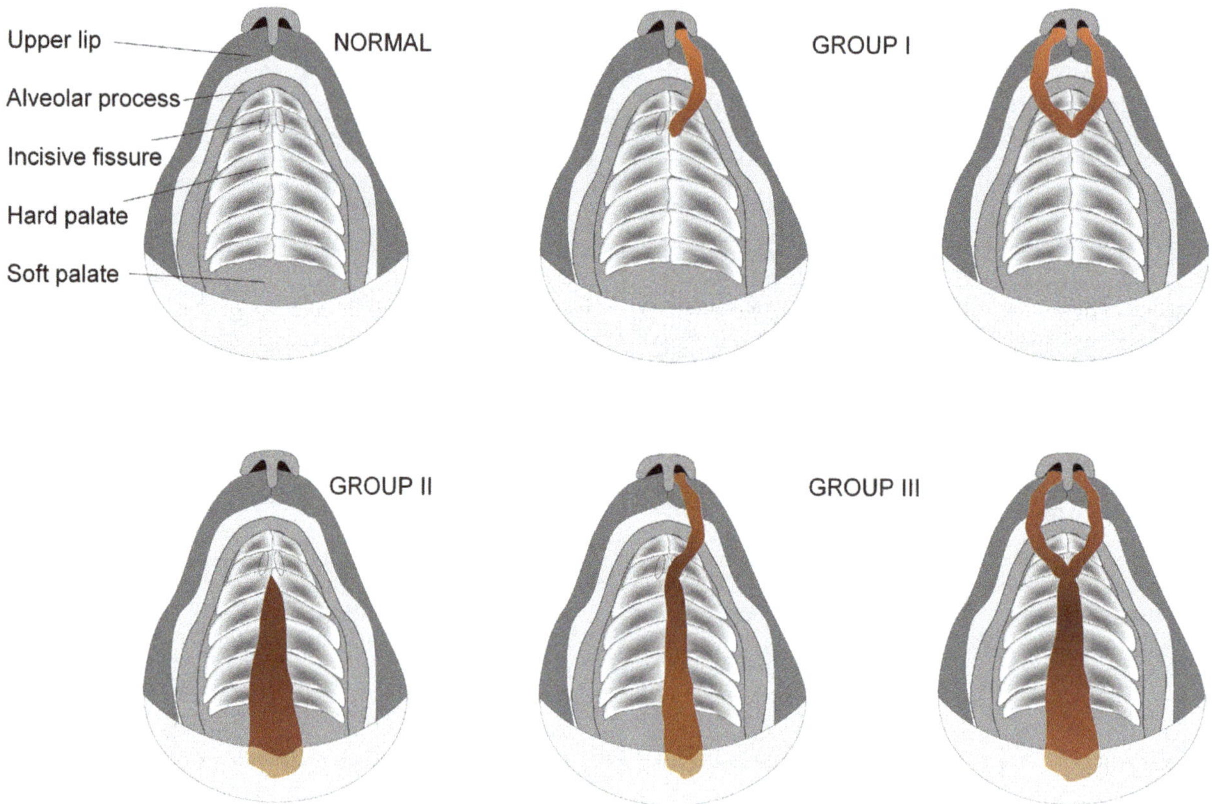

Figure 3. Types of cleft. In each group, complete unilateral or bilateral clefts are shown. However, a cleft from Group I can be left- or right-sided and affect only the lip, the lip and the alveolar process, or include the entire extension of the primary palate, as shown in the illustration. Likewise, a cleft from Group II may affect only the soft palate or the soft palate and the hard palate.

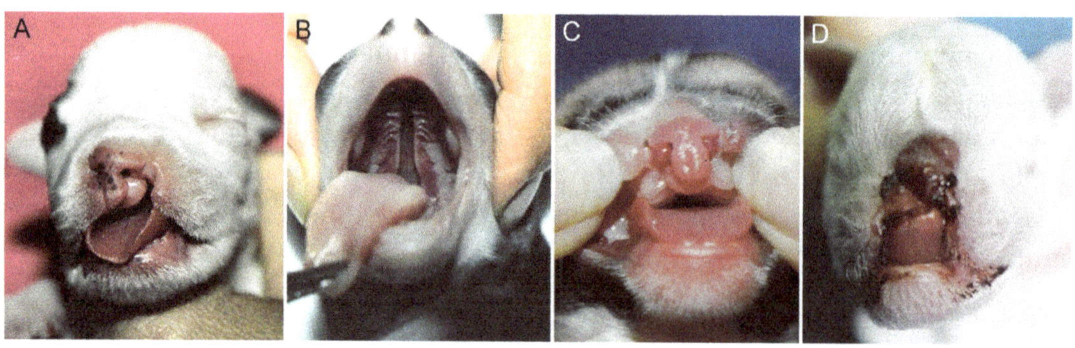

Figure 4. Dogs with nonsyndromic (A–C) and syndromic (D) clefts. (A) Left-sided unilateral cleft, affecting the upper lip, alveolar process, and incisive bone (primary palate); (B) cleft palate only; (C) bilateral cleft (upper lip, hard palate, and soft palate); (D) anophthtalmia and CLP. Photographs (A–C) reprinted from Moura and Pimpão [35].

Group I. Primary cleft palate (total or partial impairment)

1 – unilateral left or right; 2 – medial; 3 – bilateral

Group II. Secondary cleft palate only

1 – total; 2 – partial; 3 – submucous

Group III. Primary and secondary palate (total or partial impairment)

1 – unilateral left or right; 2 – medial; 3 – bilateral

The criteria for defining a cleft as partial (incomplete) or total (complete) is subjective. Thus, with broader objectives, especially for epidemiological studies and minute comparison with human clefts, we suggest using the numerical system adapted by Schwartz et al. [27] from the striped Y of Kernahan [28], known as the RPL system, or one of the others that are available.

3.3. Etiology

Cleft lip and/or palate (CL/P) in dogs, as in humans, are etiologically heterogeneous, and can be caused by genetic factors, environmental factors, or a combination of these two groups of factors [29, 30].

Mutations in different genes, both in murine models and human beings, have been associated with CL/P [29]. As these genes have the respective homologs that are also present in the canine genome, the same situation is expected to occur in dogs (see Section 4).

The environment of an embryo is represented by the amniotic sac, uterus, maternal body, and the place where the mother lives. Thus, the potentially negative influences of this environment include amniotic abnormalities, uterine abnormalities, maternal metabolic disease, viruses, chemical substances swallowed by or administered to the mother, and maternal exposure to chemical or physical environmental pollutants [31]. Few studies of dogs associate a given environmental factor to oral clefts. Furthermore, these studies focus on substances administered to the mother of the affected dogs during gestation, such as 6-diazo-5-oxo-L-norleucine, aspirin, and vitamin A [32–34]. However, it should be remembered that in the case of aspirin and vitamin A, excessive doses were used, much higher than therapeutic doses. Based on the data obtained in other species (mice, rats, cats, goats, etc.), or personal impressions, it has been suggested that maternal exposure to various substances such as hydroxyurea, griseofulvin, anabasine, metronidazole, primidone, sulphonamides, and corticosteroids can cause oral clefts in dogs [30]. Indeed, as the morphogenic processes are highly conserved [35], the same causes of oral dysmorphogenesis known in man can also be found in other species of mammals, including dogs, and vice versa (**Table 2**).

The interaction between genetic and environmental factors is a known underlying phenomenon of the development of certain phenotypes [38]. Evidence has already been found in humans, linking certain genetic markers to CL/P. For example, maternal smoking in combination with the variants of the *GSTT1* and *IRF6* genes increases the risk of clefts [29]. It should be remembered once again that dogs and humans have high genomic homology and share the same environment [1]. Therefore, similar or even identical interactions may occur.

Amoxicillin	Maternal hyperthermia
Anticonvulsants (diazepam, phenytoin, phenobarbital, topiramate)	Maternal obesity
Cholesterol deficiency	Retinoic acid
Corticosteroids	Smoking
Folate deficiency	Stress
Fluconazole	Viral infections
High parental age	Vitamin B complex deficiency
Hyperglycemia	Zinc deficiency
Ionizing radiation	
Maternal alcohol consumption	Others (occupational exposures, environmental pollutants)

Obs.: Not all the risk factors presented in this table are definitely associated with CL/P, and further studies are required. Several factors (amoxicillin, corticosteroids, maternal obesity, stress, etc.) have not shown a consistent association and there are discrepancies between the studies.

Refs. [29, 36, 37].

Table 2. Presumed or confirmed risk factors that have been associated with CL/P in humans.

3.4. Pathogenesis

Due to its etiology, a cleft lip or palate may be the result of an originally abnormal development process or negative interference in a normal development process, corresponding to the concepts of malformation and disruption, respectively, used in dysmorphology [35].

The heterogeneous etiology, in cases of malformation and disruption, assumes varied mechanisms in the development of CL/P. While some mechanisms impair the morphogenesis of various structures in addition to the palate, resulting in syndromic clefts, others act only in the palatogenesis, resulting in nonsyndromic clefts [29, 35].

Developmental field (or morphogenic field) theory aids understanding because different factors can cause the same type of defect. In the early stages, the whole embryo represents a developmental field (primary field). Later, a developmental field is a region or part of the body of the embryo which responds as a coordinated unit to embryonic induction and gives rise to multiple or complex anatomic structures [39, 40]. The induction depends on influences, both physical and chemical, that one developing tissue has on another (or others) in embryogenesis [39]. Developmental fields are systems that control the progressive differentiation of the structure and size, in addition to the temporal and spatial distribution of complex organ components [40]. During blastogenesis, the interactions of the primary field (embryo) generate the progenitor fields (primordia of the final structures) that, in turn, create the secondary fields that produce the final structures during organogenesis [41].

Defects in a structure or in part of the body result from disturbances in one or more secondary fields and are known as monotopic field defects, such as nonsyndromic oral clefts. Multiple defects are the result of disturbances in the primary field or progenitor fields, as occurs in individuals with various defects, including CL/P (syndromic clefts). Correlated defects that emerge early during blastogenesis and affecting structures in different parts of the body are polytopic field defects [41].

At any time during embryogenesis, disturbances in the developmental fields can reflect negatively on fusion mechanisms between the lateral and medial nasal processes, and the medial nasal processes with the maxillary processes (Group I clefts); and/or the mechanisms of development, elevation, and fusion of the palatal shelves and the disappearance of the midline epithelial seam (clefts in Groups II and III).

3.5. Patient evaluation

The diagnosis is conducted by visual inspection of the entire extension of the oral cavity, from the premaxilla (incisive bone) to the soft palate. Without this precaution, smaller clefts may go undetected, especially those that affect the soft palate only.

Cleft lip is evident, however, it indicates the need for a thorough and detailed examination of the oral cavity of the patient and the entire organism in search of other congenital abnormalities to determine whether the cleft is an isolated (nonsyndromic) defect or part of a larger (syndromic) condition.

In newborns, difficulty in nursing, nasal reflux of milk, and fault in development are frequent clinical signs. In older patients, in addition to delayed development, choking, coughing, and sneezing during feeding are common. Nasal discharge is also frequent, but the existence of one or more clinical signs and their intensity depends on the location and gravity of the cleft. It is important to be attentive to clinical manifestation resulting from complications, especially signs of pneumonia, a condition that requires immediate treatment.

Detailed record of the oral cleft is essential for adequate planning of treatment, evaluation of postsurgery progress, and studies with different purposes.

Evaluation of the general condition of the patient may include routine laboratory tests and X-rays. Computerized tomography may be useful for planning surgical treatment [3]. The simultaneous existence of oral cleft and other congenital defects justifies a karyotype test.

Irrespective of the existence of obvious abnormalities or clinical signs, inspection of the oral cavity should be part of the physical examination of all newborns.

3.6. Complications

Cleft lip in general means no complications or complications limited to suction problems. However, clefts that affect the incisive bone and, above all, those that affect the secondary palate cause problems of feeding, breathing, and malocclusion. They cause rhinitis, rhinosinusitis, and occasionally otitis media [42, 43]. They can also cause aspiration pneumonia with risk of death. Malnutrition, dehydration, and accumulation of food in the cleft are commonplace.

Unlike in humans and for obvious reasons, difficulty in emitting sounds is not important in dogs and speech defects do not exist.

3.7. Treatment

Cleft lip and palate require corrective surgery to enable adequate function and for esthetic reasons. However, the decision to undergo surgery falls to the owner of the dog. Although many opt for euthanasia, every day, people seek veterinary clinics to inquire about treatment for a dog born with a CL/P.

If the owner opts for treatment, it is necessary for him to be fully aware of the intensive work involved before the patient is old enough for surgery. It is also important to give the owner careful guidelines regarding feeding and cleaning procedures for his dog. He should also be warned of the need to be constantly on the lookout for possible complications. Clefts that affect only the lip or the lip and the alveolar process require little of the owner, but the more extensive clefts may require a lot of dedication.

An efficient and minimally invasive technique for feeding dogs with a cleft palate was described by Martínez-Sanz et al. [19] using baby bottle nipples and customized palatal prostheses made of dental thermoplastic plates. During the breastfeeding period, dogs were fed with a commercial maternal milk substitute using a baby bottle with a customized nipple. After weaning, which occurred during the fifth week of life, palatal prostheses were made every week in keeping with the development of the dogs. The palatal prosthesis was kept in the mouth during the day and removed at night. The technique did not impede oral development and the materials used are easily obtained from dental suppliers. The cost is relatively low and accessible to most veterinary clinics [19].

In cases of severe clefts, it is necessary for the newborn to be fed through a stomach tube to ensure its height and weight development and good nourishment. It may even be necessary to create an esophageal or gastric stoma for feeding and hospitalize the patient [30]. These procedures can be found in several textbooks of veterinary hospital techniques.

In any situation, the owner must be duly trained to deal with the patient's condition and clean the oral cavity adequately after feeding. Alternatively, the owner should take the dog to a veterinary clinic every day for adequate care. A collaborative, patient, and well-informed owner is essential for dogs with cleft lip and palate to develop and be ready for a surgical procedure.

The age that most surgeons consider appropriate for the first corrective procedure is between 4 and 6 months, i.e., it is advisable to await permanent dentition eruption. Before this time, dental development may be harmed. It is also important to consider that oral clefts tend to diminish with growth and become stable at around 6 months [30, 44, 45].

The surgery should be carefully planned and all preoperative care should be taken, including stabilization of the nutritional status and the solution of any complications that may arise. Rhinitis or rhinosinusitis should be treated with antibiotics and secretolytic agents. The same medication is used to treat aspiration pneumonia together with oxygen, bronchodilators, and, in some cases, corticosteroids [30].

Several techniques are available to correct cleft lip and cleft palate, ranging from those that use a mucosal flap or mucoperiosteal flap to autologous bone grafts and prostheses in the case of larger clefts. There are also promising procedures that use mesenchymal stem cells of the iliac bone with hydroxyapatite particles [44, 46–49]. When the correction is done in stages, the functional rehabilitation and esthetic results are better [50]. Although the main purpose is the rehabilitation of the patient, veterinary procedures in plastic surgery and dentistry are now available and would provide a really good esthetic effect in a final step.

Like all surgery, postoperative care is essential for success. Thus, supportive measures and the administration of antibiotics, analgesics, and antiinflammatory medicine should be followed strictly. Care should also be taken regarding the patient's feeding and hygiene.

3.8. Prevention

The prevention of oral clefts in dogs follows the same principles as prevention in humans. In other words, educating people regarding the risk factors and genetic counseling, with appropriate adaptations.

Pregnant dogs should be given a balanced diet and their health should be monitored. They should also be protected from viral agents. The environment where they live should be free of chemical products. Breeders and owners should be warned of the risk to the embryo/fetus from the administration of certain medicines. Before prescribing medicine, veterinary practitioners should check the teratogenic potential of the drug.

In humans, advanced parental age is linked to an increased probability of oral clefts in offspring [51]. However, in dogs, there are not studies on this aspect. Assuming that this is the case with dogs, a preventive measure is to use good sense and avoid crossing very young animals or much older ones.

As in human medicine, in veterinary medicine, mineral and vitamin supplements have been recommended, especially folic acid and vitamins B6 and B12 [52, 53]. However, the results are not definitive and there have been discrepancies between studies [29, 54].

A daily supplement of 5 mg of folic acid in pregnant French bulldogs, beginning on the 15th day and ending on the last day of pregnancy, reduced the frequency of cleft palate by 48.54% in a research period of 18 months [53]. In Boston terriers, a reduction of 76% was observed [52]. In pugs and Chihuahuas, there were reductions of 60 and 66.67%, respectively. A supplement of 5 mg/day was given to pugs and 2.5 mg/day to Chihuahuas from the beginning of estrus to the 40th day of gestation [55].

Considerations on genetic counseling will be given later in Section 4.3.

4. Genetic aspects

The genetic basis of cleft lip and palate is extremely complex due to the potential number of genes involved, their behavior (mode of inheritance, gene interaction, penetrance, expressivity, etc.), number of alleles in each gene, independent segregation (two or more genes), epistasis, and gene linkage, in addition to environmental factors that might cause phenocopies. This complexity, added to the difficulties of maintaining and handling the affected animals, has severely limited clinical and genetic studies of orofacial clefts in dogs. Consequently, few are available and these will be summarized as follows.

4.1. Syndromic and nonsyndromic clefts

Canine oral clefts may be isolated abnormalities, affecting the lip, lip and palate, or only the palate. They may also coexist with abnormalities in other areas of the body. The former are nonsyndromic clefts and the latter are syndromic clefts. The term "syndromic," as used here, is well established and corresponds to a syndrome in a general sense, i.e., a set of abnormalities that occur jointly, but does not necessarily correspond to the concept used in clinical genetics, in which a set of abnormalities can indeed be a syndrome, but also an association or sequence [39].

In dogs, there are no conclusive data on the frequency of each of these two groups. However, the clear perception of veterinary practitioners is that the nonsyndromic forms are far more common than the syndromic. In humans, approximately 70% of cleft lip and palate are isolated abnormalities, while 30% are part of multiple abnormalities due to chromosome aberrations, monogenic inheritance, teratogens, or unknown causes [56].

In veterinary clinics, the common procedure for dogs with multiple abnormalities is immediate euthanasia. This is often performed by the owners or breeders, with no records or study. Consequently, little is known about the syndromic forms of cleft lip and palate.

4.1.1. Syndromic clefts

We have seen bilateral anophthalmia and cleft lip and palate in mongrels, omphalocele, and cleft palate in Siberian huskies, and anencephaly and cleft palate in Yorkshire terriers, to name three examples. Most of the few reports available have to do with cases in which it was not possible to identify a cause. However, in four cases, a hereditary pattern was established or presumed and, in two cases, the mutation that was responsible was identified [6, 57–59].

In 2015, Wolf et al. [6] studied 13 cases of CL/P with a phenotypic spectrum ranging from bilateral cleft in the nasal wings to complete CLP in Nova Scotia duck tolling retrievers. Furthermore, 10 of the affected animals had syndactyly in the third and fourth toes, varying from incomplete in only one paw to complete in all four paws. As for the other three dogs, whether they had syndactyly was not known. These abnormalities were the result of autosomal recessive inheritance and were a syndromic form of CL/P with variable expressivity. A mutation in the *ADAMTS20* gene was associated with this phenotype. In 2014, Wolf et al. [57] had already identified another mutation in the same breed: an insertion of a LINE-1 in the *DLX6* gene, causing CP and brachygnathia with a pattern of autosomal recessive inheritance. More details on these mutations are given in the section on molecular aspects.

In 1998, Villagómez and Alonso [58] described four individuals from a litter of six Saint Bernard dogs, the offspring of normal parents. They had a cleft palate, bilateral anotia, supernumerary vertebrae and ribs, bifid tongue, and bilateral pedal preaxial polydactyly. In two of these dogs, there was also a cleft lip and one did not have polydactyly. The parents, in four previous gestations, had 28 offspring, 22 of which were normal and 6 had the same clinical phenotype as the four affected individuals. As the parents were normal and had affected male and female offspring, the authors of this report concluded that the abnormalities could be a recessive mutation of an autosomal gene, although the action of teratogens could not be discarded.

In 1985, Sponenberg and Bowling [59] studied a family of Australian shepherds in which there was a syndrome lethal only to the males. The affected animals had a cleft palate and multiple skeletal defects (scoliosis, brachygnathia, short tibia and fibula, polydactyly, syndactyly). In the females, the defects were less severe and there was no cleft palate. The authors of this report raised the hypothesis of X-linked inheritance.

There are also brief reports of omphalocele and bilateral cleft of primary palate in Yorkshire terriers [23], cleft lip and unilateral left-sided anophthalmia in a French bulldog [60], and bilateral cleft of the primary palate, anencephaly, and macroglossia in a dog of unspecified breed [61].

4.1.2. Nonsyndromic clefts

Most genetic nonsyndromic clefts occur in families in accordance with the multifactorial inheritance model. However, there are cases in which a Mendelian pattern of inheritance has been documented.

Monogenic inheritance. Monogenic inheritance is one that depends on a single gene and the type that has so far been confirmed in dogs is autosomal recessive. In other words, the phenotype only manifests if the individual has two copies of the mutant allele. Like all monogenic inheritance, it has a characteristic pattern as follows and is shown in **Figure 5** [62]:

- The phenotype occurs approximately with the same frequency in males and females;
- The parents of an affected individual are generally heterozygotes ($Aa \times Aa$) and thus phenotypically normal; although there is the possibility of an affected individual having one or both parents affected, such situations are improbable;
- The phenotype tends to skip generations;
- The risk of recurrence in descendants of the parents of an affected individual is 25%;
- There is a 50% chance of the parents of an affected having heterozygous descendants like them;
- Normal siblings of an affected individual have a chance of approximately 67% of being heterozygotes; and
- Consanguineous unions increase the chance of the phenotype occurring.

This pattern of inheritance was registered in cases of nonsyndromic CL/P in dogs of the Brittany spaniel, Pyrenees shepherd, and boxer breeds.

In Brittany spaniels, Richtsmeier et al. [63] studied dogs belonging to an intensely inbred colony. In 12 litters, 52 individuals were born, 14 of which had a cleft palate (CP). One of them also had a cleft lip (CL). In 10 of these 12 litters, the number of males and females was

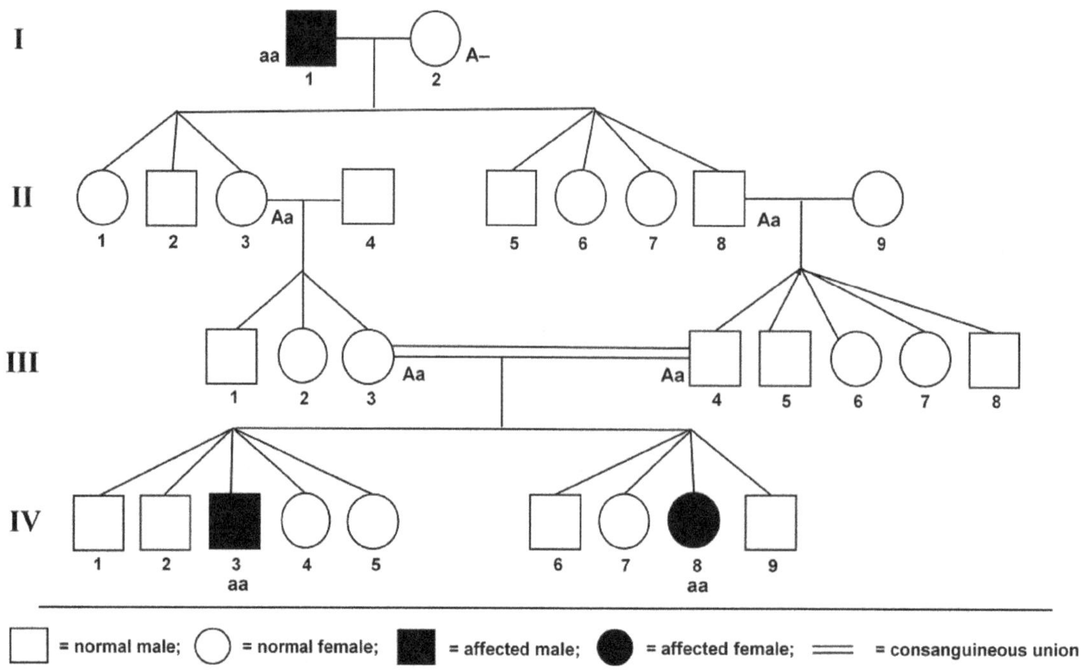

Figure 5. Autosomal recessive inheritance. Consanguineous unions increase the probability that both individuals are heterozygotes, such as couple III-3 X III-4. The risk of recurrence in the offspring of this couple is 25%. The likelihood of having more heterozygous descendants is 2/4 (50%). However, for any one of the normal descendants (male or female) that have already been born, the likelihood is 2/3 (67%).

registered (15 males and 29 females). Of those affected (11), there were more females than males (9 females and 2 males). In all crossings, the parents were normal.

In Pyrenees shepherd dogs, Kemp et al. [17] analyzed the records of a club for this breed over a 20-year period (1984–2004), corresponding to a population of 2104 dogs. They found 47 cases (24 males and 23 females) born in 37 litters with a total of 163 pups and normal parents. Some were only affected by a CP, while others had a cleft lip with or without a cleft palate (CL ± P).

In boxers, Moura et al. [64] found four affected dogs (two males and two females) in two litters with 11 pups born of a consanguineous union (uncle and niece) between normal individuals. All the dogs had essentially the same phenotype (bilateral CLP). Previously, Turba and Willer [15] had raised the hypothesis that in this breed, CLP had a monogenic autosomal recessive pattern of inheritance.

Bleicher et al. [65] reported a case of cleft palate in a beagle together with its pedigree, which is suggestive of autosomal recessive inheritance. There were five affected individuals of both sexes and, in all crossings, the parents were normal.

An older report on cleft palate is suggestive of autosomal recessive inheritance in bulldogs. It presents 33 pups (24 normal and nine affected) born in six litters of a supposedly heterozygous couple [66].

Regarding autosomal dominant inheritance, two reports have described possible cases in which there was nasal cleft, cleft lip, and cleft palate, occurring separately or in association in Bernese mountain dogs (Bernese sennenhund). An affected male that crossed with a normal female and then with a female German shepherd fathered 26 pups, 11 of which were affected [67, 68]. An abnormality with some similarity was also observed in a Portuguese pointer [69]. However, no further data were published to confirm the mode of inheritance in these dogs.

It should be remembered that, in principle, clefts with different patterns of inheritance could be present in the same lineage, which would hinder the interpretation of the gene segregation mechanism.

Multifactorial inheritance. Nonsyndromic clefts are normally distributed in families without following any monogenic pattern of inheritance, but recurrence in generations is undeniable evidence of a genetic basis. The theoretical model that explains this inheritance assumes the contribution of several genes (polygenic inheritance) with an additive effect. The presence of a determined number of liability alleles would create a critical threshold and different degrees of expression of the phenotype, which can also depend on the influence of environmental factors. For instance, if we represent four genes, segregating independently and with the liability alleles identified by the number 2, and that from five number 2 alleles the critical threshold emerges, then several genotypes would be possible (A_1A_2 B_1B_2 C_1C_2 D_2D_2; A_2A_2 B_1B_2 C_2C_2 D_1D_2; A_1A_2 B_2B_2 C_2C_2 D_2D_2; A_1A_1 B_2B_2 C_2C_2 D_1D_2; etc.). Thus, with any combination of five number 2 alleles, the cleft would occur, and the higher the quantity of these alleles, the more serious it would be, with environmental factors also contributing to this. **Figure 6** illustrates this example. There may also be a principal gene that would have a greater effect than the others. In real situations, the number involved is probably much higher than four genes.

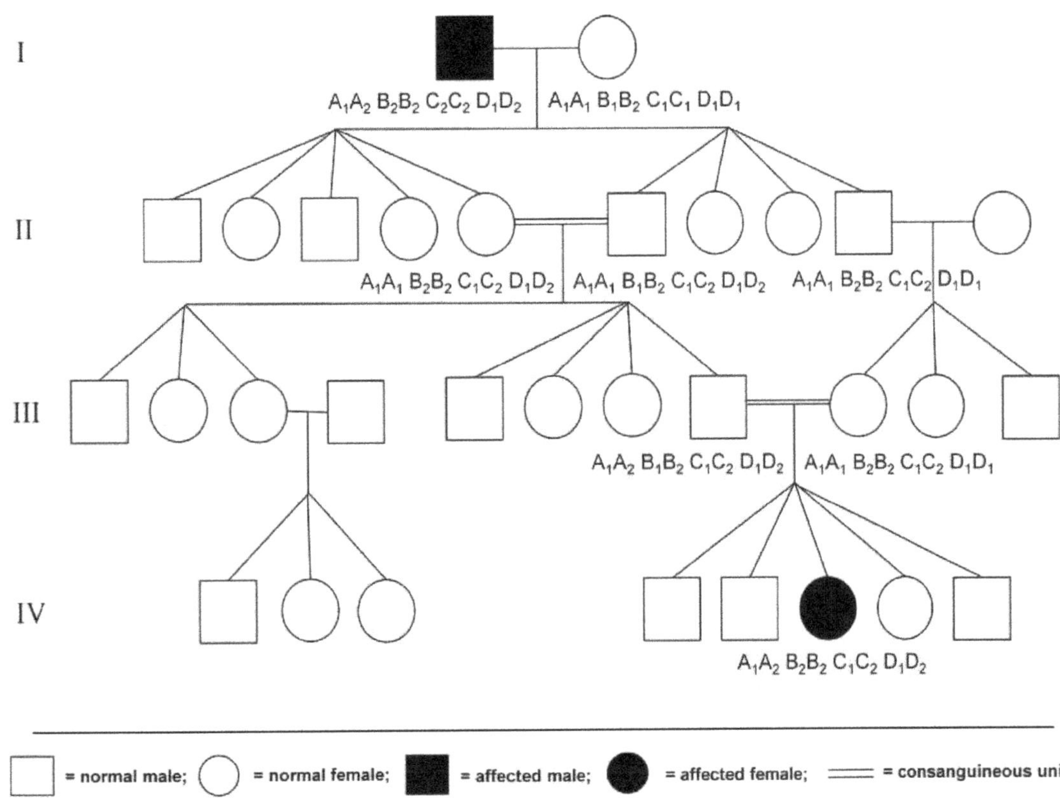

Figure 6. Polygenic inheritance. In this hypothetical pedigree, the individual who inherited at least five number 2 alleles shows the clinical phenotype.

When canine families with high degrees of consanguinity are considered, the critical threshold is more frequent than in families with less or no inbreeding (**Figure 7**). Likewise, the artificial selection process that formed certain breeds led to an increased frequency of liability alleles, making the critical threshold closer than in other breeds and, consequently, leading to a higher frequency of CL/P. As stated previously, there may be a principal gene that increases the risk, as occurs in brachycephalic breeds [70].

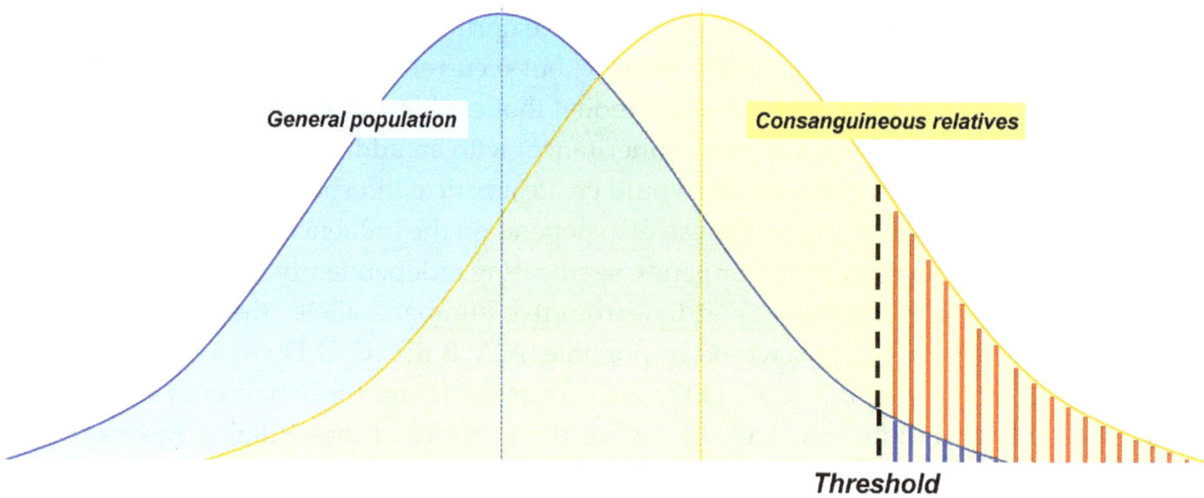

Figure 7. Distribution of genotypes in polygenic inheritance. Comparison of the threshold between the general population and consanguineous relatives or inbred lines.

4.2. Molecular aspects

Modern molecular biology techniques and the use of murine models have enabled the identification of many genes that may be associated with CL/P, and, with each new study, the number of candidate genes grows. The evidence suggests that mutations in these genes, in addition to environmental factors, can act alone or interact with several signaling pathways, negatively interfering in the development of the lip and palate [10]. These genes, and the complex signaling pathways with which they interact, are generally highly conserved in vertebrates and therefore a high degree of homology between man and dog is expected. The identification of mutations in canine genes opens up possibilities for identifying human genes and vice versa, as has happened with the discovery of mutations in mice genes [71]. **Table 3** shows several examples of candidate genes related to CL/P in humans and, potentially, in dogs.

Recently, in Nova Scotia duck tolling retrievers (NSDTR) with a cleft palate and other abnormalities, mutations have been identified in two genes: *DLX6*, located in chromosome 14 of the dog (CFA 14), and *ADAMTS20*, located in chromosome 27 (CFA 27).

In the *DLX6* gene, a LINE-1 insertion was found in the intron 2 jointly segregating with the phenotype (CP and brachygnathia) and obeying an autosomal recessive pattern of inheritance. The presence of the LINE-1 insertion disrupts the transcription of the *DLX6* gene in such a way that only 25% of the normal levels of expression occur, which is not sufficient to prevent CP and mandibular abnormalities. It is located in a noncoding region that is highly conserved,

Gene (abbrev.)	Gene name	Chromosomal assignment (human)	Chromosomal assignment (dog)
IRF6	Interferon regulatory factor 6	1	7
VAX1	Ventral anterior homeobox 1	10	28
BMP4	Bone morphogenetic protein 4	14	8
FGFR2	Fibroblast growth factor receptor 2	10	28
FOXE1	Forkhead box E1	9	11
MAFB	MAF bZIP transcription factor B	20	24
MSX1	msh homeobox 1	4	3
CRISPLD2	Cysteine rich secretory protein LCCL domain containing 2	16	5
FGF8	Fibroblast growth factor 8	10	28
GSTT1	Glutathione S-transferase theta-1-like	22	26
MTHFR	Methylenetetrahydrofolate reductase (NAD(P)H)	1	2
PDGFC	Platelet derived growth factor C	4	15
PVRL1	Poliovirus receptor-related 1 (herpesvirus entry mediator C)	11	5
SUMO1	Small ubiquitin-like modifier 1	2	37
TGFA	Transforming growth factor alpha	2	10
TGFB3	Transforming growth factor beta 3	14	8

Refs. [29, 38, 75].

Table 3. Examples of genes (human and dog orthologs) that have been associated with CL/P in humans.

disturbing a binding domain for SUZ12, a molecule that plays a significant regulatory role in the development of the embryo [57]. Dlx genes form an important family for the development of the first branchial arch, regulating genetic programs that direct the formation of the pattern of the maxilla and mandible [72]. The inactivation of *Dlx5* and *Dlx6* in mice causes serious defects in the craniofacial, axial, and appendicular skeleton, leading to perinatal death [73].

In the *ADAMTS20* gene, a deletion of two nucleotides (AA) was found, segregating together with the phenotype (CL/P and syndactyly) and adhering to an autosomal recessive pattern of inheritance. This deletion represents a frameshift mutation in the metalloprotease domain and should cause the truncation of 1461 amino acids of a protein of 1916 amino acids [6]. The *ADAMTS20* gene is a member of a gene family that encode zinc-dependent proteases. In mouse embryos, its expression is detected in the first branchial arch and between the medial nasal processes [74]. In the palatal mesenchyme, it directs the formation and extension of the palatal shelves [5].

In parallel with the study on NSDTR dogs, Wolf et al. [6] conducted a family-based genome-wide association analysis in a population of native Guatemalans. They identified a significant association between cases of CL/P and the *ADAMTS20* gene, lengthening the list of candidate genes for the etiology of oral clefts in humans.

4.3. Genetic counseling

Like any genetic abnormality, the main recommendation in cases of CLP in dogs is that affected individuals should not be crossed, nor should normal couples with affected descendants ever be crossed again. As the majority of oral clefts in dogs appear to be multifactorial or recessive, it should be noted that owners of normal dogs who have had affected offspring are not always willing to follow this recommendation, especially when the dogs have characteristics of their breed that are highly valued. Therefore, if the owners/breeders decide to cross them again, and are sure that the cleft lip or palate is genetic in nature, the risk of recurrence should be seriously taken into consideration [35].

To avoid autosomal recessive clefts, an important strategy is never to cross individuals that are known to be heterozygotes one with another, such as those that have already had affected offspring. When there is a family history of recessive cleft and the zygosity of an individual is not known, consanguineous unions should be avoided. For X-linked recessive phenotypes, normal female offspring of affected father are all carriers, i.e., heterozygotes, and should not be crossed even when the males are normal. For multifactorial clefts, the main strategy is to avoid crossing dogs that have any relationship. This will reduce the probability of reaching the critical threshold [35].

5. Final considerations

Always bearing in mind that greater knowledge results in a correct diagnosis, suitable management of each case, and definition of criteria that give consistency to guidelines for prevention of CLP, the first step to expand knowledge is appropriate details when publishing new canine cases, using one of the classifications established in human medicine. This will facilitate international communication between professionals from the different fields in question.

Breeds, lineages, or families of dogs in which CLP occurs more frequently are a valuable source of information on the molecular biology and genetics of oral clefts. Genome-wide association studies (GWAS) with genotyping using arrays based on single nucleotide polymorphisms (SNP) are powerful means for mapping of regions of interest. The current technologies of next-generation sequencing (NGS), with increasingly robust platforms and increasingly expanded panels, facilitate the identification of candidate genes, allowing studies that confirm the role of these genes in the etiology of oral clefts.

It should also be remembered that a chromosomal analysis in syndromic cases should be routine. Analyses with fluorescence *in situ* hybridization (FISH) and comparative genomic hybridization (GCH) may identify chromosomal aberrations and describe new syndromes, as well as establishing a correlation with human syndromes.

An interface of knowledge on human and canine species opens up new paths in both veterinary and human medicine. This promotes quality and more humane and competent clinical practice. It is also clearly reflected in the fields of genetics, developmental biology, and evolutionary biology.

Author details

Enio Moura[1]* and Cláudia Turra Pimpão[2]

*Address all correspondence to: enio.moura@pucpr.br

1 Service of Medical Genetics, Faculty of Veterinary Medicine, School of Life Sciences, Pontifícia Universidade Católica do Paraná (PUCPR), Curitiba, Brazil

2 Department of Animal Science, School of Life Sciences, Pontifícia Universidade Católica do Paraná (PUCPR), Curitiba, Brazil

References

[1] Shearin AL, Ostrander EA. Leading the way: canine models of genomics and disease. Dis Model Mech. 2010;**3**(1–2):27–34. doi: 10.1242/dmm.004358.

[2] Schoenebeck JJ, Ostrander EA. Insights into morphology and disease from the dog genome project. Annu Rev Cell Dev Biol. 2014;**30**:535–560. doi: 10.1146/annurev-cellbio-100913-012927.

[3] Nemec A, Daniaux L, Johnson E, Peralta S, Verstraete FJ. Craniomaxillofacial abnormalities in dogs with congenital palatal defects: computed tomographic findings. Vet Surg. 2015;**44**(4):417–422. doi: 10.1111/j.1532-950X.2014.12129.x.

[4] Wade CM, Karlsson EK, Mikkelsen TS, Zody MC, Lindblad-Toh K. The dog genome: sequence, evolution, and haplotype structure. In: Ostrander EA, Giger U, Lindblad-Toh K, editors. The Dog and Its Genome. New York: Cold Spring Harbor Laboratory Press; 2006. pp. 179–207.

[5] Enomoto H, Nelson CM, Somerville RP, Mielke K, Dixon LJ, Powell K, Apte SS. Cooperation of two ADAMTS metalloproteases in closure of the mouse palate identifies a requirement for versican proteolysis in regulating palatal mesenchyme proliferation. Development. 2010;**137**(23):4029–4038. doi: 10.1242/dev.050591.

[6] Wolf ZT, Brand HA, Shaffer JR, Leslie EJ, Arzi B, Willet CE, Cox TC, McHenry T, Narayan N, Feingold E, Wang X, Sliskovic S, Karmi N, Safra N, Sanchez C, Deleyiannis FW, Murray JC, Wade CM, Marazita ML, Bannasch DL. Genome-wide association studies in dogs and humans identify ADAMTS20 as a risk variant for cleft lip and palate. PLoS Genet. 2015;**11**(3):e1005059. doi: 10.1371/journal.pgen.1005059.

[7] Schock EN, Chang CF, Struve JN, Chang YT, Chang J, Delany ME, Brugmann SA. Using the avian mutant talpid2 as a disease model for understanding the oral-facial phenotypes of oral-facial-digital syndrome. Dis Model Mech. 2015;**8**(8):855–866. doi: 10.1242/dmm.020222.

[8] Funato N, Nakamura M, Yanagisawa H. Molecular basis of cleft palates in mice. World J Biol Chem. 2015;**6**(3):121–138. doi: 10.4331/wjbc.v6.i3.121.

[9] Lai Y, Xie C, Zhang S, Gan G, Wu D, Chen W. Bone morphogenetic protein type I receptor inhibition induces cleft palate associated with micrognathia and cleft lower lip in mice. Birth Defects Res A Clin Mol Teratol. 2016;**106**(7):612–623. doi: 10.1002/bdra.23504.

[10] Rahimov F, Jugessur A, Murray JC. Genetics of nonsyndromic orofacial clefts. Cleft Palate Craniofac J. 2012;**49**(1):73–91. doi: 10.1597/10-178.

[11] Bush JO, Jiang R. Palatogenesis: morphogenetic and molecular mechanisms of secondary palate development. Development. 2012;**139**(2):231–243. doi: 10.1242/dev.067082.

[12] Evans HE. Reproduction and prenatal development. In: Evans HE, Christensen GC, editors. Miller's Anatomy of The Dog. 2nd edition. Philadelphia: W. B. Saunders Company; 1993. pp. 13–77.

[13] Padgett GA. Control of Canine Genetic Diseases. New York: Howell Book House; 1998. 264 p.

[14] Foley CW, Lasley JF, Osweiler GD. Abnormalities of Companion Animals: Analysis of Heritability. Ames: The Iowa State University Press; 1979. 279 p.

[15] Turba E, Willer S. Studies for inheritance of the cleft lip and cleft palate in the German boxer dog (Original in German: Untersuchungen zur vererbung von hasenscharten und wolfsrachen bein deutschen boxer). Mh Vet Med. 1987; **42**:897–901.

[16] Natsume N, Miyajima K, Kinoshita H, Kawai T. Incidence of cleft lip and palate in beagles. Plast Reconstr Surg. 1994;**93**(2):439.

[17] Kemp C, Thiele H, Dankof A, Schmidt G, Lauster C, Fernahl G, Lauster R. Cleft lip and/or palate with monogenic autosomal recessive transmission in Pyrenees shepherd dogs. Cleft Palate Craniofac J. 2009;46(1):81–88. doi: 10.1597/06-229.1.

[18] Slater M. The 2005 Portuguese Water Dog Health Survey: Final Report. 2006. 38 p.

[19] Martínez-Sanz E, Casado-Gómez I, Martín C, López-Gordillo Y, González P, Rodríguez-Bobada C, Paradas I, González-Meli B, Maldonado E, Maestro C, Prados JC, Martínez-Álvarez C. A new technique for feeding dogs with a congenital cleft palate for surgical research. Lab Anim. 2011;**45**(2):70–80. doi: 10.1258/la.2010.010044.

[20] Mulvihill JJ, Mulvihill CG, Priester WA. Cleft palate in domestic animals: epidemiologic features. Teratology. 1980;**21**(1):109–112.

[21] Kirk R. A catalogue of congenital and hereditary disorders of dogs (by Breeds). In: Kirk R, editor. Current Veterinary Therapy IX. Philadelphia: W. B. Saunders Company; 1986. p. 1281–1285.

[22] Teixeira FA, Carciofi, AC. Feeding via stomach tube in a dog with cleft palate – a case report (Original in Portuguese: Alimentação via sonda orogástrica em cão com fissura palatina – relato de caso). Revista de Educação Continuada em Medicina Veterinária e Zootecnia. 2013; **11**(2):89. http://www.crmvsp.gov.br/site/revista_edu_cont.php. [Accessed: 2016-07-23]

[23] Faria JA, Alves ND; Costa VKN; Souza AHL; Feijó FMC; Rodrigues RAPF. Cleft lip in newborn dogs: a case report (Original in Portuguese: Lábio leporino em cães recém-nascidos: relato de caso). Revista de Educação Continuada em Medicina Veterinária e Zootecnia. 2014;**12**(2): 82–83, 2014. http://www.crmvsp.gov.br/site/revista_edu_cont.php. [Accessed: 2016-07-23]

[24] Calnan J. The comparative anatomy of cleft lip and palate. I. Classification of cleft lip and palate in dogs. Br J Plast Surg. 1961;**14**:180–184.

[25] Dreyer CJ, Preston CB. Classification of cleft lip and palate in animals. Cleft Palate J. 1974;**11**(0):327–332.

[26] Kernahan DA, Stark RB. A new classification for cleft lip and cleft palate. Plast Reconstr Surg Transplant Bull. 1958;**22**(5):435–441.

[27] Schwartz S, Kapala JT, Rajchgot H, Roberts GL. Accurate and systematic numerical recording system for the identification of various types of lip and maxillary clefts (RPL system). Cleft Palate Craniofac J. 1993;**30**(3):330–332.

[28] Kernahan DA. The striped Y—a symbolic classification for cleft lip and palate. Plast Reconstr Surg. 1971;**47**(5):469–470.

[29] Dixon MJ, Marazita ML, Beaty TH, Murray JC. Cleft lip and palate: understanding genetic and environmental influences. Nat Rev Genet. 2011;**12**(3):167–178. doi: 10.1038/nrg2933.

[30] Łobodzinska A, Gruszczynska J, Max A, Bartyzel BJ, Mikuła M, Mikula Jr I, Grzegrzółka B. Cleft palate in the domestic dog *Canis lupus familiaris* – etiology, pathophysiology, diagnosis, prevention and treatment. Acta Sci Pol, Zootechnica. 2014;**13**(3):5–28.

[31] Moura E. Educational Biology (Original in Portuguese: Biologia Educacional). São Paulo: Editora Moderna; 1993. 336 p.

[32] Jurkiewicz MJ, Bryant DL. Cleft lip and palate in dogs: a progress report. Cleft Palate J. 1968;**5**:30–36.

[33] Robertson RT, Allen HL, Bokelman DL. Aspirin: teratogenic evaluation in the dog. Teratology. 1979;**20**(2):313–320.

[34] Davies M. Excess vitamin A intake during pregnancy as a possible cause of congenital cleft palate in puppies and kittens. Vet Rec. 2011;**169**(4):107. doi: 10.1136/vr.d4614.

[35] Moura E, Pimpão CT. Veterinary dysmorphology. In: Perez-Marin CC, editor. A Bird's-Eye View of Veterinary Medicine. Rijeka: InTech; 2012. p. 71–98. DOI: 10.5772/32344

[36] Mossey PA, Little J, Munger RG, Dixon MJ, Shaw WC. Cleft lip and palate. Lancet. 2009;**374**(9703):1773–1785. doi: 10.1016/S0140-6736(09)60695-4.

[37] Lin KJ, Mitchell AA, Yau WP, Louik C, Hernández-Díaz S. Maternal exposure to amoxicillin and the risk of oral clefts. Epidemiology. 2012;**23**(5):699–705. doi: 10.1097/EDE.0b013e318258cb05.

[38] Zhu H, Kartiko S, Finnell RH. Importance of gene-environment interactions in the etiology of selected birth defects. Clin Genet. 2009;75(5):409–423. doi: 10.1111/j.1399-0004.2009.01174.x.

[39] Spranger J, Benirschke K, Hall JG, Lenz W, Lowry RB, Opitz JM, Pinsky L, Schwarzacher HG, Smith DW. Errors of morphogenesis: concepts and terms. Recommendations of an international working group. J Pediatr. 1982;**100**(1):160–165.

[40] Opitz JM, Zanni G, Reynolds JF Jr, Gilbert-Barness E. Defects of blastogenesis. Am J Med Genet. 2002;**115**(4):269–286.

[41] Martínez-Frías ML, Frías JL, Opitz JM. Errors of morphogenesis and developmental field theory. Am J Med Genet. 1998;76(4):291–296.

[42] Gregory SP. Middle ear disease associated with congenital palatine defects in seven dogs and one cat. J Small Anim Pract. 2000;**41**(9):398–401.

[43] White RN, Hawkins HL, Alemi VP, Warner C. Soft palate hypoplasia and concurrent middle ear pathology in six dogs. J Small Anim Pract. 2009;**50**(7):364–372. doi: 10.1111/j.1748-5827.2009.00742.x.

[44] Fiani N, Verstraete FJ, Arzi B. Reconstruction of congenital nose, cleft primary palate, and lip disorders. Vet Clin North Am Small Anim Pract. 2016;**46**(4):663–675. doi: 10.1016/j.cvsm.2016.02.001.

[45] Meijer R, Prahl B. Influences of different surgical procedures on growth of dentomaxillary complex in dogs with artificially created cleft palate. Ann Plast Surg. 1978;**1**(5):460–465.

[46] Marretta SM. Cleft palate repair techniques. In: Verstraete FJ, Lommer MJ, editors. Oral and Maxillofacial Surgery in Dogs and Cats. 1st edition. Edinburgh: Saunders; 2012. p. 351–362.

[47] Ishikawa Y, Goris RC, Nagaoka K. Use of a cortico-cancellous bone graft in the repair of a cleft palate in a dog. Vet Surg. 1994;**23**(3):201–205.

[48] Lee JI, Kim YS, Kim MJ, Lee J, Choi JH, Yeom DB, Park JM, Hong SH. Application of a temporary palatal prosthesis in a puppy suffering from cleft palate. J Vet Sci. 2006;**7**(1):93–95.

[49] Yoshioka M, Tanimoto K, Tanne Y, Sumi K, Awada T, Oki N, Sugiyama M, Kato Y, Tanne K. Bone regeneration in artificial jaw cleft by use of carbonated hydroxyapatite particles and mesenchymal stem cells derived from iliac bone. Int J Dent. 2012;**2012**:352510. doi: 10.1155/2012/352510.

[50] Bardach J, Kelly KM, Salyer KE. Relationship between the sequence of lip and palate repair and maxillary growth: an experimental study in beagles. Plast Reconstr Surg. 1994;**93**(2):269–278.

[51] Herkrath AP, Herkrath FJ, Rebelo MA, Vettore MV. Parental age as a risk factor for non-syndromic oral clefts: a meta-analysis. J Dent. 2012;**40**(1):3–14. doi: 10.1016/j.jdent.2011.10.002.

[52] Elwood JM, Colquhoun TA. Observations on the prevention of cleft palate in dogs by folic acid and potential relevance to humans. N Z Vet J. 1997;**45**(6):254–256.

[53] Guilloteau A, Servet E, Biourge V, Ecochard C. Folic acid and cleft palate in brachycephalic dogs. Waltham Focus. 2006;**16**(2):30–33.

[54] Shaw GM, Vollset SE, Carmichael SL, Yang W, Finnell RH, Blom H, Ueland PM. Nested case-control study of one-carbon metabolites in mid-pregnancy and risks of cleft lip with and without cleft palate. Pediatr Res. 2009;**66**(5):501–506. doi: 10.1203/PDR.0b013e3181b9b544.

[55] Domosławska A, Jurczak A, Janowski T. Oral folic acid supplementation decreases palate and/or lip cleft occurrence in Pug and Chihuahua puppies and elevates folic acid blood levels in pregnant bitches. Pol J Vet Sci. 2013;**16**(1):33–37.

[56] Stanier P, Moore GE. Genetics of cleft lip and palate: syndromic genes contribute to the incidence of non-syndromic clefts. Hum Mol Genet. 2004;**13** Spec No 1:R73-81.

[57] Wolf ZT, Leslie EJ, Arzi B, Jayashankar K, Karmi N, Jia Z, Rowland DJ, Young A, Safra N, Sliskovic S, Murray JC, Wade CM, Bannasch DL. A LINE-1 insertion in DLX6 is responsible for cleft palate and mandibular abnormalities in a canine model of Pierre Robin sequence. PLoS Genet. 2014;**10**(4):e1004257. doi: 10.1371/journal.pgen.1004257.

[58] Villagómez DA, Alonso RA. A distinct Mendelian autosomal recessive syndrome involving the association of anotia, palate agenesis, bifid tongue, and polydactyly in the dog. Can Vet J. 1998;**39**(10):642–643.

[59] Sponenberg DP, Bowling AT. Heritable syndrome of skeletal defects in a family of Australian shepherd dogs. J Hered. 1985;76(5):393–394.

[60] Pereira JS; Pereira ABFS. Anophthalmia and cleft lip in a dog - a case report (Original in Portuguese: Anoftalmia e lábio leporino em um cão – relato de caso). Centro de Estudos, Pesquisa e Oftalmologia Veterinária.

[61] Wammes JCS, Filadelpho AL, Birck AJ, Peres JA, Pinto e Silva JRC, Guazzelli Filho J, Barcelos RP. Anencephaly, cleft lip and macroglossia in a dog: a case report (Original in Portuguese: Anencefalia, macroglossia e fenda labial em cão: relato de caso). Revista Eletrônica de Medicina Veterinária. 2013; **21**(1):1–8. http://revistas.bvs-vet.org.br/rcemv/article/view/27833/29221. [Accessed: 2016-07-23]

[62] Moura E. Mendel's laws and inheritance patterns of genetic diseases (Original in Portuguese: Leis de Mendel e padrões de herança das doenças genéticas). In: Trevilatto PC, Werneck RI, editors. Dental Genetics (Genética Odontológica). São Paulo: Artes Médicas; 2014. p. 45–63.

[63] Richtsmeier JT, Sack GH Jr, Grausz HM, Cork LC. Cleft palate with autosomal recessive transmission in Brittany spaniels. Cleft Palate Craniofac J. 1994;**31**(5):364–371.

[64] Moura E, Cirio SM, Pimpão CT. Nonsyndromic cleft lip and palate in boxer dogs: evidence of monogenic autosomal recessive inheritance. Cleft Palate Craniofac J. 2012;**49**(6):759–760. doi: 10.1597/11-110.

[65] Bleicher N, Sloan RF, Gault IG, Ashley FL. Cleft palate in a dog. Cleft Palate J. 1965; **45**:56–61.

[66] Wriedt, 1925. Apud Hutt FB. Genetics for Dogs Breeders. San Francisco: W. H. Freeman and Company; 1979. p. 86.

[67] Weber 1955, 1959. Apud Burns M, Fraser MN. Genetics of the Dog. Philadelphia: J.B. Lippincott Company; 1966. p. 80.

[68] Weber, 1959. Apud Richtsmeier JT, Sack GH Jr, Grausz HM, Cork LC. Cleft palate with autosomal recessive transmission in Brittany spaniels. Cleft Palate Craniofac J. 1994;**31**(5):364–371.

[69] Costa-Guerreiro, 1950. Apud Burns M, Fraser MN. Genetics of the Dog. Philadelphia: J.B. Lippincott Company; 1966. p. 80.

[70] Bannasch D, Young A, Myers J, Truvé K, Dickinson P, Gregg J, Davis R, Bongcam-Rudloff E, Webster MT, Lindblad-Toh K, Pedersen N. Localization of canine brachycephaly using an across breed mapping approach. PLoS One. 2010;**5**(3):e9632. doi: 10.1371/journal.pone.0009632.

[71] Ferretti E, Li B, Zewdu R, Wells V, Hebert JM, Karner C, Anderson MJ, Williams T, Dixon J, Dixon MJ, Depew MJ, Selleri L. A conserved Pbx-Wnt-p63-Irf6 regulatory module controls face morphogenesis by promoting epithelial apoptosis. Dev Cell. 2011;**21**(4):627–641. doi: 10.1016/j.devcel.2011.08.005.

[72] Jeong J, Li X, McEvilly RJ, Rosenfeld MG, Lufkin T, Rubenstein JL. Dlx genes pattern mammalian jaw primordium by regulating both lower jaw-specific and upper jaw-specific genetic programs. Development. 2008;**135**(17):2905–2916. doi: 10.1242/dev.019778.

[73] Robledo RF, Rajan L, Li X, Lufkin T. The Dlx5 and Dlx6 homeobox genes are essential for craniofacial, axial, and appendicular skeletal development. Genes Dev. 2002;**16**(9):1089–1101.

[74] Rao C, Foernzler D, Loftus SK, Liu S, McPherson JD, Jungers KA, Apte SS, Pavan WJ, Beier DR. A defect in a novel ADAMTS family member is the cause of the belted white-spotting mutation. Development. 2003;**130**(19):4665–4672.

[75] HomoloGene. National Center for Biotechnology Information. http://www.ncbi.nlm.nih.gov/homologene. [Accessed: 2016-07-23]

6

Strategies to Optimize Global Cleft Care

Mairaj Ahmed, Yunfeng Xue and Ayisha Ayub

Abstract

Orofacial clefts represent the most common congenital craniofacial anomaly worldwide. This condition is best managed by an interdisciplinary team of specialists, often with gratifying results for both the patient and the care providers. Despite recent advances in the management, it remains a challenge today to provide cleft care in low- and middle-income countries (LMIC) due to the lack of basic health care infrastructure and long-term follow-up. International cleft mission trips have traditionally been successful in providing reconstructive plastic surgery to communities with limited resources. More recently, there has been a global effort in the cleft care community to facilitate development of sustainable local cleft care centers that are capable of providing longitudinal, comprehensive care to the indigenous population. This chapter focuses on the elements that are necessary for running a successful international cleft mission and a local cleft care facility, which include the essential personnel, operational protocols, equipment, logistics, patient selection, and follow-up. The challenges and future directions of providing cleft care in LMIC are also discussed.

Keywords: cleft, craniofacial, global health care, international missions, sustainable health care models

1. Introduction

Orofacial clefts represent the most common congenital craniofacial anomaly, with an estimated prevalence of 1.2 per 1000 people worldwide [1, 2]. Although the treatment of orofacial clefts and other craniofacial anomalies has improved dramatically in developed countries, this is not true for most low- and middle-income countries (LMIC), where the capacity of cleft treatment facilities is lacking and the overall care remains insufficient [3, 4]. More than 160,000 new patients with orofacial clefts are born globally each year [5], placing a significant economic and psychosocial burden on the individual and the families involved. The burden of care for children with orofacial clefts in LMIC is disproportionally immense due to the severely limited access to basic care. People in these resource-limited regions regularly live with untreated clefts their entire lives, battling with prejudice and social ostracism [6]. A large number of humanitarian cleft care missions have provided corrective treatments to patients in LMIC who would not otherwise have had access to such care. However, it remains difficult to provide global care to these patients due to a number of obstacles, including security issues, logistical obstruction, lack of reliable social service facilities, unsustainable or short-lived local cleft care centers, less qualified local personnel, and long-term follow-up [7].

Until recently, there had not been a set of commonly accepted standards for cleft care in less developed countries. Aiming to fill this gap, in 2006, the Volunteers in Plastic Surgery Committee of the American Society of Plastic Surgeons/Plastic Surgery Educational Foundation undertook the project of creating universal guidelines to improve quality and safety for providing reconstructive plastic surgeries in developing countries. Experienced international cleft surgeons along with representatives from Society for Pediatric Anesthesia created and published a set of guidelines, and the final document has been reviewed and approved by the boards of both organizations [8]. During the same year, Operation Smile, the largest American international cleft organization, independently convened its own conference of experts from each specialty around the world to ensure that every child receives the same first world standard of care in an international mission. The product of the conference was "Operation Smile's Global Standards of Care," which was adopted by over 60 member countries within Operation Smile network [9]. Both documents included comprehensive outlines for each aspect of cleft treatment, including site preparation, team make up, equipment, logistics and traveling, and safety standards so that every cleft child and their family can expect the same level of quality care no matter where they live [8, 9]. They have also provided foundation to the new paradigm of international cleft care, which is the creation of free-standing, sustainable cleft centers around the world, staffed, and operated year-round by both local and international personnel [10–13].

This chapter will briefly focus on the strategies that can help optimize global standards for cleft care, which should be followed when planning a cleft mission or building a self-sufficient cleft care facility to provide optimal and longitudinal care to patients with craniofacial anomalies.

2. Multidisciplinary team building

A multidisciplinary team of qualified healthcare professionals is the foundation to achieve proper cleft care anywhere in the world, as the management of orofacial cleft requires expertise from providers in various fields of medicine and dentistry.

Given the complexity and life-threatening risks inherent in performing surgical procedures, it is crucial that all team members be highly skilled and well trained in the patient care of cleft anomalies. The educational and experience requirements of each specialist on the cleft team are determined by individual specialty board, various professional associations, state licensing board, etc. These requirements change over time. The professional members should be encouraged to stay updated on all the current teachings in their respective fields by actively participating in continuing educational activities and attending professional meetings. This not only ensures that they possess appropriate and current credentials but also have the requisite experience in evaluation and treatment of patients with craniofacial anomalies [1, 7, 10].

For this purpose, large and fully articulated cleft care teams must be designed to deliver an entire range of care to the patients. This is essential in building long-term, sustainable, and self-sufficient cleft care centers. Such a team should include the following members [6, 7, 14–16]:

1. Pediatrician
2. Cleft/craniofacial surgeon
3. Cleft/craniofacial orthodontist
4. Anesthesiologist
5. Nursing staff
6. Speech pathologist
7. Psychologist
8. Medical record specialist/research coordinator
9. Other surgical specialties

If a cleft care center recruits international professionals once or twice a year during special cleft surgery camps and cleft missions, the presence of a skilled translator also becomes important because language barrier can hinder full team performance and potential. Therefore, qualified interpreters should be provided to ensure proper verbal and written communication among the team members, patients, and families. The team needs to work in a coordinated manner to provide appropriate care to any patient that comes with a cleft anomaly [10, 17].

Some cleft care centers are not able to provide all types of examinations and services required by the patients. The team in such facilities should have a mechanism for referral to the required professionals, who will be able to provide the necessary service to the patient [11].

Lastly, it is important that all members of the team are monitored regularly and their performance reviews are maintained, so that the quality of care provided to the patients is not compromised.

3. Protocols

Generally, competent surgeons, anesthesiologists, craniofacial orthodontists, and nursing staff each have their own particular way of doing things. This is especially true for professionals who work in different parts of the world. This presents a unique challenge when the team is composed of healthcare providers with diverse backgrounds. In these circumstances, setting priorities and following protocols during different phases of care can help focus the personnel into a more coherent group. Protocols also ensure consistency and decrease the margin of error in most circumstances. For instance, operative protocols could recommend certain procedures to be used by all surgeons for patients with cleft lip and palate (e.g., assuming acceptable blood reports, primary lip repair at age 10 weeks, followed by Furlow double opposing Z-plasty at the age of 10 months). Nasoalveolar molding, craniofacial orthodontic, and dentofacial orthopedic protocols could be standardized in terms of biomechanics and timing of treatment. The anesthesiologists might suggest protocols on intra- and post-operative pain management. The nursing team might recommend certain staff to patient ratio in the post-operative recovery ward. Compliance with these protocols is imperative to the success of a mission trip or permanent craniofacial care facility, and should be well articulated to each team member from the start. However, it is important to keep in mind that changes in the protocol are permissible under circumstances where it does not apply properly.

4. Equipment

In general, the equipment and supplies needed in a developing world hospital are not different from the ones needed in a modern hospital. Acquisition, preparation, shipping (in case of cleft mission), deployment, and maintenance of equipment are a big challenge for both permanent craniofacial care centers and organizations that aim to provide cleft missions. At minimum, complete surgical trays, sutures and dressings, reliable anesthesia equipment, resuscitation packs, perioperative monitors, and sterile materials are necessary for the cleft repair operations regardless of the practice setting. Care should be taken when using medications and instruments purchased in the host countries, especially if the instructions are not in English or if they are unfamiliar pharmaceutical formulations. A partial list of recommended supplies and equipment for orofacial cleft care centers are listed in **Table 1**.

Screening and assessment	• Vital sign monitors • Camera • Lights, tongue blades, and other examination material • Medical records • Lab facility for blood tests
Anesthesia	• Anesthesia machine • Resuscitation boxes with updated, unexpired drugs and dosage schedules • Airway equipment including masks, endotracheal tubes, airways, laryngoscopes, positive pressure ventilation systems, suction devices, non-invasive monitors, difficult airway management items, anesthetic agent

	• Blood supply • Defibrillator and other appropriate emergency equipment • Intravenous fluids and fluid administration sets • Equipment and soaking solutions for the sterilization of non-disposable anesthesia equipment
Post-anesthesia care	• Full resuscitation medications of appropriate doses • Arrangements for glucose level measurement • Oxygen and suction equipment at each bedside • Vital sign monitors with pulse oximetry • Suction equipment • Documentation system
Nasoalveolar molding	• Slow speed dental hand piece • Hard acrylic • Soft acrylic • Water bath • Boley gauge • Orthodontic spatula • Utility wax • Three-prong plier • Light wire plier • College plier • Scalpel • Orthodontic wire • Dental impression material and cast
Surgery	• Surgical instrument trays • Appropriate suture material • Sterilization material • Illumination • Suction machine • Electrocautery capability
Post-operative intensive care	• An appropriate ICU facility and a plan for critical patient transfer when the ICU is not within the hospital facility • Electronic monitors • Respiratory ventilators

Post-operative ward	• 24 hour nursing staff • Appropriate dressing and cleaning materials • Medications for pain management, antisepsis, nausea, and other nursing needs • Vital sign monitoring equipment • Oxygen availability

Table 1. List of minimum supplies and equipment required for proper cleft care [8, 9].

5. Logistics and transportation

Transportation of the team and equipment is an important part of cleft care during international mission trips, and should not be overlooked. Travel to and from sites can be a costly endeavor, and the logistics must be planned out well before the trip for any hope of coordinated arrival and departure of equipment and personnel. A week-long trip may require months of meticulous planning, including arrangements of passports and visas, housing, meals, social events, and security. If the mission is planned by an international healthcare organization, it is beneficial to have local partnerships or contacts to help navigate the custom regulations when bringing equipment into the host country. The equipment should also be acquired and tested prior to shipping time. Drugs and expendables should be checked for expiration dates and evidence of mishandling or breach in packaging. To further ensure successful transportation, all items should be inventoried and documented.

6. Patient screening and assessment

One of the most crucial elements in cleft care is to determine surgical priority through proper patient screening and assessment. Children in LMIC are often undernourished, and many have concomitant medical illnesses and infectious diseases, all of which can lead to a lowered healing reserve compared to children normally encountered in developing countries. Therefore, when a cleft patient first contacts a healthcare facility for treatment, he/she needs to be properly assessed by a multidisciplinary team. Blood tests should be ordered to evaluate any metabolic abnormalities and the presence of anemia. Low hemoglobin level may be a marker for poor nutrition, and thus associated with high surgical risk. Traditionally, hemoglobin value of 10 g/dl is considered the lower limit of acceptable surgical candidate; however, the data to support this are lacking [8]. During the first phase of screening, risk factors such as poor nutrition, low hemoglobin, significant airway anomalies, and young age should be considered to disqualify a child as a potential candidate for surgery. A number of studies have identified age as a significant risk factor for surgery in children using death or cardiac arrest as primary end points. These studies suggest that neonates (0–30 days) are at a risk as high as 40 times compared to older children or adults, whereas infants (1–12 months) have a 4- to 5-fold increased risk compared to older children [18–20].

For patients that have passed the initial screening phase, a final assessment and evaluation occurs before the operation, which consists of two parts. A team of surgeons first determine surgical priority of the procedure and its estimated duration. If there are any surgical contraindications to the operation, they are identified at this point and the patient will not be scheduled for surgery. Second, the pediatric anesthesiologist team determines the American Society of Anesthesiologists (ASA) patient classification and provides a second independent opinion on the suitability of patient for the surgery. Most importantly, the cardiac and respiratory status of the patient is carefully evaluated at this time [12]. A patient who has satisfied the criteria for each of these phases is selected for surgery. When indicated, a course of preoperative nasoalveolar molding therapy is advised.

Such a comprehensive and lengthy selection procedure is important to ensure patient safety, as well as to maximize the expected benefits from surgery and proper usage of time and resources. **Figure 1** shows an outline of the steps involved in patient selection.

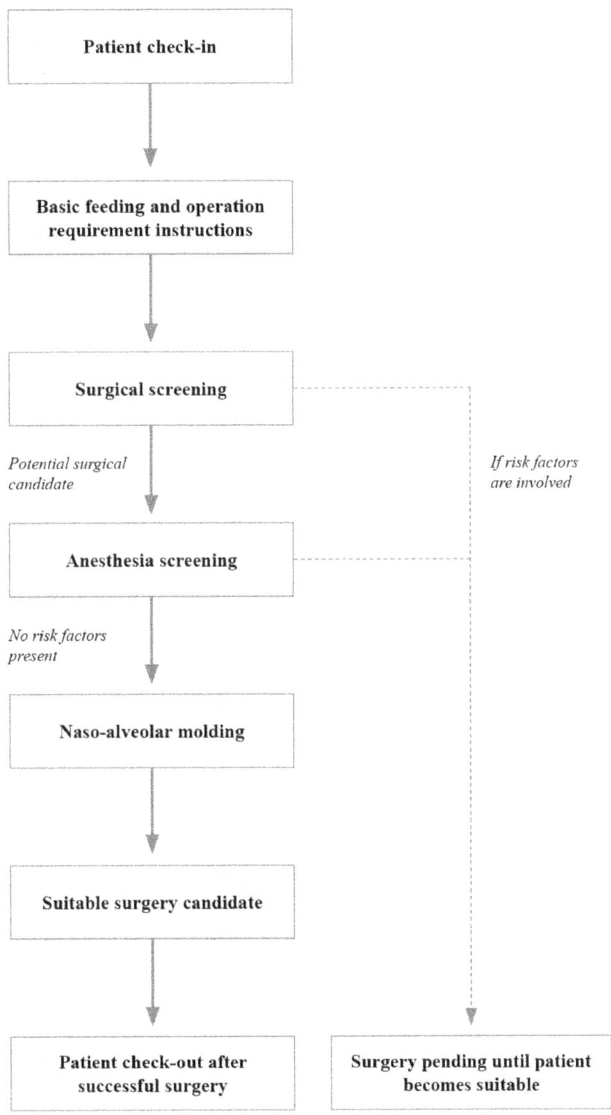

Figure 1. Steps involved in patient selection.

7. Documentation

As in all other endeavors, if it is not written it has not been done. Organizations offering optimal care ought to create detailed documentation and provide an accurate and secure record for the basis of ongoing care and outcome assessments. Documenting details of a patient at every stage makes developing the treatment plan easier for cleft patients. As shown in **Figure 2**, documentation can be divided into five vital areas.

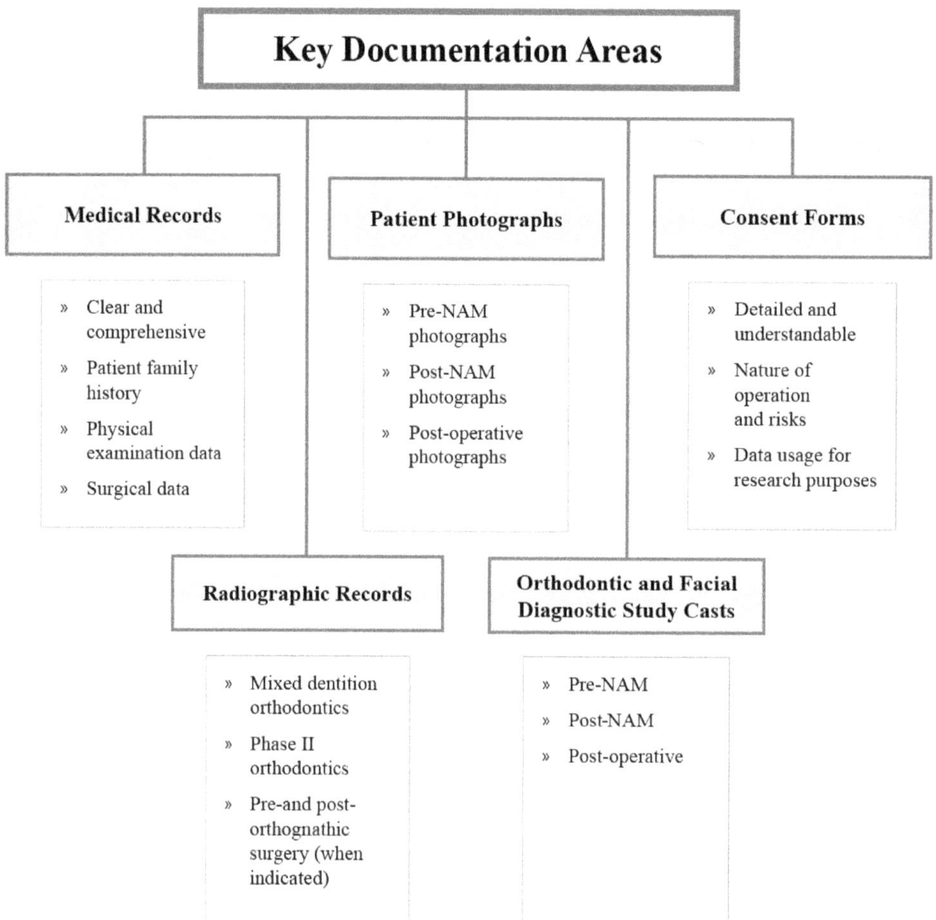

Figure 2. Key documentation areas.

• Medical records

These forms, whether written or electronic, should be identical throughout the organization. They should be comprehensive, explicit, and clear. The history section should include family background, demographic details, and previous history of cleft in the family. A complete record of physical examination and medical diagnosis of data must be entered. Multiple copies should be made for each file. This allows one copy to be left with patient's medical chart in the host country, and another copy to be used for tracking and future analysis.

- **Patient photographs**

Pre- and post-operative photographs of patients are also important as they are a key factor in analyzing results. These photographs can be further used for outcome assessment and research purposes.

- **Orthodontic and facial diagnostic study casts**

Pre-, progress, and post-nasoalveolar molding (NAM) facial and orthodontic diagnostic study casts are imperative for the fabrication of NAM appliances, orthodontic appliances, and orthopedic appliances. Additionally, they are required to evaluate treatment progress, outcomes assessment, and for research purposes.

- **Radiographic records**

Pre-, progress, and post-orthodontic and surgical imaging should be taken as indicated in order to aid in the diagnosis and treatment planning of craniofacial orthodontics, dentofacial orthopedics, and orthognathic surgery. Like photographs and diagnostic study cases, they are also useful for research purposes.

- **Consent forms**

Lastly, consent forms are an integral part of the documentation process. All patients and guardians must read and sign a consent form, which should be comprehensive and clear. The form must include the nature of the operation and its risks, use of anesthesia, potential blood transfusion, HIV, and hepatitis testing in the case of needle stick and permission for taking photographs. The families should also be informed, and oral or written consent should be taken if the data are to be used for research purposes. When language difference exists, professionals should utilize interpreters to assure informed consents are properly documented prior to delivery of care and surgery.

All members of the multidisciplinary cleft care team are responsible for documentation. The cleft care facility should work systematically to ensure that documentation tools are readily available to all health care providers, while at the same time respecting and maintaining patient confidentiality.

8. Sustainable cleft care facility

International organizations have long provided cleft care through surgical missions to selected areas in LMIC with shortage of resources and experienced personnel. The drawback of this practice model is that these health missions often provide short-term relief, making treatment available to limited amount of people for a short time period [3]. The mission trips are dependent on proper funding, grants, and resources. This model of intervention is ideal for urgent humanitarian response to disasters or epidemics, where a substantial amount of resources can be mobilized quickly for disease-specific use in LMIC. However, it is less effective for sustaining long-term care to the indigenous population and for conducting educational/preventive endeavors. This type of practice has been criticized for operating outside of the existing health care systems and structures, doing little to strengthen the primary care systems in LMIC, and compromising countries' autonomy and participation in health care initiatives [6]. Finally, most of the mission trips are not designed to deal with the complex socioeconomic disease determinants many patients face, and lack the capacity to maintain prolonged post-operative follow-up and therapy.

It has become increasingly clear that one of the most important strategies that can help optimize and increase cleft care globally is to establish effectively run, high-volume, indigenous centers of excellence, capable of serving large and wide spread populations in the LMIC [6]. The ideal long-term goal for international groups should be to prepare local surgical teams to provide the same quality care for their population without outside medical assistance [8]. Once established and maintained, such local cleft care facilities not only provide services throughout the year to its region but can also contribute to the funding needs of much poorer sites in the future.

In order to offer effective surgical and orthodontic/orthopedic interventions, these facilities must develop and maintain an environment that meets world class minimums on proper workforce, access to supplies, instrumentation, infection control, and supporting infrastructure. See **Table 2** for a list of basic requirements.

Physical space	An adequate space should be present for patient screening, assessment, operating rooms, preoperative, and post-operative wards
Laboratory	A basic clinical laboratory to perform regular blood and electrolyte tests
Equipment	The minimum number of instruments required for patient examination, anesthesia, surgery, orthodontics, nasoalveolar molding, and ward care
Staff	Administrative, management, nursing, and permanent or visiting expert surgery staff to run the facility
Donors	Various funding agencies and/or private donors to run and maintain the cleft center as well as support patients that cannot afford the treatment otherwise
Quality control	A system that ensures that quality of cleft care provided is according to international standards, assures patient/family satisfaction, conducts staff performance reports, and develop guidelines to address the problems faced in the facility

Table 2. Basic requirements for a sustainable cleft care infrastructure/facility.

9. Patient follow-up

Whether it is a cleft mission or a permanent cleft care facility, arrangements for adequate follow-up are important to maximize treatment effectiveness, access the available options for future treatment, and monitor outcomes. As shown in **Figure 3**, a basic post-operative follow-up has two intervals.

However, such a simplified follow-up regimen is rarely adequate for most cleft patients. From birth throughout childhood and adolescence, a cleft patient requires coordinated care among surgeons, orthodontists, and other health care providers. Even after surgery, most cleft patients require regular ear examinations during infancy. Approximately 75% of cleft patients require two to three additional orthodontic/dentofacial orthopedic interventions and continued speech therapy throughout childhood and adolescence to achieve satisfactory growth, speech, and language competence. Coordination of various dental procedures is crucial from the period of mixed dentition through adolescence. Furthermore, overall health and the psychosocial impact of having a cleft also need to be monitored routinely [1, 12, 21].

To achieve such a prolonged follow-up plan, it is the responsibility of the cleft team to maintain communication with the patients and families, extensively educate them on the importance of follow-up and maintain appropriate documentation and record keeping.

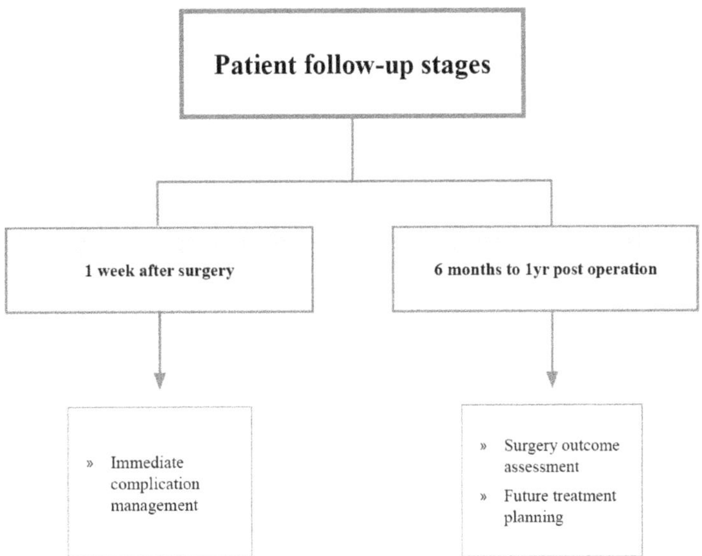

Figure 3. Patient follow-up stages.

10. Education and research

Finally, education and awareness regarding orofacial clefts are key factors in achieving better long-term global access to cleft care. Education in cleft care is conducted at two levels:

(a) Education of parents and caregivers

Educating the care givers of cleft patient is crucial in achieving proper care and satisfactory future outcomes. On the initial visit, caretakers of the children should be given instructions on feeding assistance, airway maintenance, and other basic cleft care information to help the patient prepare for surgical intervention. After the operation, families should be given strict instructions regarding the remainder of their post-operative care at home prior to discharge. Families must be educated on the need for follow-up after operations and the importance of regular visits to the craniofacial orthodontist, pediatrician, speech therapist and feeding specialist for the long-term.

(b) Training and education of local professionals

It has long been the aim of global health care organizations to provide educational and training opportunities to health care professionals of LMIC, who can thereafter deliver high quality, team-based care in their local regions. A number of approaches have been outlined and proven to be effective in accomplishing this goal:

- **On-site education**

Delivering knowledge to local professionals on-site during cleft missions is effective in transmitting small, focused, and discrete areas of knowledge and experience. Although enormously enriching, such short-term programs provide a rather limited introduction to cleft care and surgery to local professionals present at the time [6].

- **Long-term education and training**

Long-term partnerships between local hospitals and academic institutions in wealthy countries help to provide proper, professional education, and experience. This can either be achieved by allowing fully credentialed visiting surgeons to stay with a host hospital and teach for an extended period of time or by bringing a limited number of host country participants to educational programs in regions with well-established craniofacial centers. More robust academic partnerships can also promote local academic leaders and would enhance training for health care providers in other fields, including speech pathology and surgical technicians. Such training programs aim to provide much needed local cleft care experts, who can contribute to the development of sustainable, self-sufficient cleft care centers.

(c) Clinical research

Collection of prospective, standardized data can yield high quality information that can be used to improve overall knowledge, cleft care processes, and outcomes. In addition to contributing to the field, research results can be presented to local health care professionals and the general population. Research can broadly be categorized as: epidemiological, genetic, prevention/risk factors, clinical presentation, outcomes assessment, and quality of life.

11. Conclusion

Orofacial clefts are a correctable condition with proper treatment resulting in a dramatic improvement of function and quality of life. Providing universal cleft care in LMIC still faces numerous challenges today due to a lack of basic health care infrastructures [22]. Traditionally, international health missions have been very successful in providing reconstructive plastic surgery to people in resource-limited regions. Largely due to the success of cleft missions, the cleft care community is now in position to increase surgical capacity and promote development of sustainable local cleft care centers that are capable of providing comprehensive, longitudinal care to the indigenous population [6]. With the shift in global cleft care delivery, many organizations have started to incorporate efforts to expand local facility, increase human capital, and foster interdisciplinary quality health care by local providers [22]. As we move toward the future of accessible, sustainable cleft care in LMIC, it will continue to rely on concerted efforts from both international aid groups and local governments to invest in the local health care system.

Author details

Mairaj Ahmed[1]*, Yunfeng Xue[2] and Ayisha Ayub[3]

*Address all correspondence to: mairaj.ahmed@mountsinai.org

1 Cleft/Craniofacial Center, Icahn School of Medicine at Mount Sinai, New York City, NY, USA

2 University of Texas McGovern Medical School, Houston, TX, USA

3 Cleft Hospital, Gujrat, Pakistan

References

[1] Parameters for the evaluation and treatment of patients with cleft lip/palate or other craniofacial anomalies. American Cleft Palate-Craniofacial Association. Cleft Palate-Craniofacial Journal 1993; 30 (Suppl 1): S1–S16.

[2] Mossey PA, Modell B. Epidemiology of oral clefts 2012: an international perspective. Front Oral Biol. 2012;16: 1–18.

[3] Magee WP. Evolution of a sustainable surgical delivery model. J Craniofac Surg. 2010;21(5): 1321–1326.

[4] Donkor P,Bankas DO, Agbenorku P, Plange-Rhule PG,Ansah SK. Cleft lip and palate surgery in Kumasi, Ghana: 2001–2005. J Craniofac Surg. 2007;18(6): 1376–1379.

[5] Lee ST. International surgical missions in cleft lip and palate. In Wyszynski DF, editor. Cleft Lip and Palate from Origin to Treatment. New York: Oxford University Press; 2002. 424p.

[6] Patel PB, Hoyler M, Maine R, Hughes CD, Hagander L, Meara JG. An opportunity for diagonal development in global surgery: cleft lip and palate care in resource-limited settings. Plast Surg Int. 2012;2012: 892437.

[7] Sherman R, Magee WP. Global aspects of cleft care. In Loose J, Kirschner RE, editors. Comprehensive cleft care.2nd edition. CRC Press, Boca Raton, Florida, USA; 2015.

[8] Schneider WJ, Politis GD, Gosain AK, et al. Volunteers in plastic surgery guidelines for providing surgical care for children in the less developed world. Plast Reconstr Surg. 2011;127(6): 2477–2486.

[9] Global standards of care [Internet]. 2015. Available from:https://www.operationsmile.org/sites/default/files/Operation%20Smile%20Global%20Standards%20of%20Care.pdf [Accessed: 2016-11-1]

[10] Wexler A. So you want to run a mission. Now what? Planning and safety for international cleft missions [Internet]. Available from: http://www.thepsf.org/Documents/So%20you%20want%20to%20run%20a%20mission.pdf [Accessed: 2016-10-30]

[11] Roldán JC, Pape HD, Koch H, Koller M. Ten-Year cleft surgery in Nepal: achievements and lessons learned for better cleft care abroad. Plast Reconstr Surg Glob Open. 2016;4: e711.

[12] Eberlin KR, Zaleski KL, Snyder HD, Hamdan US, Children MM. Quality assurance guidelines for surgical outreach programs: a 20-year experience. Cleft Palate Craniofac J. 2008;45: 246–55.

[13] Politis GD, Schneider WJ, Van Beek AL, et al. Guidelines for pediatric perioperative care during short-term plastic reconstructive surgical projects in less developed nations. Anesth Analg. 2011;112: 183–90.

[14] Semer NB, Sullivan SR, Meara JG. Plastic surgery and global health: how plastic surgery impacts the global burden of surgical disease. J Plast Reconstr Aesthet Surg. 2010;63: 1244–48.

[15] Bearn D, Mildinhall S, Murphy T, et al. Cleft lip and palate care in the United Kingdom—the Clinical Standards Advisory Group (CSAG) Study. Part 4: outcome comparisons, training, and conclusions. Cleft Palate Craniofac J. 2001;38: 38–43.

[16] Maine RG, Hoffman WY, Palacios-Martinez JH, Corlew DS, Gregory GA. Comparison of fistula rates after palatoplasty for international and local surgeons on surgical missions in Ecuador with rates at a craniofacial center in the United States. Plast Reconstr Surg. 2012;129: 319e–26e.

[17] Patel KG, Eberlin KR, Vyas RM, Hamdan US. Use of safety measures, including the modified world health organization surgical safety checklist, during international outreach cleft missions. Cleft Palate Craniofac J. 2014;51: 597–604.

[18] Tiret L, Desmonts JM, Hatton F, Vourc'h G. Complications associated with anaesthesia—a prospective survey in France. Can Anaesth Soc J. 1986;33: 336–44.

[19] Tiret L, Nivoche Y, Hatton F, Desmonts JM, Vourc'h G. Complications related to anaesthesia in infants and children. A prospective survey of 40240 anaesthetics. Br J Anaesth. 1988;61: 263–9.

[20] Cohen MM, Cameron CB, Duncan PG. Pediatric anesthesia morbidity and mortality in the perioperative period. Anesth Analg. 1990;70: 160–7.

[21] Standards for cleft palate and craniofacial teams [Internet]. 2016. Available from: http://www.acpa-cpf.org/team_care/standards/[Accessed: 2016-11-1]

[22] Fayyaz GQ, Gill NA, Ishaq I, et al. A model humanitarian cleft mission: 312 cleft surgeries in 7 days. Plast Reconstr Surg Glob Open. 2015;3: e313.

7

Surgical Techniques for Treatment of Unilateral Cleft Lip

Mustafa Chopan, Lohrasb Sayadi and
Donald R. Laub

Abstract

A surgeon intending habilitation of a child with cleft lip should be familiar with the normal anatomy of the lip and nose, the distortions introduced by the cleft deformity, and the many techniques available to employ those best suited to correction of that child's deformity.

Keywords: surgical techniques, cleft lip, cleft surgery

1. Introduction

"Whatever is worth doing at all is worth doing well."

—Philip Stanhope, 4th Earl of Chesterfield

The treatment of children with cleft lip deformity has long challenged surgeons. Numerous surgical techniques have been developed to restore function, symmetry, and aesthetics. Early surgical techniques in treatment of cleft lip deformity involved straight-line repairs were limited in restoring symmetry to the lip of a child with unilateral cleft lip. LeMesurier and Tennyson developed the use of flaps that allowed reconstruction of the cupid's bow of the lip. Millard's technique of "rotation-advancement" brought about the modern era of cleft lip reconstruction. Later refinements by Salyer, Noordhoff, Cutting, and others have allowed the surgeon to more effectively restore function, symmetry, and aesthetics

2. Normal anatomy

"All cleft surgery is merely applied embryology."

—Victor Veau [1]

The pathologic origins of a cleft lip are traceable to distinct embryological events. The fusion failure during gestational weeks 4–7 of facial primordia: the central frontonasal prominence and two lateral maxillary prominences result in a typical cleft lip of a newborn. Advances in developmental science have promoted our knowledge and understanding of this phenomenon, helping to guide diagnosis and surgical reconstruction; however, craniofacial embryology is beyond the scope of this chapter.

It is important to note that cleft lip and palate is considered a distinct entity from isolated cleft palate, the difference chiefly characterized by the location of the cleft palate anterior or posterior to incisive foramen, respectively. Soft-tissue and bony deficiencies are variable with accompanying nasal distortion (**Figure 1**). Surgical management hinges upon the accurate identification of involved structures and methodical attention to detail in surgical techniques in reconstruction.

A B

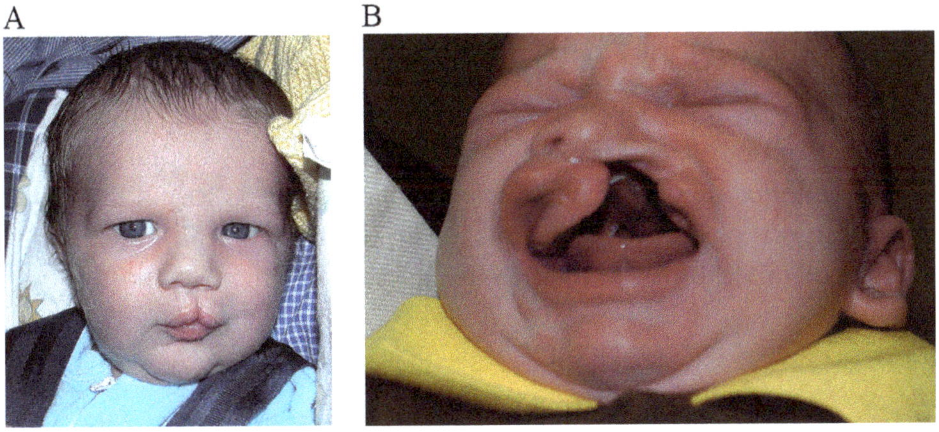

Figure 1. (A) A child with a microform or "forme fruste" cleft lip, demonstrating vermilion notching, scar-like depression. (B) A child with a complete unilateral cleft lip, demonstrating tissue hypoplasia and asymmetry.

2.1. Normal anatomy of the lip

The layers of the lip include the skin, a thin layer of subcutaneous tissue, orbicularis oris and other facial muscles, and mucosa. The vermillion is a unique tissue consisting of modified mucosa, and the white roll is a ridge at the junction of the vermillion and the lip skin. The lips are divided into four aesthetic subunits: the philtrum, two lateral wings (from the philtral columns to the nasolabial folds), and the entire lower lip.

Muscles of the upper lip include orbicularis oris, levator labii superioris alaeque nasi, zygomaticus major and minor, levator labii superioris, and nasalis. The orbicularis oris consists of superficial and deep layers. The deep fibers run circumferentially between modioli and function as the primary sphincter in feeding. The superficial fibers originate from the ipsilateral modiolus and run obliquely toward midline, interdigitating with the other muscles of facial expression and inserting into the dermis. The superficial fibers are further distinguished into either superior fibers (pars peripheralis) or inferior fibers (pars marginalis) of the upper lip. The pars marginalis courses along the vermillion border connect with the contralateral pars marginalis fibers at midline and inserts into the region of the vermilion tubercle. The pars peripheralis has a flat-fan shape diffusing out from each modiolus, and inserting into the skin of the contralateral philtral ridge [2]. Two other distinct fibers of the pars peripheralis have also been identified using micro-computed tomography [3]. One bundle terminates at the tissue below the ipsilateral anterior nasal spine, in continuation with depressor septi. The other bundle crosses midline and continues with the alar portion of nasalis muscle. The decussation of fibers creates the philtral columns, and lack of insertion at the midline creates the philtral depression.

Superficial layers of the levator labii superioris alaeque nasi, zygomaticus minor, and levator labii superioris cross the nasolabial groove and migrate toward the superficial orbicularis. The levator labii superioris alaeque nasi originates from the upper face, enters the upper lip superior and lateral to the ipsilateral philtral column, and descends on the medial side of the column. A bundle of fibers terminate in the dermis of the lateral aspect of the ipsilateral philtral column. Another bundle of short and long fibers terminates in the skin of the vermillion border; however, the long fibers interlock with the pars marginalis before their insertion. Thus the lip peak of the vermillion border, which creates cupid's bow, is due to a balance of muscular tension between the pars marginalis and levator labii superioris alaeque nasi.

Superficial reticular fibers of the levator labii superioris alaeque nasi, zygomaticus major and minor, levator labii superioris, and orbicularis oris insert into the medial philtrum ridge. The intersection of these fibers and the contralateral orbicularis oris forms the philtral column. The bulging appearance of the region lateral to the philtral column, however, results from a greater number of muscle insertions into the lateral skin than to the philtral dimple [4] (**Figure 2A**).

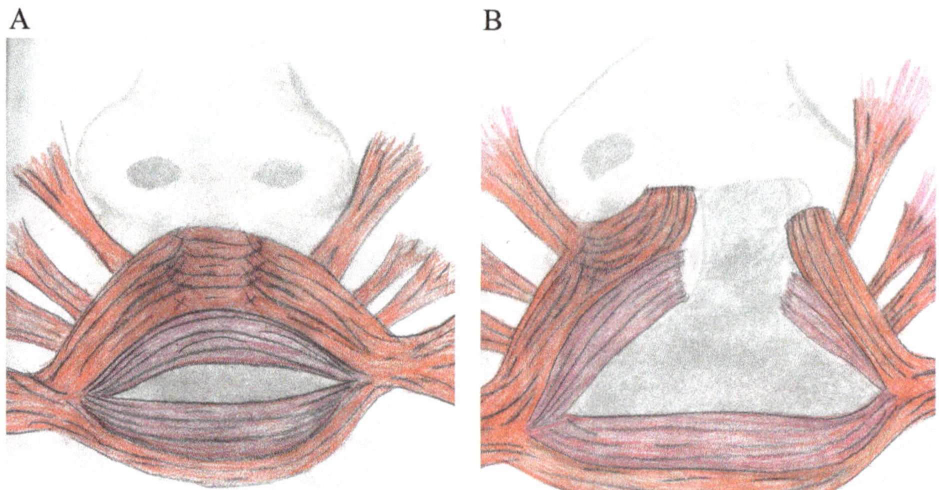

Figure 2. (A) A schematic representation of the orbicularis oris, demonstrating symmetry and continuity. (B) A schematic representation of the orbicularis oris affected by a cleft, demonstrating asymmetry and discontinuity.

2.2. Normal anatomy of the nose

The nose can be divided into anatomical thirds. The proximal third consists of the paired nasal bones and bony septum (vomer, perpendicular plate of ethmoid, nasal crest of maxilla and palatine bone). Upper lateral cartilages and cartilaginous septum comprise the middle third. Lower lateral cartilages, the tip, and caudal cartilaginous septum form the lower third of the nose. The lower lateral cartilages consist of the medial, middle, and lateral crura

(**Figure 3A**). The scroll area refers to the overlapping of lateral crura with the caudal edge of upper lateral cartilages. The nasalis muscle originates at the incisive fossa and inserts into four different regions. The transverse part courses past the alar base around the lateral side of the nose, and ascends medially to join procerus and the contralateral transverse fibers at midline. Fibers that course around the alar rim and above the lower lateral cartilages are the alar portion of nasalis. The columella and basal parts insert in the membranous septum, medial crura, and nostril sill skin. The columellar part of nasalis is synonymous with depressor septi.

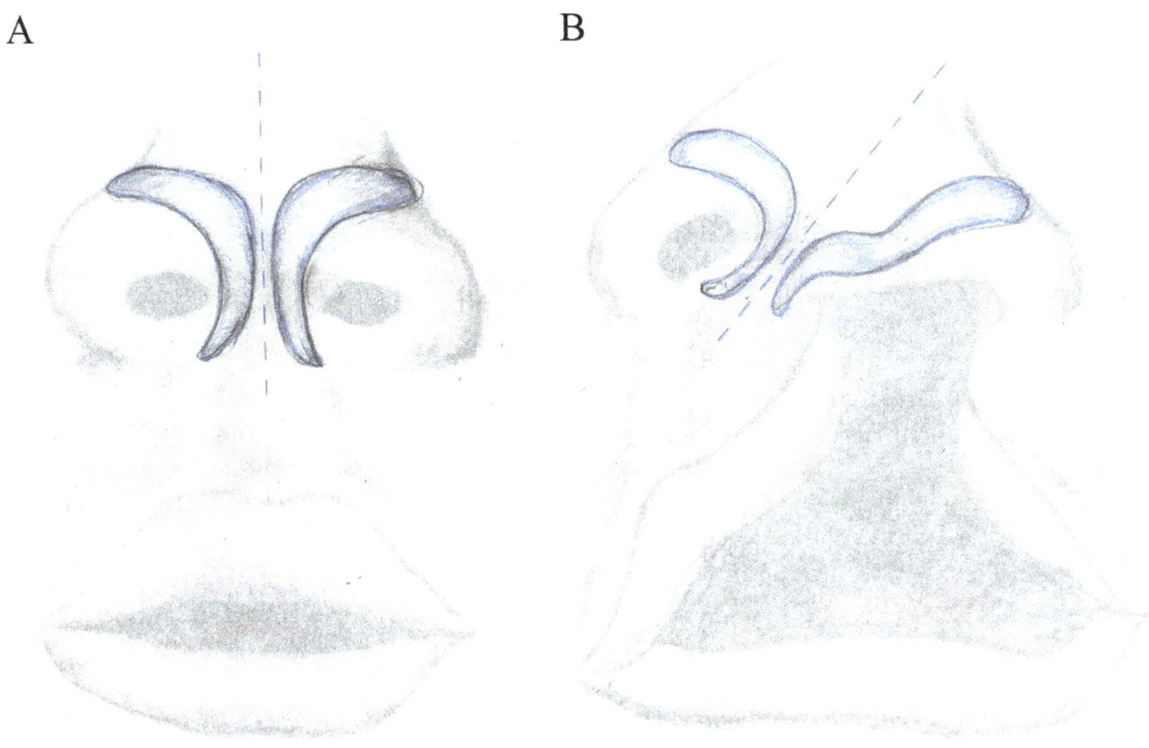

Figure 3. (A) A schematic representation of the lower lateral cartilages demonstrating symmetry. (B) A schematic representation of the lower lateral cartilages demonstrating asymmetry: a short medial crus, an obtuse genu, and a lateral crus that is longer and drawn into an S-shaped fold on the cleft side.

The facial artery is the main blood supply to the upper and lower lips. The facial artery travels through the cheek beneath zygomaticus major and superficial to buccinator muscles, giving rise to the inferior and superior labial arteries. Once the superior labial artery emerges from the zygomaticus major, it may dive into the substance of the orbicularis oris, giving rise to the ipsilateral columellar artery. After giving rise to the superior labial artery, the facial artery terminates as the angular artery. The lateral nasal artery is a branch of the angular artery.

3. Abnormal anatomy of unilateral cleft deformity: muscle imbalance, tissue hypoplasia, and skeletal asymmetry

"If you can articulate a problem, it is 98% solved."

—Edwin Land

The severity of a unilateral cleft lip varies from the microform (**Figure 1A**) to a complete cleft extending into the nasal sill (**Figure 1B**). Varying degrees of nasal deformity and alveolar deficiency may also be present [5, 6]. There is varying degree of absence of central lip, philtral and nasal columella tissue [7].

The unilateral cleft typically results in a disruption of cupid's bow and the absence of one philtral column. The continuity of the orbicularis oris circumferentially is compromised, with abnormal insertions. In the lateral lip element, the upper part of cutaneous orbicularis (Pars Superficialis) inserts in the lateral aspect of the alar base and the nasolabial fold, while the lower part inserts into the nostril base periosteum of the pyriform rim. In the medial lip element, the cutaneous orbicularis (pars superficialis) inserts into the anterior nasal spine and columella. The deep orbicularis (pars marginalis) is simply interrupted by the cleft deficiency and results in a diminished vermillion-cutaneous ridge at the cleft margin (**Figure 2B**).

Anatomical characteristics of unilateral cleft lip include nasal deformities of the tip, columella, nostril, alar base, septum, and skeleton. The lower lateral cartilages on the cleft side have a short medial crus, an obtuse genu, and a lateral crus that is longer and drawn into an S-shaped fold (**Figure 3B**). The caudal septum is deviated toward the noncleft side. The nasal tip it typically directed toward the noncleft side [8]. In addition, the columella is shorter on the cleft side with deviation toward the noncleft side due to the unopposed action of the orbicularis oris. The alar base is more horizontal on the cleft side with deviation of the nasal septum toward the noncleft side. The alar base on the cleft side is positioned laterally, inferiorly, and posteriorly.

Nasal deformities in a unilateral cleft lip-nose arise from this cartilage deformity, muscle imbalance, and skeletal hypoplasia [5]. The various deformities are listed here:

1. Alar base displacement posteriorly and inferiorly, causing a flattening of the dome
2. Lateral crus of the alar cartilage and underlying skin is drawn to an S-shaped fold
3. Short medial crus of the alar cartilage on the cleft side
4. Columellar deviation toward the noncleft side and shortening on the cleft side
5. Nasal tip displacement and asymmetry
6. Caudal septum and anterior nasal spine displacement toward the noncleft side, with deviation to the cleft-side airway causing obstruction
7. Inferior turbinate hypertrophy of the cleft side
8. Hypoplastic maxillary segment and displacement on the cleft side
9. Nasal floor is lowered or absent
10. Nasal pyramid asymmetry

4. Goals of surgical repair

"If you know what you value, then making a decision is easy."

—Walt Disney

The goals of unilateral cleft lip repair are both functional and aesthetic. In order to address these goals, one must understand the anatomical characteristics of unilateral cleft lip. Aesthetically the goals of surgical intervention include formation of lip continuity, establishing symmetry of the cupid's bow and the nose in a manner that places scars in less discernable areas. Recreation of the orbicularis muscle to circumferentially surround the opening of the oral cavity is important for long-lasting cosmetic outcomes and lip and mouth function. Patients with isolated cleft lip rarely have feeding problems, unlike those with cleft palate. However, enrolling the child in a multidisciplinary clinic is advised to address the needs of each patient and family.

5. Preoperative tissue mobilization

"Success depends on preparation, and without preparation, there is failure."

—Confucius

The goal of preoperative tissue mobilization is to lessen the soft tissue and bony cleft and accompanying deformities prior to definitive surgical treatment. Preoperative improvement facilitates surgical repair and results in better outcomes.

5.1. Adhesive tape

Pool and Farnworth advocated the use of adhesive tape for soft tissue mobilization prior to surgical repair of unilateral and bilateral clefts Long strips were applied from cheek to cheek for 6 weeks prior to surgery (**Figure 4**). They found a 53% average reduction in alveolar gaps, and lip segment narrowing from 40% to complete apposition [9].

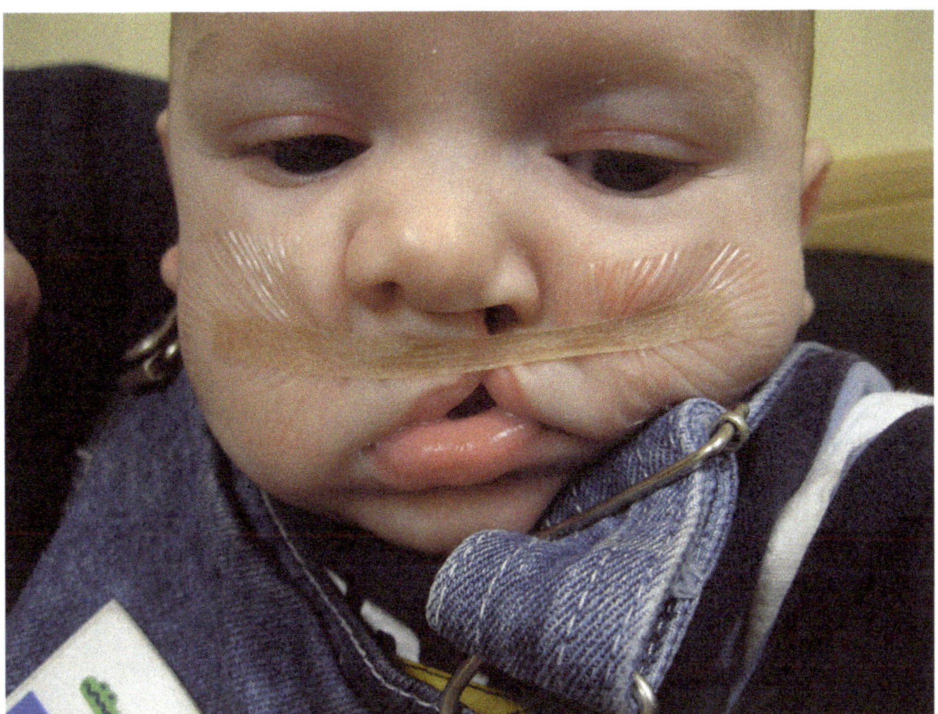

Figure 4. A child with a complete unilateral cleft lip, with adhesive tape therapy in place. This is the same child in **Figure 1B**. Note the mobilization of soft tissue.

5.2. Nasoalveolar molding

Alveolar molding is performed with an intraoral appliance to align the maxillary alveolar segments and narrow the cleft. Latham developed an active orthopedic device consisting of methyl methacrylate bases attached to the palatine bone with metal pins, and connected by a screw [10, 11]. Turning of the screw exerts an anterior force on the cleft-side segment, narrowing the gap.

Grayson and the NYU group employ presurgical molding, using the nasoalveolar molding (NAM), a passive orthodontic appliance [12, 13]. An acrylic orthodontic plate is fitted to cover the entire maxillary arch, with two buttons placed at 45° angle to the occlusal plane. Circular elastics are attached from the buttons and to steristrips on the face bilaterally (**Figure 5**). Every 1–2 weeks the orthodontist adjusts the device small amounts by removing and adding acrylic. Once the alveolar gap measures less than 5 mm, a nasal stent is added to the appliance by wire extending from the plate. The stent is positioned under the soft triangle, and periodically augmented by adding soft acrylic. This tissue-expansion effect molds the alar cartilage and lengthens the columella with the goal of increasing tip projection.

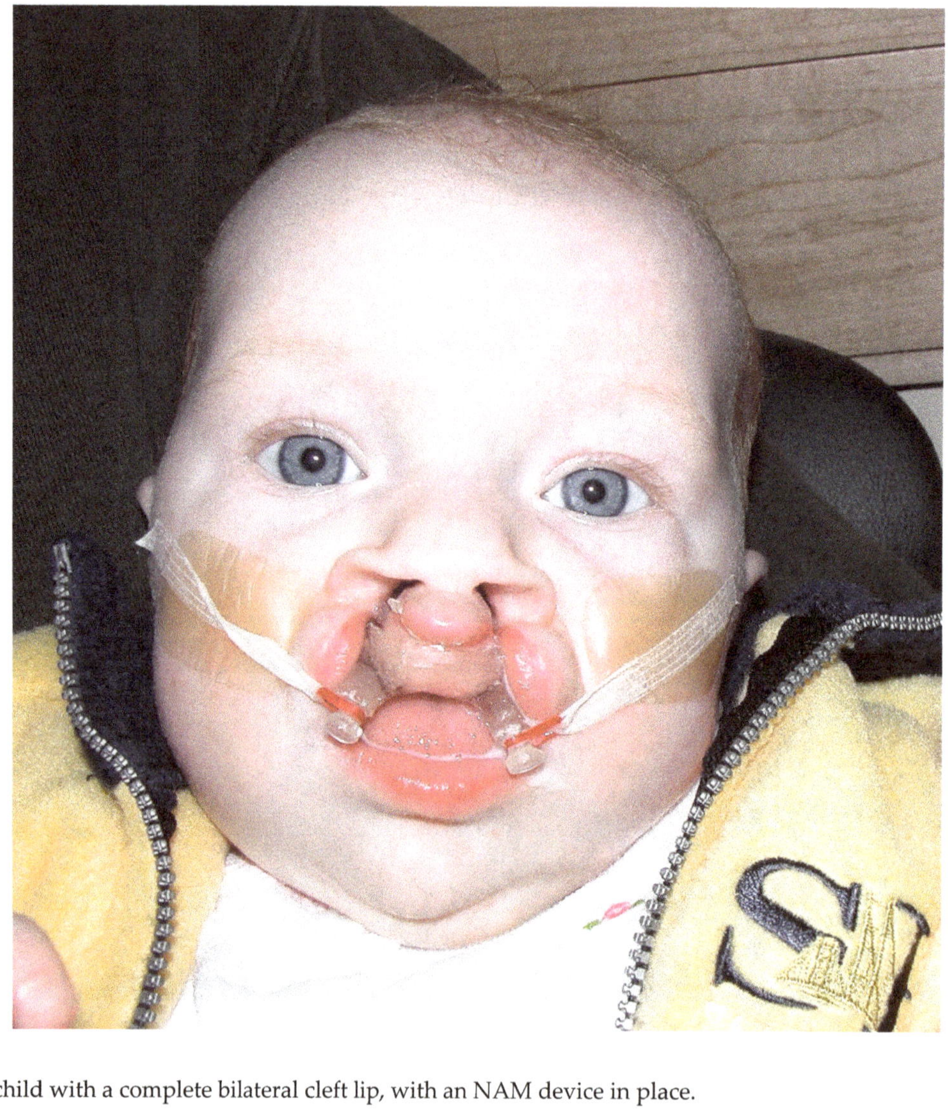

Figure 5. A child with a complete bilateral cleft lip, with an NAM device in place.

5.3. Surgical lip adhesion

Lip adhesion is a first surgical stage in a two-stage reconstruction developed by Randall [14]. A lip after adhesion not only molds the alveolar segments, but also improves nasal contour and vertical lip height of both medial and lateral segments. The disadvantages of a two-stage surgical repair include an additional procedure and scarring, possibly making dissection more difficult during the second, definitive surgery. Randall made incisions on the vermillion of the medial and lateral lip elements. On the lateral lip element, supraperiosteal dissection is performed through a buccal incision. Subcutaneous dissection is performed on the medial segment to the nasal tip, allowing for mobilization of the cleft-side lower lateral cartilage independent from rest of the nose. Mattress sutures are passed through the medial cleft margin incision, through the orbicularis oris and buccal mucosa. The mucosal flaps are then closed in layered fashion.

6. Surgical techniques of unilateral cleft lip repair

"Things done well, and with a care, exempt themselves from fear."

—William Shakespeare

In unilateral cleft repairs, regardless of the name assigned, except for straight-line techniques, have an oblique medial incision to correct the nasal malposition and drop the cupid's bow into a horizontal posture [15]. If the lateral segment is contoured to interpolate a congruent tissue flap, the repair can be conceptualized as a Z-plasty. We have categorized lip repairs in this chapter by the level at which in the tissue is interpolated.

6.1. Straight-line repairs

6.1.1. Early repairs [16, 17]

Ambroise Paré described a straight-line repair for cleft lip in 1575. He excised the skin margins of the cleft with a razor, freeing the lip elements from the upper jaw and joining them together by transfixing the edges of the cleft with a needle and securing the needle with thread in a figure of eight pattern. In 1570 Gaspar Tagliacozzi of Bologna described excoriating the cleft edges and using interrupted sutures to close the cleft.

6.1.2. Rose-Thompson (et al.) principle

Some of the earliest changes in cleft lip repair were based on modifications to the straight line repair to increase the vertical length of the lip. In 1879, William Rose developed a design for cleft lip closure using curved incisions mutually concave from nostril to vermilion at a 60° angle [18]. This method was significant as it lengthened the union of the two cleft margins (**Figure 6**).

Later, James E. Thompson who aspired to reproduce a natural cupid's bow designed his paring procedure in a shape of a diamond excision. He emphasized the need for accurate markings for precise matching of the cleft sides when brought together [19]. In addition, when the vermilion thickness varied, Thompson altered the angle of his incisions to balance the vermilion closure [20]. Victor Veau performed a modified straight-line closure, where on the noncleft side he excised the mucosa just distal to the mucocutaneous junction line to achieve a normal length [1]. He was successful in approximation of the muscular elements but rarely achieved a symmetric cupid's bow. The British surgeon Thomas Kilner described a technique of straight-line closure combining methods used by Rose, Thompson, and Veau. Kilner's technique, known for its simplicity, lengthened the lip, and reapproximated the muscle. Kilner believed that a superior cosmetic result could be achieved by secondary surgery to perfect the initial repair. Nakajima and others utilized curved incisions on the noncleft side and but straight incisions on the cleft side to equalize the length and allow a straight line repair [21].

Straight-line repairs have grouped together as the "Rose-Thompson principle." While these techniques have the advantage of simplicity and speed, they often result in an asymmetric cupid's bow, a prominent scar and retrusion of the maxilla.

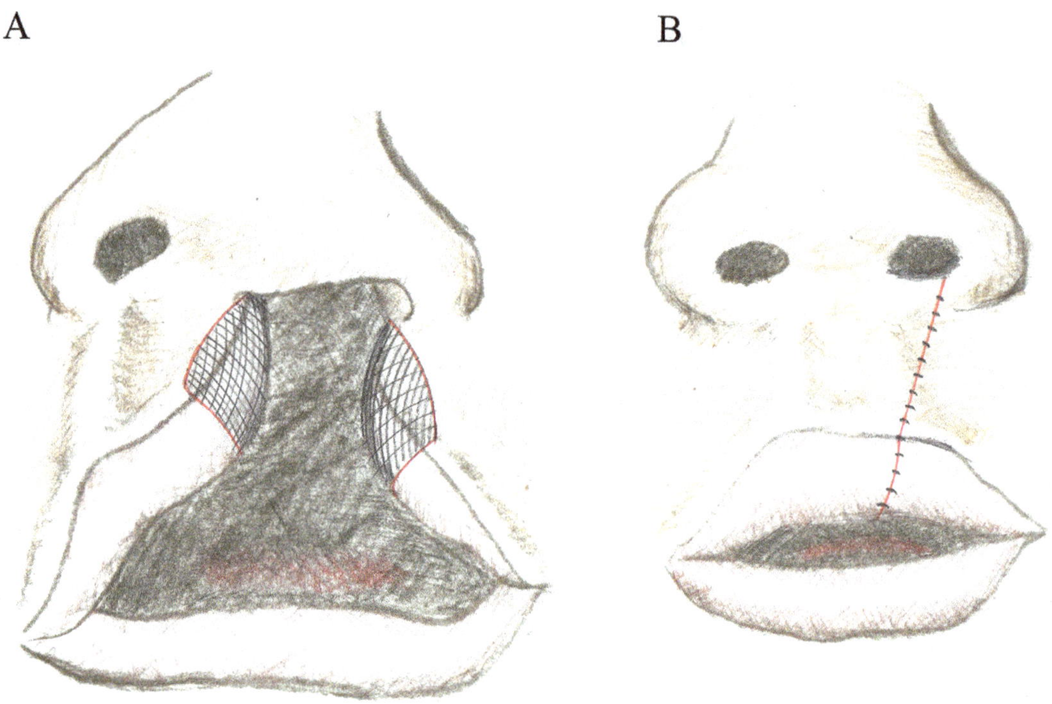

Figure 6. (A) Schematic representation of the incisions for a Rose repair. (B) Schematic representation of the closure of a Rose repair.

6.2. Upper lip flaps

6.2.1. Millard technique

Millard conceptualized his rotation-advancement technique while serving in Korea and first published in 1957 [22]. His technique is the most widely used by cleft surgeons, but has been modified since its inception. Its principles serve as the foundation of many unilateral repairs today.

Millard preserved anatomical landmarks: the cupid's bow and the philtral column. Downward rotation of the medial lip element restores vertical lip height and advancement of the lateral lip element repositions the alar base.

Millard marked the nadir and peaks of cupid's bow on both the lateral and medial lip with methylene blue. The distance from the alar base and the point selected for cupid's peak on the lateral segment should equal that of the noncleft side. His medial segment incision extends from the lateral cupid's peak of the medial element through the columellar-labial junction to the philtral column of the noncleft side. The lateral advancement flap extends from the nasal sill around the alar base. The medial segment with cupid's bow is rotated downward, and the lateral segment flap is advanced into the defect created.

Millard felt that markings served as a guide only, with the actual repair being "cut-as-you-go" individualized surgery (**Figure 7**).

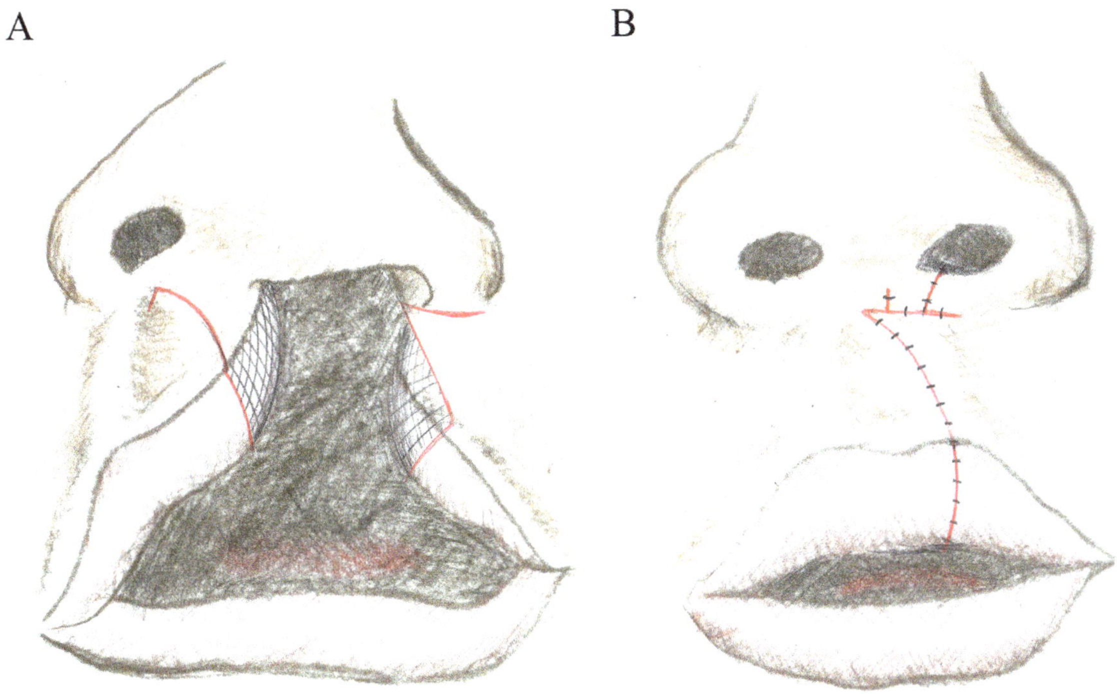

Figure 7. (A) Schematic representation of the incisions for a Millard repair. (B) Schematic representation of the closure of a Millard repair.

6.2.2. Salyer's modification

Salyer modified the rotation advancement with many improvements, most notably by making the transverse incision of the lateral segment B-flap not below the alar rim, but instead intranasally [23].

6.2.3. Mohler technique

Whereas the scar runs obliquely across the philtral column in Millard's repair, Mohler modified the technique to create a "mirror image" of the philtral column on the noncleft side [24]. He accomplished a straight-line closure of the lip by moving the rotation flap up into the columella. His technique used a back-cut that terminated at the midpoint of the philtral depression. The defect created by the downward rotation was filled by tissue from the lateral element.

6.2.4. Cutting technique ("Extended Mohler")

Mohler's technique was modified by Cutting who moved the upper end of the incision to just beyond the midline of the columella (about 4/7th of the width on the noncleft side), and extended the back-cut down to the noncleft philtral column [25]. This left a enough columellar tissue to fill in the defect created by downward rotation. A straight-line closure symmetric to the noncleft side philtral ridge is the result. There is then abundant lateral segment tissue that may be used to provide nasal lining, as shown in **Figure 8A** and **B**.

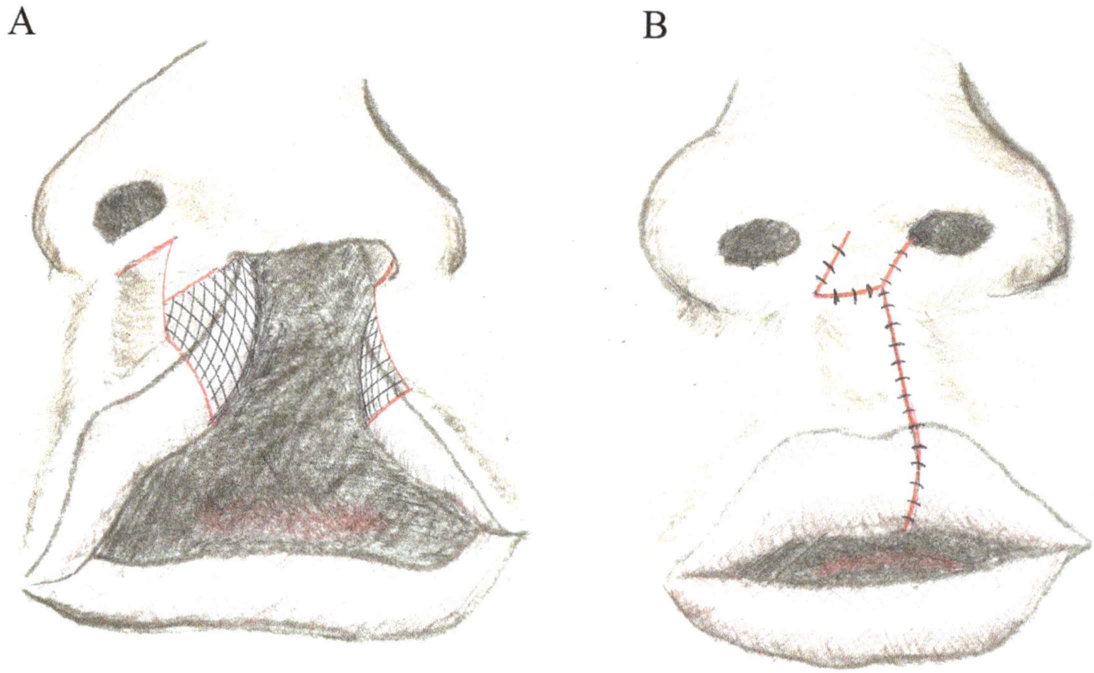

Figure 8. (A) Schematic representation of the incisions for a Cutting repair. (B) Schematic representation of the closure of a Cutting repair.

6.3. Middle lip flaps

6.3.1. LeMesurier technique

In the LeMesurier technique, a quadrilateral shape flap is created on the lateral side of the cleft lip which is rotated to the medial side where a notch is formed by a back cut, as shown in **Figure 9A** and **B** [26].

In addition to creating fullness in the lower lip, an advantage of this technique includes the placement of the suture line down the center of the lip. Thus, the cupid's bow can be made symmetrical. The scar that develops from the LeMesurier technique is a "step line" scar which is unlike most scars associated with cleft lip repair. This may overcome the characteristic appearance of a cleft lip repair and can look like an accidental wound to the observer [27].

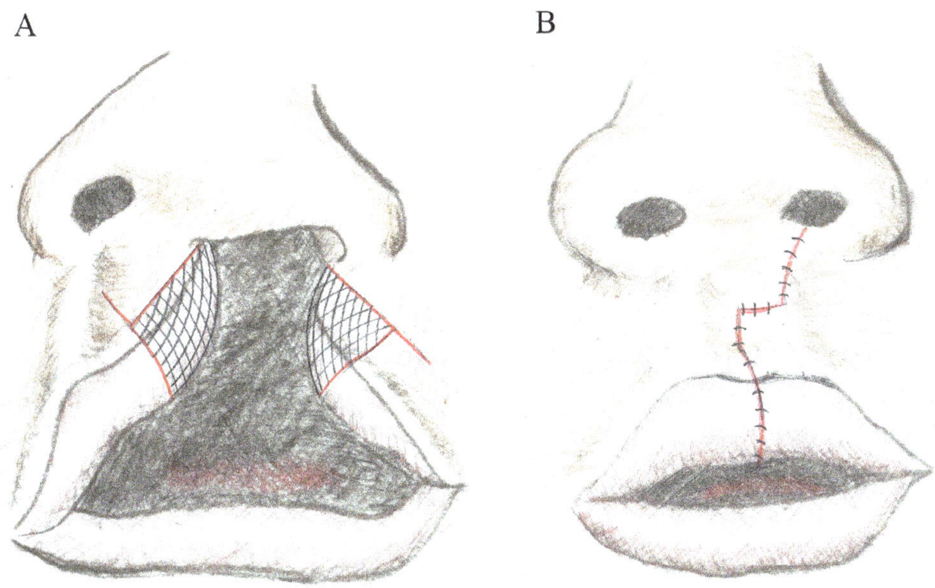

Figure 9. (A) Schematic representation of the incisions for a LeMesurier repair. (B) Schematic representation of the closure of a LeMesurier repair.

6.3.2. Pool repair

Pool placed the transverse limb of his Z-plasty repair of the lip approximately 3–4 mm below the alar bases [28]. He found that positioning the incision of the medial segment allowed for complete caudal rotation and proper horizontal positioning of the cupid's bow without the need for back-cuts or secondary flaps, see **Figure 10A** and **B**. He also found that this

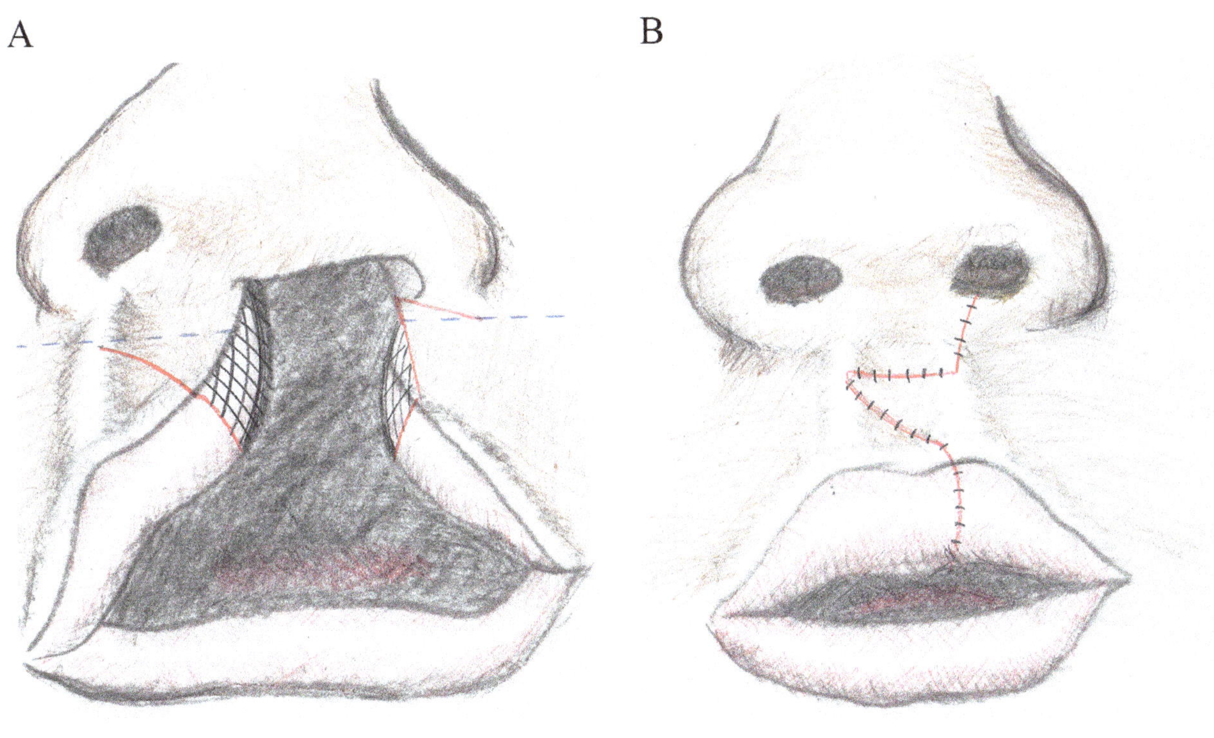

Figure 10. (A) Schematic representation of the incisions for a Pool repair. The blue dotted line represents a horizontal approximately 3 mm below the alar bases for planning the Z-plasty. (B) Schematic representation of the closure of a Pool repair.

technique allowed a better contour of the lip, especially the curve of the columellar-labial juncture, which may be distorted by the transverse scar in higher rotation advancement techniques. The incisions also allow a "cut as you go" adjustment to the alar base for symmetry.

6.4. Lower lip flaps

6.4.1. Tennison-Randall repair

In 1952, Charles Tennison proposed a repair based on the Z-plasty principle to gain vertical lip length [29]. His technique, in particular, has proven to be advantageous in wide complete clefts. Peter Randall devised a mathematical system for designing the lip operation [30].

The base of the isosceles triangle of the lateral element is determined by the difference in lengths between the noncleft cupid's peak to the alar base and to the base of the columella. The isosceles triangle side length should equal the length of the 90° back cut of the medial element, as shown in **Figure 11A** and **B**.

A B

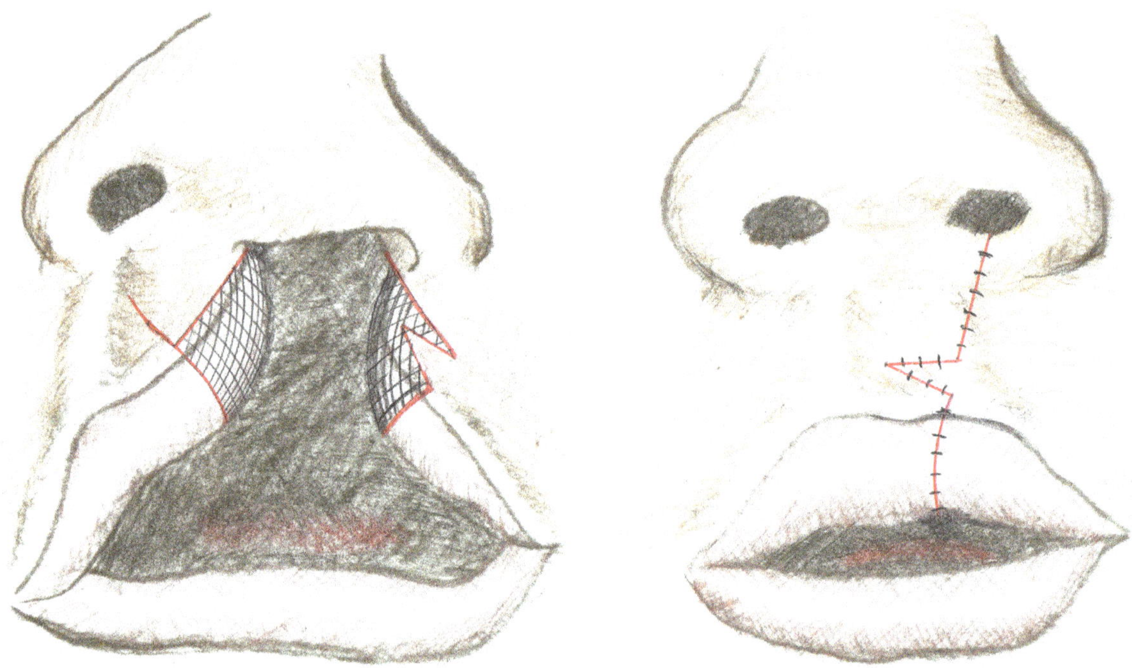

Figure 11. (A) Schematic representation of the incisions for a Tennison-Randall repair. (B) Schematic representation of the closure of a Tennison-Randall repair.

6.4.2. Fisher "anatomic subunit" repair

Fisher designed a repair utilizing the Rose-Thompson principle with close attention to the borders of aesthetic subunits of the lip, as well as a small lower lip triangular interpolation flap [31]. Many have found that this technique yields esthetic scars and achieves a natural contour of the upper lip (**Figure 12**).

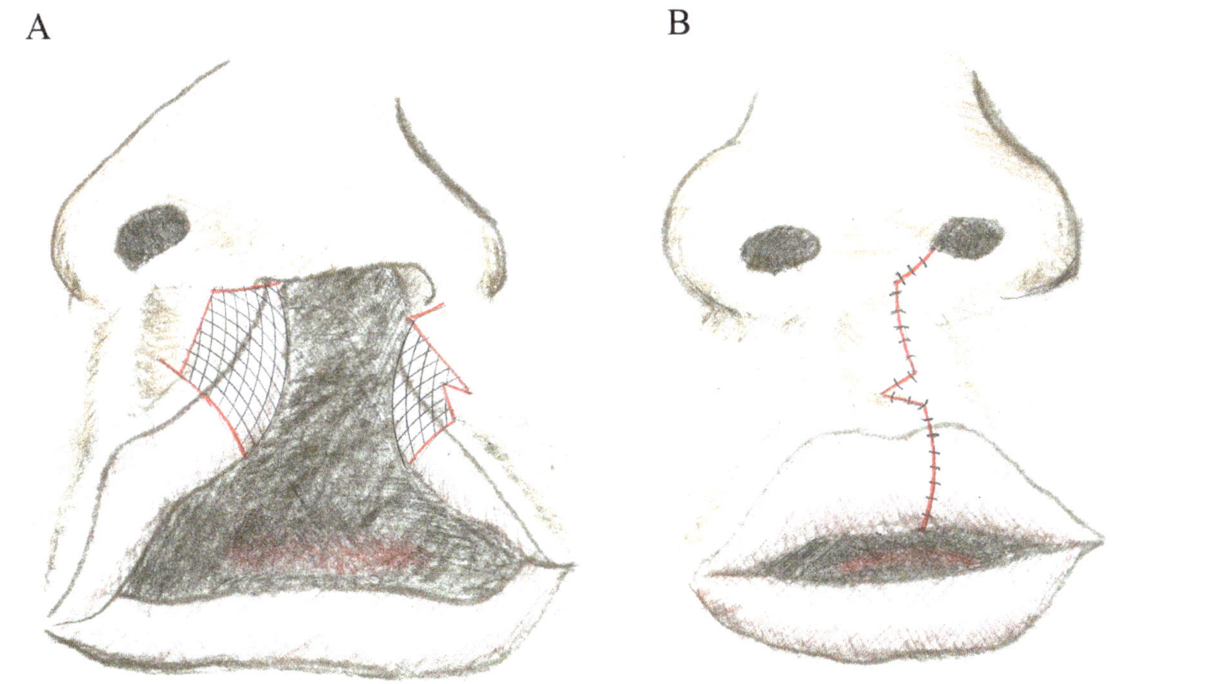

Figure 12. (A) Schematic representation of the incisions for a Fisher repair. (B) Schematic representation of the closure of a Fisher repair.

6.5. Vermilion flaps

6.5.1. Noordhoff technique

The Noordhoff technique utilizes a lateral lip triangular flap to reconstruct the dry vermilion [32]. A triangular flap is made on the lateral side of the cleft, where the vermilion height is the greatest, just before the red line converges to meet the white roll at the cleft edge (Noordhoff's point). The vermilion tissue medial to this triangular marking is used to augment the deficient vermilion underneath the cupid's bow. A straight cut is made on the medial side of the cleft to fit the inset of the lateral triangular flap (**Figure 13**).

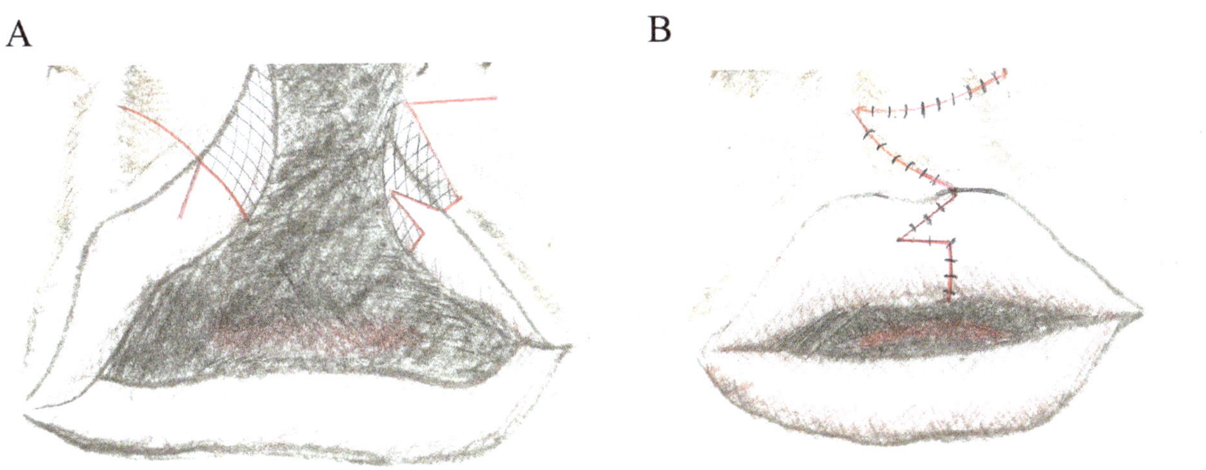

Figure 13. (A) Schematic representation of the incisions for a Noordhoff flap. (B) Schematic representation of the closure of a Noordhoff flap.

6.5.2. *Powar technique*

The Powar Technique for unilateral cleft lip repair is a modification of the Noordhoff's lateral vermilion flap. The Powar technique not only maintains the parallel relationship of the muco-vermillion "red line" with the white roll but also more accurately matches the vermilion on the noncleft side [33]. In Power's modification, the vermilion deficiency is measured on the medial cleft segment and a custom matching triangular flap is created above the muco-vermilion junction on the lateral slide (**Figure 14**). This avoids the mucosal bulge that often is the result of the Noordhoff triangular flap inset.

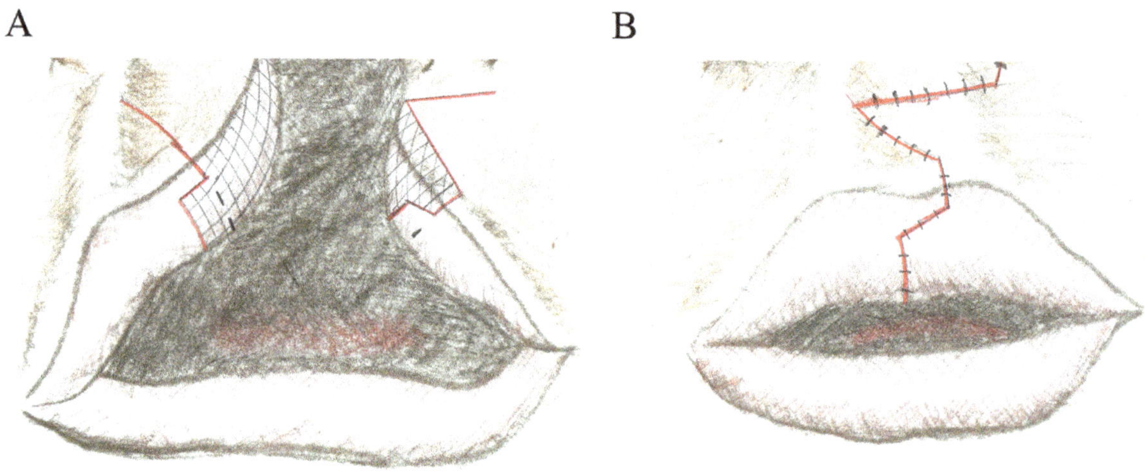

Figure 14. (A) Schematic representation of the incisions for a Powar flap. (B) Schematic representation of the closure of a Powar flap.

6.6. Adjuntive flaps

Creation of the cupid's bow is a critical aesthetic concern in cleft lip surgery and has two major elements: continuity of the white roll and sufficient caudal rotation. It is tempting for the surgeon, when faced with a wide cleft, to preserve as much tissue width as possible. However, preserving lip tissue with attenuated or absent white roll yields unsatisfactory outcomes. The vast majority of patients who present for a revision of cleft lip scar benefit from excision of scar to an accurately determined Noordhoff's point and meticulous suture approximation of the white roll.

A cleft lip repair may be unacceptable if the cupid's bow is not horizontal due to insufficient caudal rotation of the lip. A great advantage in the Pool technique is that it easily provides sufficient caudal rotation. In the case of insufficient rotation, enlarging the Z-plasty flaps, a flap "back cut," or a second Z-plasty may bring cupid's bow horizontal. A second smaller Z-plasty just above the white roll is a very useful tool: the tightness caused by the Z-plasty enhances the prominence of the white roll, and small flaps also break up a long linear scar (**Figure 15**). The Tennison and Fisher techniques employ this principle as part of their initial design.

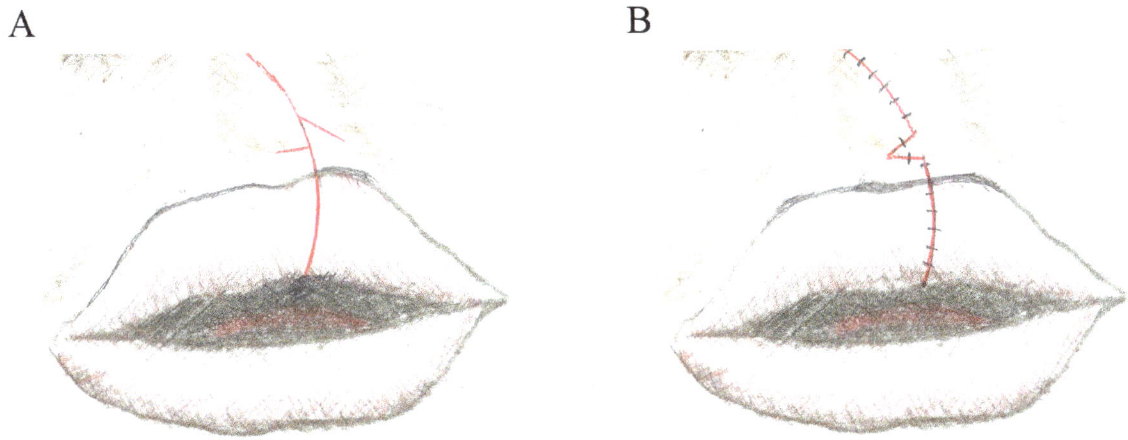

Figure 15. (A) Schematic representation of closure of a cleft repair with the cupid's bow under-rotated. The incisions for a second, smaller Z-plasty above the white roll are planned. (B) Schematic representation of the closure of Z-plasty.

6.7. Hard palate repair at the time of lip repair

Sommerlad advocates the Oslo Protocol for closure of the hard palate: a single-layer mucoperichondral flap of the vomarine septum simultaneous with primary cleft lip repair [34]. While the lip is incised and retracted, tissue exposure is optimal to the anterior palate. This technique seems not to have unfavorable outcome on maxillofacial growth [35].

6.8. Primary nasal repair

Early nasal reconstruction is important for the patient's self-esteem from a young age, and eliminates the need for correction of worsening nasal deformities as one matures and grows. The reparative success of cleft nasal deformity is dependent on dissection that frees the alar cartilage and its translocation into normal position.

6.8.1. McComb's technique

McComb's technique lifts the alar cartilage with its vestibular lining to shorten the cleft-side nose [36]. Dissection in a subcutaneous plane is performed from the upper buccal sulcus and also through the columella to release the medial and lateral crura. The dissection then is extended from the nostril rim to the tip, dorsum, and nasion. The alar lift is achieved with either one or two mattress sutures through the nasal lining at the intercrural angle, raising the cleft side lower lateral alar cartilages to a symmetrical position.

6.8.2. Anderl's technique

The Anderl technique utilizes the incisions made for cleft lip repair and wide undermining of the nasal skin. The Anderl technique has extensive mobilization by undermining of the nasal dorsum, supraperiosteal dissection on the surface of maxilla from the vestibule to the infraorbital rim and from the piriform aperture to the maxillary tuberosity [37]. This maneuver allows for greater medial excursion of the lateral element during repair of the lip and nose. The cartilaginous septum is also released from its base attachment to the hard palate, straightened and sutured to the anterior nasal spine.

6.8.3. Salyer's technique

Salyer also uses extensive subcutaneous freeing of all elements and floating them above an abnormal skeletal base. He uses two intranasal-transdermal sutures to create the genu of the ala [38]. In the completion of the lip and nasal repair, additional sutures may be used to contour the alar base.

7. Outcomes assessments repair

"It is very difficult to understand the effectiveness of our actions without measurements."

—Steve Killelea

Most outcome studies for unilateral cleft lip-nose repair are single-surgeon experiences with their preferred techniques [39]. Outcomes are measured with postoperative photographs that assess various anatomic landmarks and features. Other studies compare results as surgeon's technique change over time [40, 41].

AmeriCleft, a large, multicenter study in the U.S., validated the use of the Asher-McDade rating scale, to audit four different institutions each with their own protocols [42]. The Asher-McDade system stratifies cleft patients on a seven-point scale in each of the following nasolabial characteristics [43]:

a. Nasal form
b. Symmetry of the nose
c. Shape of the vermillion
d. Nasal profile including upper lip

The EuroCleft, a large multicenter European study, found that physical metrics correlated poorly with satisfaction [44]. Furthermore, there are few studies that examine the functionality and quality of life of cleft patients postoperatively [45]. Future metric systems should be comprehensive, incorporating all patient-related outcomes in a cleft population.

8. Author's experience

"It is life's tragedy that we get old too soon and wise too late"

—Benjamin Franklin

The senior author (DL) was trained in plastic surgery residency, as many were, to repair unilateral cleft lips with the Millard rotation-advancement technique. Later, while on surgical missions to developing world countries, I had the opportunity and honor to work with Dr. Robert Pool, and learn his midlip Z-plasty technique of lip repair. Moreover, I also observed his meticulous surgical technique and attention to detail that brought the children on whom he operated such excellent results. When I began practice with the Vermont State Cleft/Craniofacial Center, I used the Pool technique.

Still later in my practice, I was quite intrigued by the extended Mohler technique advocated by Dr. Court Cutting. While in New York City attending Dr. Barry Grayson's excellent workshop on nasoalveolar molding, Dr. Cutting graciously invited me to observe him operating on an infant with unilateral cleft lip. I observe his similar scrupulous attention to detail and excellent technique. I then began using this technique for a period of time. For reasons discussed below, I have returned to a midlip Z-plasty technique for surgical reconstruction of children with unilateral cleft lip.

In my experience, the upper lip techniques of lip reconstruction have the disadvantage of a transverse scar across the columellar-labial junction. The columellar-labial junction naturally has a gentle curved shape, but a transverse scar across this curve will frequently result in a tight, noncurved junction.

Linear scars the entire height of the lip often results in scar hypertrophy (**Figure 16**). The linear Cutting/Mohler surgical linear scar line mimics a natural philtral ridge, however may result in a hypertrophic scar of the vertical limb.

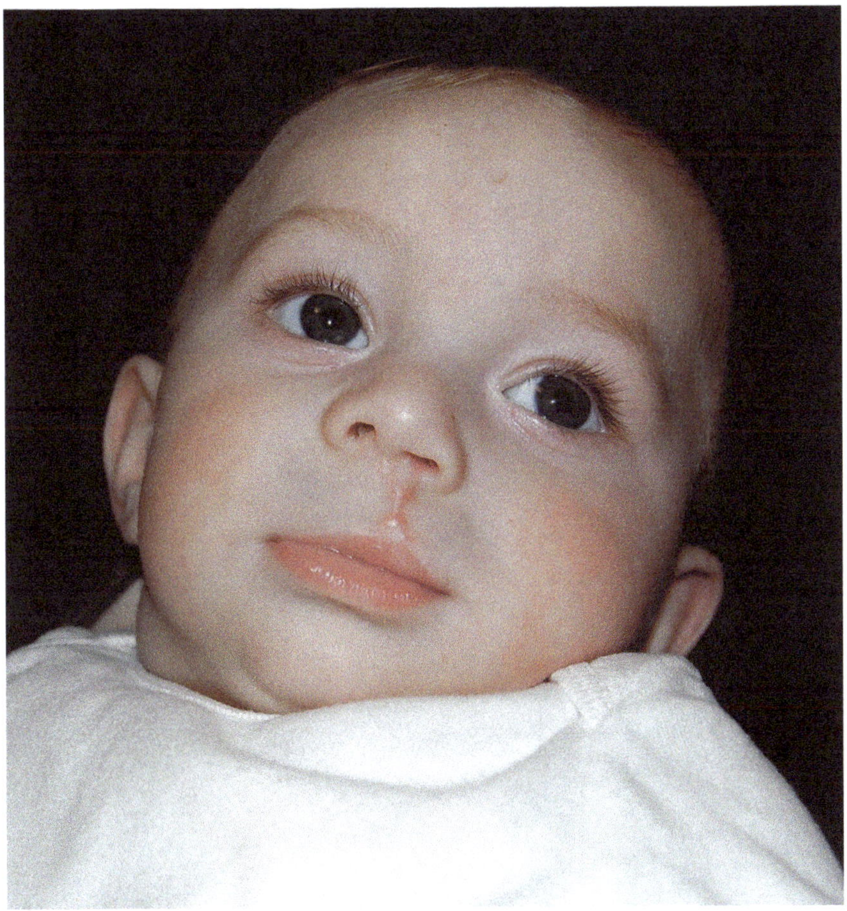

Figure 16. A child 5 months after cleft lip repair by the Cutting "Extended Mohler" technique and Powar vermillion flap. This is the child from **Figure 1B** and **Figure 4**. Note the somewhat hypertrophied straight-line vertical limb of the scar.

Continuity of orbicularis oris is the critical functional concern of cleft lip surgery. Midlip surgical techniques have a great advantage in that the incisions are made over the abnormal muscle bundles, and flap transposition redirects those muscle bundles with less extensive dissection (**Figure 17**).

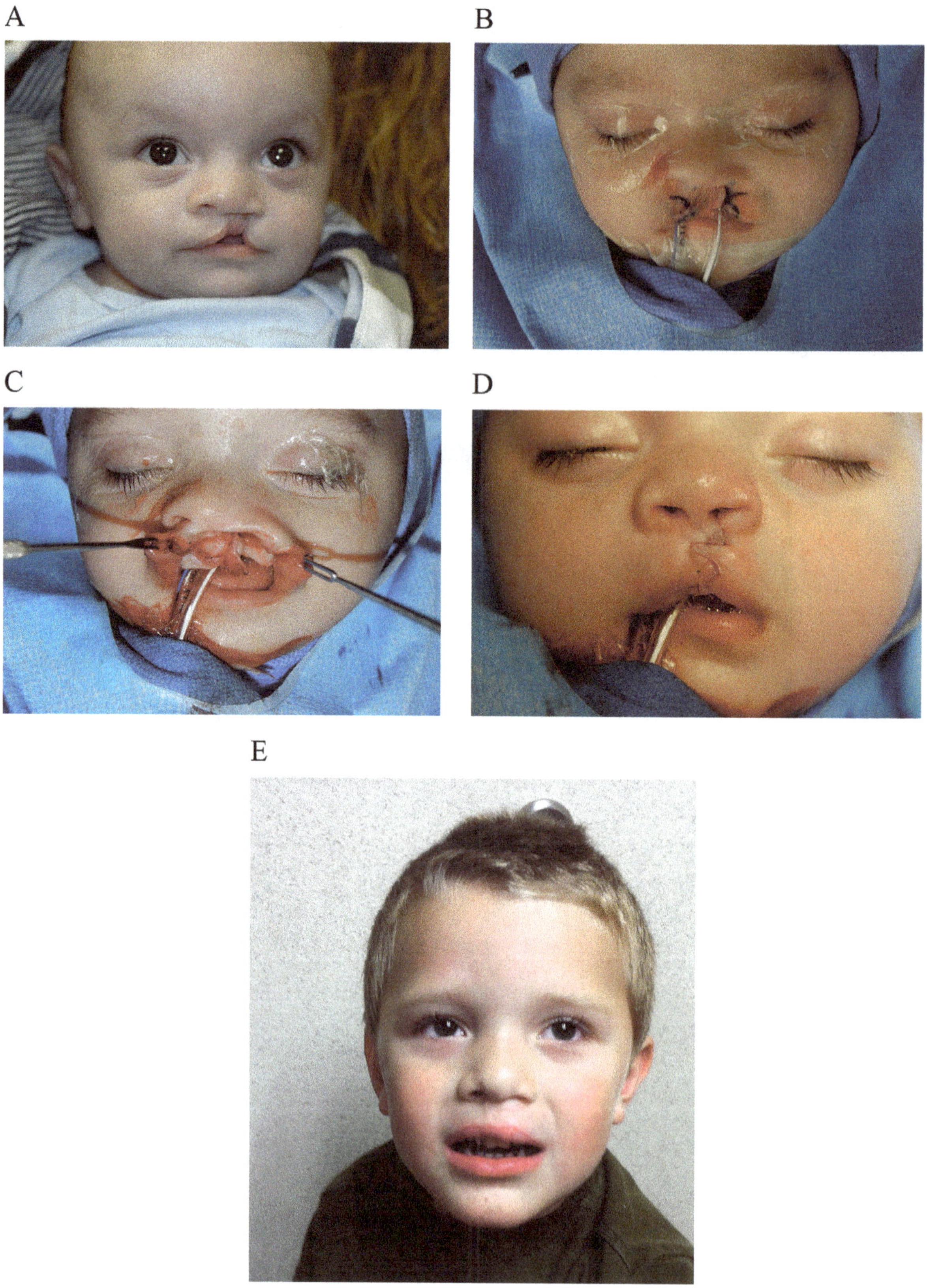

Figure 17. (A) An infant with a complete unilateral cleft lip. (B) The infant in the operating room with markings for a Pool midlip Z-plasty and Noordhoff vermillion flap repair. (C) The infant in the operating room with dissection completed. Because the Z-plasty design and muscles are freed from their abnormal insertions without as much undermining of the skin. (D) The infant in the operating room with surgical repair completed. (E) This child at 3 years of age.

In my opinion, this technique yields very satisfactory results (**Figure 18**).

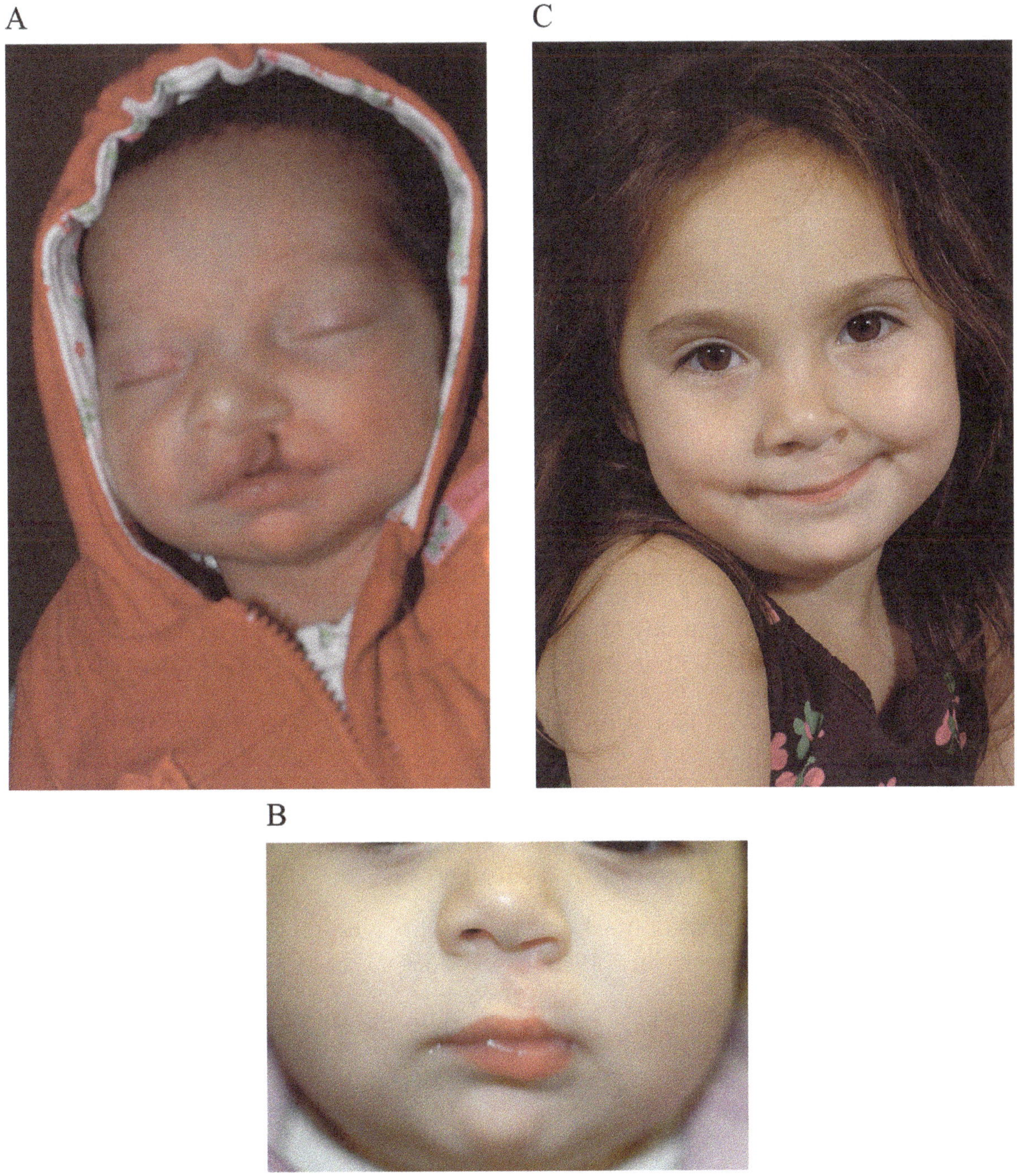

Figure 18. (A) An infant with a wide, yet incomplete unilateral cleft lip. Note the narrow Simonart's band. (B) The infant after a Pool midlip Z-plasty and Powar vermillion flap repair. (C) The same child at 5 years of age.

At Vermont State Cleft/Craniofacial Center, we perform formal NAM presurgical orthopedics only on children with bilateral clefts who have premaxillary protrusion (**Figure 5**). Unfortunately, we have found that the frequent visits and lack of insurance coverage for NAM result in a high burden of care for families in Vermont. Because of this, we have not adopted this modality for children with unilateral clefts. We have found presurgical taping (**Figure 4**) to be an efficacious yet inexpensive modality and it offers an opportunity for parents to play an active role in their child's care.

Thoughtful selection of a surgical method and careful attention to detail in the execution of surgical technique will yield the best results. We hope that this chapter will help surgeons in the care of children with cleft lip.

Author details

Mustafa Chopan, Lohrasb Sayadi and Donald R. Laub*

*Address all correspondence to: Donald.Laub@uvmhealth.org

University of Vermont College of Medicine, Burlington, Vermont, USA

References

[1] Veau V RJ. Bec-de-lièvre: formes cliniques, chirurgie [Hare-lips: clinical forms, surgery] Paris: Masson et Cie; 1938.

[2] Bo C, Ningbei Y. Reconstruction of upper lip muscle system by anatomy, magnetic resonance imaging, and serial histological sections. J Craniofac Surg. 2014; 25(1): 48–54.

[3] Wu J, Yin N. Detailed anatomy of the nasolabial muscle in human fetuses as determined by micro-CT combined with iodine staining. Ann Plast Surg. 2016; 76(1): 111–116.

[4] Yin N, Wu J, Chen B, Song T, Ma H, Zhao Z, et al. Muscle tension line concept in nasolabial muscle complex-based on 3-dimensional reconstruction of nasolabial muscle fibers. J Craniofac Surg 2015; 26(2):469–472.

[5] Huang MHS, Lee S, Lee, S. Anatomy of Cleft Lip and Palate. In: Losee JE, Kirshner RE, editor. Comprehensive Cleft Care. 2nd ed. New York: McGraw-Hill; 2009. pp. 223–239.

[6] Pool R. The configurations of the unilateral cleft lip, with reference to rotation advancement repair. Plast Reconstr Surg. 1966. 37:558–565.

[7] Liau JY, van Aalst JA, Sadove AM. Understanding and caring for children with cleft lip and palate. In: Coran AG, editor. Pediatric Surgery. Philadelphia: Elsevier Saunders; 2012. pp. 699–706.

[8] Wang TD, Milczuk, H.A. Cleft lip and palate. In: Paul WF, editor. Cummings Otolaryngology. Philadelphia: Elsevier Saunders; 2015. pp. 2915–32.e3.

[9] Pool R. Farnworth TK. Preoperative lip taping in the cleft lip. Ann Plast Surg. 1994; 32(3):243–249.

[10] Cruz C. Presurgical orthopedics appliance: the Latham technique. Oral Maxillofac Surg Clin North Am. 2016; 28(2): 161–168.

[11] Millard DR, Jr., Latham RA. Improved primary surgical and dental treatment of clefts. Plast Reconstr Surg. 1990; 86(5): 856–871.

[12] Aminpour S, Tollefson TT. Recent advances in presurgical molding in cleft lip and palate. Curr Opin Otolaryngol Head Neck Surg. 2008; 16(4): 339–46.

[13] Grayson BH, Santiago PE, Brecht LE, Cutting CB. Presurgical nasoalveolar molding in infants with cleft lip and palate. Cleft Palate Craniofac J. 1999; 36(6): 486–498.

[14] Randall P. A lip adhesion operation in cleft lip surgery. Plast Reconstr Surg. 1965; 35:371–376.

[15] Demke JC, Tatum SA. Analysis and evolution of rotation principles in unilateral cleft lip repair. J Plast Reconstr Aesthet Surg. 2011 Mar; 64(3): 313–8.

[16] Millard DR, Jr. Paring and approximation with needles and/or sutures. Cleft Craft: The Evolution of its Surgery. I. Boston: Little & Brown; 1976. pp. 82–87.

[17] Randall P, Jackson, O. A short history of cleft lip and cleft palate. In: Losee JE, Kirshner RE, editors. Comprehensive Cleft Care. 2nd ed. New York: McGraw-Hill; 2009. pp. 187–209.

[18] Rose, W. On Harelip and Cleft Palate. London: HK Lewis; 1891.

[19] Thompson, JE. An artistic and mathematically accurate method of repairing the defects in cases of harelip. Surg Gynecol Obstet. 1912(14): 498–502.

[20] Millard DR, Jr. Increasing vertical length of cleft edges. Cleft Craft: The Evolution of its Surgery. I. The Unilateral Deformity. Boston: Little & Brown; 1976. pp. 90–92.

[21] Nakajima T, Yoshimura Y, Yoneda K, Nakanishi Y. Primary repair of an incomplete unilateral cleft lip: avoiding an elongated lip and achieving a straight suture line. Br J Plast Surg 1998; 51(7): 511–516.

[22] Millard DR, Jr. A radical rotation in single harelip. Am J Surg. 1958; 95(2): 318–322.

[23] Salyer K, Marchac, A, Cheng, MS, Michienza JW, Genecov, E. Unilatera cleft lip/nose repair. In: Losee JE, Kirshner R, editor. Comprehensive Cleft Care. 2 ed. New York: McGraw-Hill; 2009. pp. 299–329.

[24] Mohler LR. Unilateral cleft lip repair. Plast Reconstr Surg. 1987; 80(4): 511–7.

[25] Cutting C. The extended mohler unilateral cleft lip repair. In: Losee JE KR, editor. Comprehensive Cleft Care. 2nd ed. New York: McGraw-Hill; 2009. pp. 286–97.

[26] LeMesurier A. A method of cutting and suturing the lip in the treatment of complete unilateral clefts. Plast Reconstr Surg. 1949; 4(1): 1–12.

[27] Bauer TB, Trusler HM, Glanz S. Repair of unilateral cleft lip; advantages of LeMesurier technique use of mucous membrane flaps in maxillary clefts. Plast Reconstr Surg. (1946). 1953; 11(1): 56–68.

[28] Pool R. Cleft lip. In: Stark RB, editor. Plastic Surgery of the Head and Neck. 1st ed. New York: Churchill-Livingstone; 1987. pp.1179–1189.

[29] Tennison CW. The repair of the unilateral cleft lip by the stencil method. Plast Reconstr Surg. (1946). 1952;9(2): 115–120.

[30] Randall P. A triangular flap operation for the primary repair of unilateral clefts of the lip. Plast Reconstr Surg. 1959; 23(4): 331–347.

[31] Fisher DM. Unilateral cleft lip repair: an anatomic subunit approximation technique. Plast Reconstr Surg. 2005; 116: 61–71.

[32] Noordhoff MS. Reconstruction of vermilion in unilateral and bilateral cleft lips. Plast Reconstr Surg. 1984; 73(1): 52–61.

[33] Powar RS, Patil S, Kleinman ME. A geometrically sound technique of vermilion repair in unilateral cleft lip. J Plast Reconstr Aesthet Surg. 2007; 60(4): 422–425.

[34] Sommerlad BC. Surgery of the cleft lip and nose—the GOStA approach. B-ENT. 2006; 2 Suppl. 4: 29–31.

[35] Ferdous KM, Salek AJ, Islam MK, Das BK, Khan AR, Karim MS. Repair of cleft lip and simultaneous repair of cleft hard palate with vomer flap in unilateral complete cleft lip and palate: a comparative study. Pediatr Surg Int. 2010 Oct; 26(10): 995–1000.

[36] McComb H. Primary correction of unilateral cleft lip nasal deformity: a 10-year review. Plast Reconstr Surg. 1985; 75(6):791–799.

[37] Anderl H, Hussl H, Ninkovic M. Primary simultaneous lip and nose repair in the unilateral cleft lip and palate. Plast Reconstr Surg. 2008; 121(3): 959–970.

[38] Salyer KE, Genecov ER, Genecov DG. Unilateral cleft lip-nose repair: a 33-year experience. J Craniofac Surg. 2003;14(4): 549–558.

[39] Al-Omari I, Millett DT, Ayoub AF. Methods of assessment of cleft-related facial deformity: a review. Cleft Palate Craniofac J. 2005; 42(2): 145–156.

[40] Lazarus DD, Hudson DA, van Zyl JE, Fleming AN, Fernandes D. Repair of unilateral cleft lip: a comparison of five techniques. Ann Plast Surg. 1998 Dec; 41(6): 587–594.

[41] Chang CS, Liao YF, Wallace CG, Chan FC, Liou EJ, Chen PK, Noordhoff MS: Long-term comparison of the results of four techniques used for bilateral cleft nose repair: a single surgeon's experience. Plast Reconstr Surg. 2014 Dec; 134(6): 926e–36e.

[42] Mercado A, Russell K, Hathaway R, Daskalogiannakis J, Sadek H, Long RE, Jr., et al. The Americleft study: an inter-center study of treatment outcomes for patients with unilateral cleft lip and palate part 4. Nasolabial aesthetics. Cleft Palate Craniofac J. 2011; 48(3):259–64.

[43] Asher-McDade C, Roberts C, Shaw WC, Gallager C. Development of a method for rating nasolabial appearance in patients with clefts of the lip and palate. Cleft Palate Craniofac J.1991;28(4):385–90; discussion 90–1.

[44] Semb G, Brattstrom V, Molsted K, Prahl-Andersen B, Zuurbier P, Rumsey N, et al. The Eurocleft study: intercenter study of treatment outcome in patients with complete cleft lip and palate. Part 4: relationship among treatment outcome, patient/parent satisfaction, and the burden of care. Cleft Palate Craniofac J.. 2005; 42(1): 83–92.

[45] Eckstein DA, Wu RL, Akinbiyi T, Silver L, Taub PJ. Measuring quality of life in cleft lip and palate patients: currently available patient-reported outcomes measures. Plast Reconstr Surg. 2011; 128(5): 518e–26e.

8

Debridement of Lower Lateral Cartilages in Cleft Lip–Nose Cases along with Management of Skin and Fibrotic Traction

Nikolay P. Serdev

Abstract

Rhinoplasties in case of cleft lip–nose and palate are difficult and may include: primary repair of nasal deformities at the time of cleft lip repair; secondary staged repair of cleft lip–nasal deformities; separation of the quadrangular cartilage of the septum from the maxillary crest and securing it to the midline; removal of deviated portions, strut grafts, transplants to project the radix and dorsum, cartilage grafts, multidisciplinary care, etc. Results can vary widely, from excellent in primary corrections to very poor in late surgery cases. In some secondary rhinoplasties, based on skin and fibrotic tractions and deviations, the author offers a more simple method of debridement of the normally formed cartilages. It includes closed approach T-excision with releasing the alar cartilages from their attachments, columella sliding and sutures for stabilization of the columella, nasal tip refinement, dorsal augmentation, and overall symmetry. Such approach could be sufficient in selected cases. In other cases, additional steps may be necessary.

Keywords: Rhinoplasty, cleft lip and nose, debridement, T-excision, transcutaneous Serdev Sutures®, symmetrization, parallel medial crura suture, columella sliding for tip projection

1. Introduction

The goal of surgical treatment of cleft nasal deformity is not only rhinoplasty but includes normal speech, aesthetic facial appearance, normal occlusion, unobstructed nasal passages, and absence of psychological pathology. Surgical correction of nasal deformities removes the abnormal appearance and improves the opportunities for normal social integration.

2. Secondary rhinoplasty

Despite the move toward primary correction of cleft nasal deformities, secondary rhinoplasty procedures are often necessary. It is advisable that the patient has reached bony maturity. Maxillary deficiencies have to be treated appropriately prior to surgery.

Open approach is often used, because it provides exposure. Autologous cartilage grafts are often used to provide structural support and to restore contours and grafts – to project and support.

3. Surgical technique

Having in mind that deformations depend mostly on skin/fibrotic traction, the author uses the closed rhinoplasty approach. Its main goals, by steps, are:

1. Using retrocolumellar incision and eventually T-excision technique to correct hanging columella or elongated (mostly deviated) caudal septum.
2. To release the lower lateral cartilages from the skin/fibrotic lateral attachments and reposition them. Usually, alar cartilages show minimal deformations.
3. To redefine the dome and tip defining points, using transcutaneous Serdev Sutures® (described in the next chapter): a. for tip refinement and symmetrization of the tip and tip defining points of projection; b. transmucosal domal and columellar sutures for refinement of the nasal tip and stabilization of the columella. In cases of equal projection of both sides of the tip, the needle should penetrate horizontally. The trick to get symmetry in unequal projection of both sides is to place the needle and suture parallel to the asymmetric tip (Figure 1).

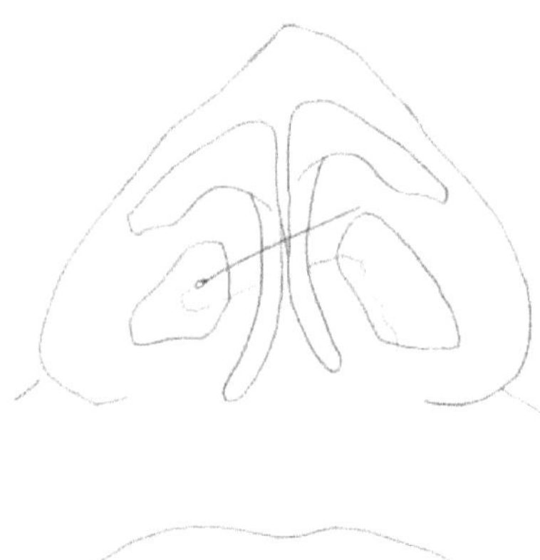

Figure 1. Transmucosal sutures have to be parallel to the symmetry or asymmetry of the tip defining points; 2–3 sutures can equalize the dome projection on both sides.

4. To project the nasal tip. Instead of a columellar strut graft, the author uses columella sliding for nasal tip projection. Note that columella sliding cannot be used in most Asian, Afro-American, and some Latino-American patients, where the columella is typically soft and unstable and is the main reason for the low projection in these ethnic groups. Caucasian septum and columella are very stable and in most cases do not need additional support.

Repositioning of the lower lateral cartilage and some of the described mini-invasive techniques can be sufficient to restore the columella, refine the nasal tip, get tip projection, and achieve overall symmetry (Figure 2).

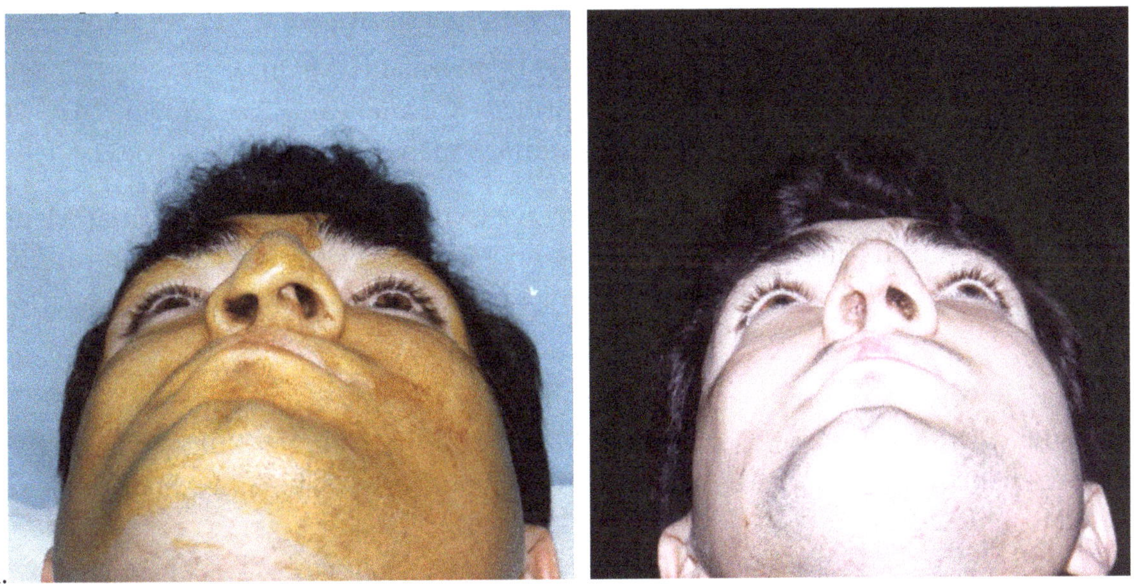
A. B.

Figure 2. A. Before. The lower lateral cartilages in cleft lip and nose cases are exposed to skin/fibrotic pressure and/or traction. The chin is deviated to the right. **B**. After author's secondary rhinoplasty: retrocolumellar incision and T-excision technique to deal with hanging columella and elongated deviated caudal septum; debridement, release of lower lateral cartilages from the skin/fibrotic lateral attachments and their repositioning; transmucosal domal and columellar sutures to reposition the lower lateral cartilages and obtain symmetry at the domal tip **defining** points (as shown in Figure 1), for refinement of the tip and stabilization of the columella; redefining the dome and tip defining points using transcutaneous Serdev Sutures® (described in the next chapter) for tip refinement and **symmetrization** of the tip and tip defining points of projection; columella sliding for nasal tip projection. Additional Serdev Suture® technique is performed for transcutaneous chin soft tissue fixation to the left-side menton periosteum. The result is equalization and stabilization of the nose and overall facial symmetry.

More severe cases require additional procedures and local flaps for correction.

4. Conclusion

In selected cases, more atraumatic and mini-invasive techniques such as debridement and release of the lower lateral cartilages, author's suture techniques, and columella sliding can be enough to stabilize, equalize, and get overall symmetry of the nose and the whole face.

Author details

Nikolay P. Serdev*

Address all correspondence to: serdev@gmail.com

New Bulgarian University, Sofia, Medical Centre "Aesthetic Surgery and Aesthetic Medicine," Sofia, Bulgaria

References

[1] Serdev NP. Mentoplastia sin implantes. IX Journadas Mediteraneas de Confrontationes Terapeuticas an Medicina y Cirurgia Cosmetica, Sitges, Spain, May 2001. Available from: http://ijcs.org/7/23/135/index.php?pageFrom=1&pageTo=21

[2] Serdev NP. Principios basicos para el rejuvenecimiento facial. IX Journadas Mediteraneas de Confrontationes Terapeuticas an Medicina y Cirurgia Cosmetica, Sitges, Spain, May 2001. Available from: http://ijcs.org/7/23/128/index.php?pageFrom=1&pageTo=60

[3] Serdev NP. Suture Suspensions for Lifting or Volume Augmentation in Face and Body (English version), 2nd Annual Meeting of the National Bulgarian Society for Aesthetic Surgery and Aesthetic Medicine, Sofia, March 18, 1994, *Int J Aesth Cosm* 2001; 1(1):2561-2568

[4] Serdev NP. Principles of Face Beautification, Third World Congress of the International Society of Aesthetic Surgery, Tokyo April 8-10, 2000, 9W58

[5] Serdev NP. Serdev sutures for: Nasal tip refinement, nasal tip rotation, Nasal alar base narrowing. *Int J Cosm Surg* 2007; 7(1):328- 386

[6] Serdev NP. Serdev techniques in beautification rhinoplasty: T-zone excision, columella sliding, Serdev sutures. *Int J Cosm Surg* 2008; 8(1):388-469

[7] Serdev NP. Nasal tip refinement, rotation, projection, alar base narrowing In: Serdev NP, Ed. *Serdev Sutures® Face and Body Lifts and/or Volumising*. Marllor editions, Italy, 2013: 75-81

[8] Serdev NP. Serdev Sutures® in middle face 4. Beautification rhinoplasty – tip rotation and refinement, alar base narrowing. In: Serdev NP, Ed. *Miniinvasive Face and Body Lifts – Closed Suture Lifts or Barded Thread Lifts*. Intech, Rijeka, 2013. Available from http://www.intechopen.com/books/miniinvasive-face-and-body-lifts-closed-suture-lifts-or-barbed-thread-lifts/serdev-sutures-in-middle-face.

[9] Serdev NP. Live on TV Rhinoplasty, Brow Suture Lift, Chin Enhancement 10.01.2013 r. http://www.youtube.com/watch?v=H73PTB2xyKU

9

Tympanostomy Tube Placement for Otitis Media with Effusion in Children with Cleft Lip and Palate

Chin-Lung Kuo and An-Suey Shiao

Abstract

The condition of cleft lip/palate (CLP) in children is psychologically stressful for family members and debilitating for the patients themselves. These children must undergo a series of major invasive surgeries following birth, including cleft lip repair surgery, cleft palate repair surgery, bone grafting surgery, and dental implant surgery. Unfortunately, the clinical significance of otitis media with effusion (OME), a complication associated with CLP, is often overlooked, and very few studies have explored this condition in depth. This chapter reviews pathogenesis, clinical manifestations, consequences, examination, and diagnosis related to OME in children with CLP. Controversies surrounding the treatment of OME in CLP children are also discussed. We also provide a flowchart for management guidance in OME in children with CLP.

Keywords: otitis media, middle ear effusion, cleft lip and palate, conductive hearing loss, grommet tube, children

1. Introduction

Cleft lip/palate (CLP) is a congenital orofacial anomaly that is debilitating for patients and psychologically stressful for family members. Children with CLP are forced to undergo a series of major invasive surgeries, including surgery for cleft lip repair, bone grafting, and dental implants [1].

Otitis media with effusion (OME), also called serous/secretory otitis media or glue ear, is a collection of nonpurulent fluid within the middle ear space. OME is a common condition among infants and children between the ages of 1 and 3 years [2]. Compared to healthy children, children with CLP are more susceptible to OME [3]. Despite the fact that the vast majority of patients (about 80%) do not have OME at birth [4], statistics show that OME occurs at least once before the first birthday in as many as 90% of the infants born with CLP [2]. In addition, as many as 97% of the infants born with CLP suffer concurrent OME within the first two years of life [5].

The clinical significance of OME is often overlooked, and very few studies have explored this condition in depth, despite it being a complication commonly associated with CLP. This chapter reviews pathogenesis, clinical manifestations, consequences, examination, and diagnosis related to OME in children with CLP. Controversies surrounding the treatment of OME in CLP children are also discussed. We also provide a flowchart for management guidance in OME in children with CLP. It is our hope that the results of this study will provide clinicians and patients/parents with a valuable reference.

2. Pathogenesis

Numerous factors have been cited in the development of OME in children suffering from CLP, including (1) immature development of the Eustachian tube, (2) abnormalities in the muscle associated with the Eustachian tube, and (3) craniofacial bone abnormalities [3].

2.1. Immature development of the Eustachian tube

The Eustachian tube of children is not yet fully developed and therefore shorter than that of adults. It is positioned at a more horizontal angle, and the opening to the nasopharynx is narrower. When upper respiratory tract infection causes swelling and inflammation of the respiratory mucosa, the narrow opening of the Eustachian tube can easily be clogged, leading to negative pressure in the middle ear. In addition, the position and length of the Eustachian tube allow viruses and bacteria from the upper respiratory tract to easily pass into the middle ear cavity, which can cause middle ear infection with effusion. Even after infection has been controlled, it is difficult to discharge fluid from the middle ear through the Eustachian tube to the throat, because the Eustachian tube is shorter and more horizontal with a narrow opening. The remaining fluid can lead to OME [6–9].

2.2. Abnormalities of Eustachian tube-associated muscle

Anatomical or structural defects associated with cleft palate can affect velopharyngeal function. In children with CLP, the abnormal reflux of food and fluid from the mouth into the nasal cavity due to velopharyngeal insufficiency can result in inflammation and edema of the Eustachian orifices and hypertrophy of adenoid pads, leading to tubal obstruction and secondary OME [6]. In addition, abnormal development of the tensor veli palatini (TVP) muscle and levator veli palatini muscle in children with CLP can cause maladjustment in the regular opening of the Eustachian tube [10, 11]. When the atmospheric pressure of the environment changes (e.g., during descent in an airplane) or the gas in the middle ear is absorbed by mucosa, the Eustachian tube is unable to open and thereby relieve pressure in the middle ear. The resulting negative pressure can cause the eardrum to retract, leading to the collection of fluid in the middle ear, which can again lead to OME [6].

2.3. Craniofacial bone abnormalities

Other abnormalities in the structure of the Eustachian tube in children with CLP have also been associated with the pathogenesis of OME. These abnormalities include increased nasopharyngeal space, alterations to the medial pterygoid plate and hamulus, a shorter tube, larger angle between the cartilage and TVP, higher cartilage cell density, a smaller ratio of lateral and medial lamina area in the cartilage, less curvature of the lumen, less elastin in the hinge portion of the cartilage, and a lower insertion ratio of TVP to the cartilage [12, 13]. Kemaloglu et al. evaluated clinical and cephalometric data of 37 Japanese children with unilateral complete CLP or isolated cleft palate and compared them to 40 non-cleft children. They found that differences in the mastoid-middle ear-Eustachian tube system are associated with a tendency toward OME in CLP children. This fact helps to elucidate the pathogenesis of OME in children with CLP [14].

3. Clinical manifestations

Aside from mild conductive hearing loss, OME does not cause any other symptoms of discomfort and is therefore easily overlooked. In infants, OME combined with hearing loss may continue for weeks or even months without being detected. A child with OME may also suffer poor sleep quality [15]. Parents of children with CLP should pay particular attention to how their children interact with others and how they react to sound. If any abnormality is observed, the child should undergo expert evaluation. More importantly, children should visit an otolaryngologist for a regular otologic examination to ascertain whether they are suffering from OME. Early diagnosis and treatment are invaluable in preventing or alleviating future hearing loss.

4. Consequences of OME in CLP

Children with CLP may suffer recurrent or continuous OME, causing atelectasis, ossicular fixation, and tympanosclerosis [2, 16, 17], which can result in conductive hearing loss of up to 30 decibels (dB). Researchers have previously shown that, regardless of whether they have undergone cleft palate repair surgery, as many as 90% of children with CLP suffer from OME or conductive hearing loss, while 50% suffer from recurrent otitis media [2, 5, 18–20]. In comparison, the prevalence of conductive hearing loss among children without CLP is 12.9%. Although the likelihood of developing OME is reduced after reaching adulthood, it is estimated that 50% of these children suffer from permanent conductive hearing loss [21, 22]. Additionally, 0.9–5.9% of patients with CLP develop primary acquired cholesteatoma, the probability of which is 100–200 times higher among those without CLP [23, 24].

In addition, sensorineural losses have been ascribed to pathologic changes in the inner ear resulting from inflammation in the middle ear and presumably mediated via the round or oval window [3]. Toxins produced by long-term inflammation can pass through the round window or the oval window into the inner ear, causing permanent sensorineural hearing loss [17, 25].

Many studies have indicated that although reconstructive surgery for CLP improves linguistic ability, language development depends on the extent to which hearing ability is maintained [23, 26]. If OME is not treated properly, long-term hearing loss can negatively influence the language development of children [27]. Hearing loss in children suffering from CLP can also affect their academic comprehension and learning performance [20, 27, 28]. Bess et al. indicated that even if children suffer hearing loss in only one ear, academic performance can still be seriously affected in up to 33% of patients and up to 40% of patients are unable to participate in regular activities or interactions due to hearing loss [29]. It has been found that children with cleft palate are prone to specific psychological problems [30, 31]. Children suffering from this condition may also display behavioral difficulties due to feelings of isolation [29].

5. Examination and diagnosis

Up to 90% of infants born with CLP suffer from OME before their first birthday [2]; therefore, it is recommended that otologic tests be conducted as soon as possible after birth to ascertain whether fluid has collected in the middle ear [21, 32]. The use of a pneumatic otoscope is the fastest and most direct method used for the inspection of the eardrum for color and contour and determining whether fluid has collected in the middle ear. It should be noted that the effectiveness of a pneumatic otoscope to test for OME depends on the experience and skill of the clinicians, the patient's full cooperation, and the anatomical structure of the ear canal [2].

Another method for inspecting the eardrum is videotelescopy. A telescope is placed against the eardrum through the external ear canal, and a charge-coupled device (CCD) camera captures images of the eardrum. The resulting magnified images can be presented on a monitor, thereby allowing clinicians to accurately diagnose middle ear effusion [33]. Guo and Shiao conducted a prospective study on the diagnostic efficacy of videotelescopy, pneumatic otoscopy, and tympanometry for the detection of pediatric OME. Their results demonstrate that the sensitivity, specificity, and accuracy of the videotelescopy were 97.8, 100, and 98.0%, respectively. These values significantly exceed the accuracy of conventional tests using pneumatic otoscope and tympanometry [33]. Videotelescopy provides clinicians with visual information with which to validate the accuracy of the pneumatic otoscopy.

Pneumatic otoscopy and even videotelescopy are difficult to administer on newborns and small infants with CLP. Thus, objective acoustic immittance testing plays an important role in the diagnosis of OME in CLP patients [34]. Tympanometry is the most commonly used acoustic immittance test to measure pressure changes in the middle ear and the compliance of the eardrum [27]. Chen et al. found that the specificity of tympanometry, when used to test for OME in infants with CLP, was relatively low (only 59.6%). When used to test infants within 9 months of age, specificity dropped to only 37.5% [28]. Furthermore, when infants are crying or unable to cooperate during testing, it can be difficult to maintain airtight conditions in the ear, thereby preventing successful completion of the examination.

Pure tone audiometry can also be used to facilitate the diagnosis of OME; the results may reveal conductive or mixed hearing loss. The cooperation of children is required for this procedure, which means that it may be unsuitable for children under 3 years of age [35]. For patients in this age group, spectral gradient acoustic reflectometry (SGAR) may be an effective alternative to pure tone audiometry in the diagnosis of OME. SGAR transmits ultrasound waves to the eardrum, whereupon a microcomputer is used to filter, record, and analyze the ultrasound waves reflected back. SGAR is an efficient diagnostic tool for the detection of OME, requiring less than one second to complete the procedure. Although the sensitivity and specificity are somewhat low, SGAR is a noninvasive test that is unaffected by crying, cerumen, client cooperation, or the quality of the air seal in the ear, thereby making it useful for testing difficult infants [28, 36–38].

6. Watchful waiting for OME

Alt first identified the relationship between CLP and hearing impairment in 1878, and OME has since been the subject of investigation [39]. The severe complications caused by OME in CLP children can have far-reaching consequences; therefore, determining the optimal treatment strategy is a topic worthy of in-depth exploration.

Many researchers have recommended watchful waiting as a treatment of choice for OME among children with CLP, particularly when parents prefer to avoid or postpone surgery. Muntz reported that more than 50% of CLP children who develop OME naturally recover from OME and have no need to undergo ventilation tube surgery after 3 years of age [40]. Flynn et al. studied the longitudinal prevalence of OME in CLP children between 7 and 16 years of age and found that middle ear problems gradually dissipate between 7 and 13 years of age [41]. Rynnel-Dagoo et al. found that 82% of the CLP children with or without OME had a normal hearing at 3–4 years of age, indicating recovery from OME [42]. Smith et al. found that the Eustachian tube function of most children with CLP significantly improved by 6–7.5 years of age [43].

A number of researchers have reported that OME and Eustachian tube function improve as the patient grows older [41, 43, 44], recommending watchful waiting for CLP children with OME for a period of 3–6 months from the diagnosis of effusion [41, 43–45]. During the observation period, patients can wear hearing aids to attain the same hearing performance of children with ventilation tubes [45]; however, it should be noted that children may find hearing aids inconvenient or may worry about the social stigma associated with wearing such aids [27, 46].

7. Ventilation tube insertion (VTI) for OME

Previous studies have shown that 90% or more of the children who undergo palatoplasty for CLP still suffer recurrent OME [20], which is a reflection of persistent poor Eustachian tube function after repair surgery [47]. Thus, many doctors prefer to perform the repair of cleft palate and ventilation tube surgery simultaneously when the child is 1 year old [2, 17, 48–50]. This combined surgical approach is done in the hope of overcoming the problem of middle ear effusion and improving the hearing ability of children, thereby enhancing their long-term linguistic development.

This chapter summarizes previous studies that addressed the effectiveness of VTI for OME in CLP children aged 18 years or less. Each of the studies we summarize below measured outcomes using a variety of methods. We attempted to normalize those measurements. As for hearing outcomes, the natural effect measure refers to the difference in hearing ability. For studies using outcome measures on different scales, we summarized the findings as the percentage of ears presenting hearing loss or improvement. For the frequency of grommet insertion, measurements were summarized as the percentages of ears that underwent one or more grommet insertions and the number of times that insertion was performed. For complications or sequelae, the main summary measure was the occurrence of complications. For middle ear status, the effect measures included the rates of OME recurrence and resolution and the percentage of ears presenting various types of tympanogram.

7.1. Comparative effectiveness for hearing outcome

7.1.1. CLP children versus age-matched non-CLP children

Two studies compared CLP children with age-matched healthy children with regard to hearing outcomes after VTI for OME [51, 52]. One prospective study with an excellent study design reported similar hearing outcomes between children with and without palate conditions (CLP group 10.5 dB versus control group 10.9 dB, $p > 0.05$, follow-up 5–7 years) over the short term [51]. The other retrospective study of moderate study design reported a significantly higher percentage of ears with hearing loss (CLP group 24% versus control group 0%, follow-up 3–5 years) [52]. However, 64% of children in the CLP group underwent VTI, while only 6% in the non-CLP group underwent VTI ($p < 0.0005$).

7.1.2. Pre-VTI versus post-VTI hearing outcomes

Hearing outcomes were evaluated in several case-series studies [16, 23, 43, 53–57]. Over the long term, between 50 and 94% of CLP children recovered normal hearing after being administered VTI in conjunction with palatoplasty (follow-up 5.5–15.4 years) [16, 43, 54–57]. Furthermore, children requiring a higher number of VTIs were at increased significant risk for long-standing hearing loss [16, 23].

7.1.3. VTI versus non-VTI

Zheng et al. conducted a randomized controlled trial to determine the effectiveness of grommets on hearing recovery among CLP children with OME [58]. The authors reported hearing improvement in only 22 of 39 CLP children with VTI; however, no hearing results were obtained from those that did not undergo VTI. Furthermore, the authors reported hearing outcomes over the short term (6 months of observation); however, little emphasis was placed on the long-term outcomes, which makes it difficult to interpret their results.

Several prospective [51, 59, 60] and retrospective [20, 44, 46, 52, 61–68] cohort studies evaluated hearing outcomes. Among these cohort studies, several studies compared VTI with non-VTI (i.e., myringotomy alone, hearing aids, watchful waiting) [44, 60, 62, 64–68]. It has been reported that the improvements in hearing afforded by VTI over the short term (within 18 months after VTI) are more pronounced than those of myringotomy, watchful waiting, or HA [64–66]. Potsic et al. found that, compared with CLP children without VTI for OME, those with VTI had a lower percentage of ears presenting hearing loss over the short term (less than 5 years) [68]. As for long-term hearing outcomes, Hubbard et al. reported that early VTI (3 month of age) could have a greater effect on hearing than that achieved when adopting a conservative approach to treatment [60].

Despite the fact that most studies on hearing outcomes have advocated VTI for CLP children, a number of researchers have expressed reservations, based on conflicting results. Some cohort studies observed that CLP children that had undergone VTI for OME presented worse hearing outcomes over the short term (less than 5 years) [44] or a higher percentage of ears with hearing loss after surgery over the long term (9–21 years), compared to children that did not undergo the procedure [62, 67].

7.1.4. Summary of evidence on hearing outcome

More than half (50–94%) of CLP children recovered normal hearing 5–15 years after VTI [16, 43, 54–57]. Moreover, compared with conservative management, most studies have shown that VTI is beneficial to hearing recovery over the short as well as long term [60, 64–66, 68]. There remains a belief that early VTI at the time of palatoplasty is beneficial; however [69], there is little evidence indicating the optimal timing for grommet insertion.

7.2. Comparative effectiveness for speech and language outcomes

7.2.1. CLP children versus age- and sex-matched non-CLP control

One article compared CLP children with age- and sex-matched non-CLP controls with regard to post-VTI speech and language outcomes [69]. Normal or near-normal speech intelligibility ratings were similar in CLP (90%) and non-CLP children (96%).

7.2.2. VTI versus non-VTI

Several studies have assessed speech and language outcomes in CLP patients with OME, including prospective [60] and retrospective cohort studies [44, 69–72]. Five articles compared children that were or were not administered VTI for OME [44, 60, 70–72]. No differences in speech or language development were observed in short-term (0–5 years) [44, 72] or long-term (8–10 years) [70, 71] follow-ups. With one exception, all investigators used the same number of CLP children matched for cleft type, age, sex, socioeconomic status, and birth order. After a 9-year follow-up, consonant articulation was found to be better after early VTI ($p = 0.03$) [60]. However, the authors performed myringotomy on the control group (when deemed necessary), which prevented the clear elucidation of differences in functional outcome between children that did or did not undergo VTI for OME.

7.2.3. Summary of evidence on speech and language outcomes

No differences in speech or language development were observed between CLP children that underwent conservative observation and those that underwent aggressive VTI, over the short term (0–5 years) [44, 72] or long term (8–10 years) [70, 71]. Further, assessments of speech by Merrick et al. revealed a similar percentage of children with normal or near-normal speech intelligibility ratings in the CLP and non-CLP groups [69]. These findings appear to indicate that speech and language skills do not depend on the VTI approach to OME treatment, but rather on the timing of palatoplasty.

7.3. Complications of VTI for OME

7.3.1. CLP children versus age-matched healthy children

Two studies compared age-matched healthy control children with regard to VTI complications [51, 52]. One study showed that the prognosis of children with CLP that undergo early VTI is comparable to that of children without CLP [51]; however, the other study reported contradictory results with higher rates of complications among CLP children [52].

7.3.2. VTI versus non-VTI

Several retrospective cohort studies compared children with and without VTI (i.e., hearing aids or watchful waiting) with regard to post-VTI complications [44, 46, 61, 62, 66, 67, 72]. Those studies reported higher complication rates among children with VTI than among those without, over the short term (<5 years of follow-up) [44, 46, 61, 66, 72] as well as long term (9–21 years of observation) [62, 67]. All results were statistically significant; however, differences were not calculated in two of the studies [62, 72].

Among the various types of complications, tympanosclerosis and otorrhea generally present transient but common sequelae following VTI [73, 74], with other studies reported permanent perforations and cholesteatoma [73, 75, 76]. As for the occlusion of grommets, infection, and the presence of granulation tissue, the evidence was too limited and blurred to determine the direction of effects between VTI and adverse events in CLP children with OME.

7.3.3. Tympanosclerosis

Tympanosclerosis has little influence on hearing [16, 72, 77]; however, this is the most common VTI-related complication, the rates of which were in the range of 0–52% [4, 20, 44, 46, 52–54, 57, 58, 61, 65, 67, 72, 78]. Tympanosclerosis can, albeit rarely, cause conductive hearing loss if it extensively involves the ossicle chain [72].

7.3.4. Otorrhea

Otorrhea is a complication of the tympanostomy tubes in children who are otherwise healthy [79]. However, otorrhea has not been systematically studied in CLP children after VTI. Some studies have reported a low probability (4–11.5%) of post-VTI otorrhea in CLP children [44, 50, 66, 79], whereas others reported inconsistent results (55–68%) [31, 57, 78]. The evidence is inconclusive due to conflicting results among these studies. Otorrhea appeared to be more common in ears that underwent VTI than in those that did not [66]. However, the evidence is insufficient to reveal an association between the long-term use of grommets and otorrhea. Only one study on post-VTI otorrhea reported the management of otorrhea [72]. Freeland et al.

found that although 68% of infants developed otorrhea following the use of grommets over a mean duration of 3.9 months, the otorrhea usually responded promptly to antibiotic-corticosteroid drops or systemic antibiotic treatment in more resistant cases.

7.3.5. Eardrum perforation

In CPL children, eardrum perforation occurred in 0–19% of VT-treated ears in follow-ups of 1–15 years [4, 16, 20, 43, 44, 46, 50–54, 56–58, 60, 61, 66, 67, 70, 72, 78]. In a study by Shapiro, the rate of eardrum perforation was found to be as high as 50% after VTI [80]; however, the number of children with VTI (only six children) was too small to be of reference value (low-quality study design). In contrast, eardrum perforation was observed in only 0–7% of non-VT-treated ears (i.e., observation or hearing aids) during follow-ups of 1–4 years [61, 66, 72]. In non-CLP children with OME, only one study reported a 3% incidence of post-VTI eardrum perforation within a 5-year follow-up [51].

7.3.6. Cholesteatoma

Grommet insertion has been reported to be an iatrogenic cause of secondary acquired cholesteatoma [81–86]. The development of the disease is quite uncommon, with a reported rate of approximately 1% in non-CLP children with VTI [73, 87]. However, evidence has shown that the CLP children were at increased risk of developing cholesteatoma [66, 73], with a higher rate of 0–6.9% within 12 years after VTI [16, 23, 58, 62, 66, 67, 73, 80, 88].

It should be noted that Hornigold et al. reported an incidence of 29% for CLP children 21 years after VTI for OME [62], Similarly, Spilsbury et al. conducted a retrospective cohort study on the relationship between CLP and secondary cholesteatoma following VTI in children [73]. They examined the complete hospital in-patient history of a large unselected population (869 CLP children versus 56080 non-CLP children) over a 29-year period. The authors reported that children with CLP developed cholesteatoma 7.5 (95% confidence interval, 3.8–18.2) times faster after the first VTI, compared to children without CLP.

7.3.7. Summary of evidence on VTI complications

CLP children with VTI generally have a higher risk of complications than do those without, over the short-term (less than 5 years) [44, 46, 61, 66, 72] as well as long-term (9–21 years) follow-up [62, 67]. However, compared to non-CLP children with OME, there is insufficient evidence to draw any conclusions due to conflicting results among these studies on CLP and non-CLP children [51, 52].

7.4. Comparative effectiveness for middle ear status

Previous studies have compared the effect of VTI on middle ear by using outcome measurements including the rates of OME resolution, persistent OME, and OME recurrence. The rates of OME resolution were reported in three high-quality studies, including a randomized control trial, a prospective cohort study, and a retrospective cohort study [50, 51, 58]. The rates of OME resolution ranged from 48.7 to 86% within the first 6.5 years. These results were supported by Goudy et al., who reported a median resolution time of conductive hearing loss of approximately 5 years [23]. Kuscu et al. observed that normal otoscopic examination findings were higher in CLP children without VTI than in those with VTI [89].

Persistent OME was observed in 29–52% of CLP children 4–7 years after VTI [20, 44, 68, 72]. Gordon et al. [67] found that only 5% of CLP children had persistent OME 9 years or more after palatoplasty with VTI, concluding that Eustachian tube function may be adequate by age of 9 years. These results are supported by Smith et al. [43], who found that Eustachian tube function eventually returned to normal in most CLP children and that the age of Eustachian tube normalization was approximately 8 years (1.5–17.3). As for OME recurrence, a number of studies have reported that 17–45% of CLP children had OME recurrence 3–6 years after VTI, at a mean age of approximately 7 years [20, 56, 57, 61].

7.4.1. CLP children versus non-CLP control

Four articles reported in post-VTI middle ear function in CLP and non-CLP children [51, 52, 59, 69], three of which included an age-matched non-CLP control group [51, 52, 69]. The results in studies by Ovesen and Blegvad-Andersen [52] and Broen et al. [59] were not considered for further interpretation because only 6 and 31% of the non-CLP children with OME underwent VTI, respectively. Merrick et al. reported comparable rates of persistent OME in children with and without cleft palate (24% versus 14%, $p = 0.31$) [69]. Valtonen et al. reported similar OME resolution rates in CLP and non-CLP children (64.1% versus 60.6%) [51]. In summary, the prognosis for middle ear recovery among CLP children with early VTI is comparable to that of children without CLP.

7.4.2. VTI versus non-VTI

Zheng et al. performed a randomized controlled trial comparing OME resolution rates between CLP children with and without VTI [58]. They reported a significantly higher OME resolution rate (48.7%) in children undergoing palatoplasty and VTI than in those undergoing palatoplasty alone (24.5%, $p < 0.01$). Children with VTI had a shorter observation period (6 months versus 20 months); however, the authors expected that the OME resolution rate would have been higher if the children had been followed up for the same period as those without VTI, such that the difference in resolution rate between the groups would become increasingly pronounced. In another study by Potsic et al., [68] the authors found that CLP children that did not undergo VTI had a significantly higher rate of persistent OME at the age of 5 years than did those with VTI. Freeland et al. [72] obtained the same result for CLP children at the age of 4 years. However, two other studies reported conflicting results, i.e., a higher rate of persistent OME in CLP children with VTI [44, 67].

7.4.3. Summary of evidence on middle ear status

Three high-quality studies reported that more than half (48.7–86%) of the CLP children that underwent VTI presented OME resolution within the first 6.5 years [50, 51, 58]. The median resolution time of conductive hearing loss was found to be approximately 5 years [23]. The high OME resolution rates were supported by four other studies, in which persistent OME was observed in less than half (29–52%) of the CLP children in the first 4–7 years after VTI [20, 44, 68, 72]. Eustachian tube function began to normalize by 7–9 years of age [20, 43, 44, 50, 51, 58, 67, 68, 72]. In addition, fewer than half of the CLP children (17–45%) presented OME recurrence within the first 3–6 years of follow-up [20, 56, 57, 61]. Importantly, the prognosis for CLP children that undergo early VTI was comparable to that of the children without CLP.

7.5. Frequency of grommet insertion

A significant proportion (53.2–98%) of CLP children with OME required VTI [4, 51, 54, 61, 78] with an average of between 0.55 and 2.2 VTIs per patient in the first 7 years of observation [20, 44, 59, 66]. Cleft defects play an important role in OME formation; therefore, it would be reasonable to assume a higher need for grommets in children with more overt palatal malformations. This assumption is supported by several studies [67, 71, 88], in which a relationship was established between the degree of clefting and the frequency of VTI, with severe or complete clefts more likely to involve grommet insertion. Children with cleft palate had a significantly higher frequency of VTIs than those without [51, 59]. However, this issue requires further investigation. Lithovius et al. reported that the severity of the cleft was not a significant factor related to the number of ventilation tubes required [90]. Surgical techniques used to repair the cleft palate are not significantly associated with the number of VTI required [90]; however, palatoplasty may indeed decrease the rate of ventilation tube reinsertion in children with cleft palate, as evidenced by a recent population-based study [91].

7.6. Summary of evidence pertaining to effectiveness of VTI for OME

Compared with a conservative approach, early VTI was shown to improve hearing, and this improvement was maintained in more than half of the CLP children 5–15 years after surgery. Nonetheless, VTI does not necessarily lead to improvements in speech or language development in CLP children, and the CLP children with VTI had a higher risk of complications than did those without. It appears that VTI is beneficial for the recovery from OME in CLP patients. There is insufficient evidence to suggest the optimal timing of VTI (e.g., at the time of repair of lip/palate); however, it may be convenient for surgeons to combine these procedures.

7.7. Limitations of previous studies

Despite considerable research into subgroups of CLP children with regard to the effectiveness of grommets for OME, heterogeneity in the design of studies has proven a formidable barrier to the synthesis of evidence [92, 93]. Most previous studies failed to clearly describe their criteria in the definition of OME. Previous studies included subjects of different ages with different types of cleft who had undergone different procedures and employed different criteria for VTI. Grommet insertion (unilateral or bilateral) was treated as a single procedure in some studies or as two procedures in other studies. The measures used in the studies were nonuniform; different time points were used for the determination of outcomes, and baseline measures were not always provided. Studies also varied in the length of observation periods.

Most studies in this review were retrospective studies. Only otologic findings during a particular month, or interpolation from examinations in adjoining months, were used in arriving at the monthly status of each ear. Thus, patient history was of limited value because it was difficult to determine when grommets had been extruded and if ear drainage was occurring. Due to mixed results, statistical differences could not be calculated for each complication, such that it is unclear whether the differences reached statistical significance. Finally, the issue of missing data was not taken into account.

8. Debate concerning selection of treatment strategy

A review of previous studies shows that there is currently no consensus as to the optimal method of treating OME, and many researchers are at odds regarding their views on the subject [46]. Most previous studies are based on retrospective analysis and vary widely in their design; therefore, it is difficult to make an informative comparison. Even in prospective studies on OME in CLP children [51, 58, 59], there remains a lack of high-quality, adequately powered randomized controlled trials. One reason may be that most parents require recommendations pertaining to treatment, rather than allowing their child to be randomly included in an experimental or control group, particularly children who have undergone or will undergo a series of major invasive surgeries. Thus, it is currently impossible to conduct a meta-analysis of previous research, which could be used to summarize treatment methods and/or provide guidance with regard to treatment choices [2, 45].

9. Clinical guidelines

9.1. NICE clinical guideline

The UK National Institute for Health and Clinical Excellence has published clinical guidelines for the surgical treatment of OME in children with or without CLP [45]. Those guidelines indicate that there is currently insufficient evidence to prove that simultaneous cleft palate repair surgery and ventilation tube surgery are effective approaches to the alleviation of OME. Thus, the simultaneous insertion of a ventilation tube during the surgical repair of a cleft palate is not recommended unless careful otological and audiological assessments have been performed. The guidelines recommend that treatment be based on the needs and desires of children and their parents and that ventilation tube surgery be viewed as an alternative to hearing aids in CLP children with persistent bilateral OME and hearing loss.

9.2. Clinical guidelines of AAO-HNSF, AAP, and AAFP

Updated clinical guidelines have recently been published for OME. These guidelines were codeveloped by the American Academy of Otolaryngology-Head and Neck Surgery Foundation (AAO-HNSF), the American Academy of Pediatrics (AAP), and the American Academy of Family Physicians (AAFP) [94]. The guideline update group claims that it may be appropriate to offer tympanostomy tubes on an individualized basis for cleft palate infants with OME that persists after failing hearing tests. They claim that resolving the issue of middle ear effusion could facilitate the assessment of hearing status.

It is also recommended that clinicians evaluate children with cleft palate for OME and hearing loss at the time at which cleft palate is first diagnosed. Monitoring for OME and hearing loss should continue throughout childhood, including after palate repair. Specifically, the guideline update group recommends that middle ear status be assessed at 12–18 months of age, considering that this is a critical period in the development of language skills, speech, balance, and coordination. By 18 months of age, delays in language and speech development are easily identified.

In these guidelines, it is recommended that VTI be considered when type B tympanogram or OME persists for 3 months or longer. These recommendations are based on the assumption that the likelihood of spontaneous resolution is low. For children who do not receive tympanostomy tubes, the follow-up schedule to monitor OME and hearing loss until OME resolves should be more frequent than the 3- to 6-month intervals recommended for children without cleft palate.

9.3. PRISMA-compliant systematic review

Many clinical guidelines fail to provide clear recommendations with regard to treatment approaches, due to a lack of conclusive studies [27, 95]. Despite the fact that a number of reviews have been published on treatment choices for the management of OME in CLP children, a number of these are narrative reviews [3, 6, 96–98], whereas others are systematic reviews pertaining mainly to otherwise healthy children [27, 45, 77, 95, 99–105]. The lack of research on the CLP subgroup of children means that there is currently no evidence-based information for clinicians or parents with regard to the effectiveness of grommets for OME in CLP children.

Ponduri et al. performed a systematic review on the routine early insertion of grommets for OME in CLP children [2]. The authors concluded that there is currently insufficient evidence on which to base recommendations pertaining to clinical practice in this area. However, they did not perform data synthesis with regard to patient-centered outcomes, nor did they provide a detailed, well-described protocol, such as The Cochrane [106] and PRISMA [107]. A systematic review based on predefined eligibility criteria conducted in accordance with a predefined methodological approach could facilitate the appraisal of review methods and reveal modifications to methods and selective reporting in completed reviews [108].

A recent systematic review by Kuo et al. published in *Pediatrics* addressed the effects of VTI in children with cleft palate and OME with regard to patient-centered outcomes [109]. The review followed the protocol outlined in Preferred Reporting Items for Systematic Reviews and Meta-analyses (PRISMA) to enable full and transparent assessment of the existing literature, in order to provide evidence-based information pertaining to the management of OME in children with cleft palate.

That review indicated that 38–53% of CLP children underwent VTI for OME and that more severe cases were more likely to undergo grommet insertion. Compared with a conservative approach, it appears that VTI may improve hearing outcomes in CLP children and that these improvements could remain for at least 1–9 years after surgery. In addition, children who have undergone VTI face a higher risk of complications than do those who have not received this form of treatment. The most common post-VTI complications include eardrum retraction and tympanosclerosis, with incidence rates of 11–37%. Of particular importance is the need to perform grommet insertion within a highly specified time frame. The authors concluded that existing evidence is insufficient to support any assertions with regard to the use of grommets, either therapeutically or prophylactically, at the time of palatoplasty or afterward.

9.4. Future research needs

In the future, there may be a need to develop rigorous methodologies for the examination of functional outcomes in CLP children after VTI. Further multi-institute prospective studies or well-designed randomized controlled trials are needed to develop a comprehensive base of evidence sufficient to clarify the effectiveness of VTI for OME in CLP children.

10. Recommendations for management

Strategies related to the treatment of OME in CLP children are still under debate, and there is insufficient evidence with which to establish absolute guidelines. We believe that the lack of consensus regarding the optimal treatment for OME in CLP children should prompt a relatively conservative approach. Patients and parents should also be given a range of treatment options based on their individual needs and desires.

Figure 1 presents a flowchart of recommended OME management in CLP children. From the time of birth, children with CLP should undergo continual and regular otologic examinations and audiological monitoring for the assessment of OME. Children with delayed speech and/or language development should be suspected of having OME, such that otolaryngology referral is indicated. Once OME is confirmed, the coexisting sensorineural component of hearing loss should be further investigated. It is recommended that children suffering from middle ear effusion without significant hearing loss (hearing threshold ≤30 dB) remain under observation [45]. Children with hearing loss exceeding 30 dB can be managed through active observation for 3 months or alternatively referred for surgery, in accordance with the child's developmental, social, and educational status. If a patient suffers OME in only one ear, the observation period may be extended to 6 months [49]. During the observation period, hearing aids could be considered [110]. Patients suffering from recurrent OME following surgery may undergo repeated ventilation tube surgery, and those in whom the disease persists after an observation period of 3–6 months may be referred for surgery.

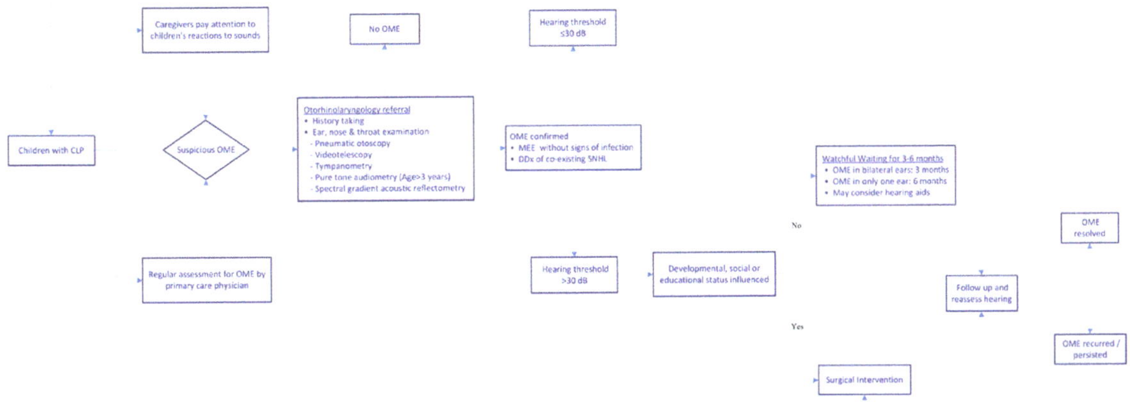

Figure 1. Flowchart of recommended management guidance for OME in CLP children. OME, otitis media with effusion; CLP, cleft lip/palate; MEE, middle ear effusion; DDX, differential diagnosis; dB, decibel; SNHL, sensorineural hearing loss.

11. Summary

Otitis media with effusion associated with Eustachian tube dysfunction can seriously affect hearing in children with CLP, which can lead to linguistic and speech disorders, and ultimately to the disruption of learning and development. Compared with watchful waiting or hearing aids, VTI has been shown to improve hearing in more than half of CLP children 5–15 years after surgery. VTI and the conservative approach do not appear to differ with regard to speech and language outcomes. CLP children that undergo VTI present a higher risk of complications than do children without VTI. It has been shown that VTI is beneficial in helping CLP patients to recover from OME. There is insufficient evidence with regard to the timing of VTI (e.g., prophylactic insertion during repair of lip or palate). This summary is based on underpowered studies, and the evidence for each outcome is inconclusive. The lack of concrete evidence regarding the optimal treatment for OME in CLP children should prompt a relatively conservative approach. Most importantly, the needs of children and their parents must be taken into consideration. Only a consensus between patients/parents and surgeons regarding the most suitable treatment strategy for OME can ensure the greatest benefits.

Disclosures

Competing interests: None

Funding/support: This study was sponsored by grants from Taoyuan Armed Forces General Hospital (No. 10507 and No. 10626), Taoyuan, Taiwan, ROC.

Acknowledgements

The chapter partly borrows from the authors' earlier publications [Refs. 3 and 109].

Author details

Chin-Lung Kuo[1, 2, 3, 4*] and An-Suey Shiao[1, 2*]

*Address all correspondence to: asshiao@gmail.com; drkuochinlung@gmail.com

1 Department of Otolaryngology-Head and Neck Surgery, Taipei Veterans General Hospital, Taipei, Taiwan, ROC

2 Department of Otolaryngology, National Yang-Ming University, School of Medicine, Taipei, Taiwan, ROC

3 Institute of Brain Science, National Yang-Ming University, Taipei, Taiwan, ROC

4 Department of Otolaryngology, Taoyuan Armed Forces General Hospital, Taoyuan, Taiwan, ROC

References

[1] Lilja J. Cleft lip and palate surgery. *Scand J Surg* 2003; 92:269–273.

[2] Ponduri S, Bradley R, Ellis PE, Brookes ST, Sandy JR, Ness AR. The management of otitis media with early routine insertion of grommets in children with cleft palate – a systematic review. *Cleft Palate Craniofac J* 2009; 46:30–38.

[3] Kuo CL, Lien CF, Chu CH, Shiao AS. Otitis media with effusion in children with cleft lip and palate: a narrative review. *Int J Pediatr Otorhinolaryngol* 2013; 77:1403–1409.

[4] Szabo C, Langevin K, Schoem S, Mabry K. Treatment of persistent middle ear effusion in cleft palate patients. *Int J Pediatr Otorhinolaryngol* 2010; 74:874–877.

[5] Dhillon RS. The middle ear in cleft palate children pre and post palatal closure. *J R Soc Med* 1988; 81:710–713.

[6] Sharma RK, Nanda V. Problems of middle ear and hearing in cleft children. *Indian J Plast Surg* 2009; 42(Suppl):S144–S148.

[7] Bluestone CD, Klein JO. Pediatric otolaryngology. In: Bluestone CD, Stool SE, Alper CM (eds). Philadelphia: Saunders, 2003:474–685.

[8] Kuo CL, Wang MC, Chu CH, Shiao AS. New therapeutic strategy for treating otitis media with effusion in postirradiated nasopharyngeal carcinoma patients. *J Chinese Med Assoc* 2012; 75:329–334.

[9] Chang CW, Yang YW, Fu CY, Shiao AS. Differences between children and adults with otitis media with effusion treated with CO_2 laser myringotomy. *J Chin Med Assoc* 2012; 75:29–35.

[10] Takasaki K, Sando I, Balaban CD, Ishijima K. Postnatal development of eustachian tube cartilage. A study of normal and cleft palate cases. *Int J Pediatr Otorhinolaryngol* 2000; 52:31–36.

[11] Stool SE, Randall P. Unexpected ear disease in infants with cleft palate. *Cleft Palate J* 1967; 4:99–103.

[12] Bluestone CD. Studies in otitis media: children's hospital of Pittsburgh-University of Pittsburgh progress report–2004. *Laryngoscope* 2004; 114:1–26.

[13] Rajion ZA, Al-Khatib AR, Netherway DJ, et al. The nasopharynx in infants with cleft lip and palate. *Int J Pediatr Otorhinolaryngol* 2012; 76:227–234.

[14] Kemaloglu YK, Kobayashi T, Nakajima T. Analysis of the craniofacial skeleton in cleft children with otitis media with effusion. *Int J Pediatr Otorhinolaryngol* 1999; 47:57–69.

[15] Rosenfeld RM, Goldsmith AJ, Tetlus L, Balzano A. Quality of life for children with otitis media. *Arch Otolaryngol Head Neck Surg* 1997; 123:1049–1054.

[16] Sheahan P, Blayney AW, Sheahan JN, Earley MJ. Sequelae of otitis media with effusion among children with cleft lip and/or cleft palate. *Clin Otolaryngol Allied Sci* 2002; 27:494–500.

[17] Robinson PJ, Lodge S, Jones BM, Walker CC, Grant HR. The effect of palate repair on otitis media with effusion. *Plast Reconstr Surg* 1992; 89:640–645.

[18] Sheahan P, Miller I, Sheahan JN, Earley MJ, Blayney AW. Incidence and outcome of middle ear disease in cleft lip and/or cleft palate. *Int J Pediatr Otorhinolaryngol* 2003; 67:785–793.

[19] Chu KM, McPherson B. Audiological status of Chinese patients with cleft lip/palate. *Cleft Palate Craniofac J* 2005; 42:280–285.

[20] Phua YS, Salkeld LJ, de Chalain TM. Middle ear disease in children with cleft palate: protocols for management. *Int J Pediatr Otorhinolaryngol* 2009; 73:307–313.

[21] Viswanathan N, Vidler M, Richard B. Hearing thresholds in newborns with a cleft palate assessed by auditory brain stem response. *Cleft Palate Craniofac J* 2008; 45:187–192.

[22] Bluestone CD, Beery QC, Cantekin EI, Paradise JL. Eustachian tube ventilatory function in relation to cleft palate. *Ann Otol Rhinol Laryngol* 1975; 84:333–338.

[23] Goudy S, Lott D, Canady J, Smith RJ. Conductive hearing loss and otopathology in cleft palate patients. *Otolaryngol Head Neck Surg* 2006; 134:946–948.

[24] Harris L, Cushing SL, Hubbard B, Fisher D, Papsin BC, James AL. Impact of cleft palate type on the incidence of acquired cholesteatoma. *Int J Pediatr Otorhinolaryngol* 2013, http://dx.doi.org/10.1016/j.ijporl.2013.01.020.

[25] D'Mello J, Kumar S. Audiological findings in cleft palate patients attending speech camp. *Indian J Med Res* 2007; 125:777–782.

[26] Schonweiler R, Lisson JA, Schonweiler B, et al. A retrospective study of hearing, speech and language function in children with clefts following palatoplasty and veloplasty procedures at 18–24 months of age. *Int J Pediatr Otorhinolaryngol* 1999; 50:205–217.

[27] Rosenfeld RM, Culpepper L, Doyle KJ, et al. Clinical practice guideline: Otitis media with effusion. *Otolaryngol Head Neck Surg* 2004; 130:S95–S118.

[28] Chen YW, Chen KT, Chang PH, Su JL, Huang CC, TJ. L. Is otitis media with effusion almost always accompanying cleft palate in children? The experience of 319 Asian patients. *Laryngoscope* 2012; 122:220–224.

[29] Bess FH, Klee T, Culbertson JL. Identification, assessment, and management of children with unilateral sensorineural hearing loss. *Ear Hear* 1986; 7:43–51.

[30] Smith RM, McWilliams BJ. Creative thinking abilities of cleft palate children. *Cleft Palate J* 1966; 3:275–283.

[31] Paradise JL, Bluestone CD. Early treatment of the universal otitis media of infants with cleft palate. *Pediatrics* 1974; 53:48–54.

[32] Luthra S, Singh S, Nagarkar AN, Mahajan JK. The role of audiological diagnostics in children with cleft lip & palate (CLP). *Int J Pediatr Otorhinolaryngol* 2009; 73:1365–1367.

[33] Guo YC, Shiao AS. Diagnostic methods for otitis media with effusion in children. *Zhonghua Yi Xue Za Zhi (Taipei)* 2002; 65:372–377; discussion 363–374.

[34] Wimmer E, Toleti B, Berghaus A, Baumann U, Nejedlo I. Impedance audiometry in infants with a cleft palate: the standard 226-Hz probe tone has no predictive value for the middle ear condition. *Int J Pediatr Otorhinolaryngol* 2010; 74:586–590.

[35] Halloran DR, Hardin JM, Wall TC. Validity of pure-tone hearing screening at well-child visits. *Arch Pediatr Adolesc Med* 2009; 163:158–163.

[36] Schwartz DM, Schwartz RH. Validity of acoustic reflectometry in detecting middle ear effusion. *Pediatrics* 1987; 79:739–742.

[37] Oyiborhoro JM, Olaniyan SO, Newman CW, Balakrishnan SL. Efficacy of acoustic otoscope in detecting middle ear effusion in children. *Laryngoscope* 1987; 97:495–498.

[38] Pellett FS, Cox LC, MacDonald CB. Use of acoustic reflectometry in the detection of middle ear effusion. *J Am Acad Audiol* 1997; 8:181–187.

[39] Alt A. Heilunger Taubstummheit erzielte durch Bersitung einer otorrhooe einer angibornen Gaummenspalte. *Arch Augenheilkd* 1878; 7:211–213.

[40] Muntz HR. An overview of middle ear disease in cleft palate children. *Facial Plast Surg* 1993; 9:177–180.

[41] Flynn T, Lohmander A, Moller C, Magnusson L. A longitudinal study of hearing and middle ear status in adolescents with cleft lip and palate. *Laryngoscope* 2013; 123:1374–1380.

[42] Rynnel-Dagoo B, Lindberg K, Bagger-Sjoback D, Larson O. Middle ear disease in cleft palate children at three years of age. *Int J Pediatr Otorhinolaryngol* 1992; 23:201–209.

[43] Smith TL, DiRuggiero DC, Jones KR. Recovery of eustachian tube function and hearing outcome in patients with cleft palate. *Otolaryngol Head Neck Surg* 1994; 111:423–429.

[44] Robson AK, Blanshard JD, Jones K, Albery EH, Smith IM, Maw AR. A conservative approach to the management of otitis media with effusion in cleft palate children. *J Laryngol Otol* 1992; 106:788–792.

[45] NICE Clinical Guideline: *Surgical Management of Otitis Media with Effusion in Children*: National Collaborating Centre for Women's and Children's Health (UK), 2008, http://www.ncbi.nlm.nih.gov/pubmedhealth/PMH0009526/.

[46] Gani B, Kinshuck AJ, Sharma R. A review of hearing loss in cleft palate patients. *Int J Otolaryngol* 2012; 2012:548698.

[47] Alper CM, Losee JE, Mandel EM, Seroky JT, Swarts JD, Doyle WJ. Pre- and post-palatoplasty Eustachian tube function in infants with cleft palate. *Int J Pediatr Otorhinolaryngol* 2012; 76:388–391.

[48] Andrews PJ, Chorbachi R, Sirimanna T, Sommerlad B, Hartley BE. Evaluation of hearing thresholds in 3-month-old children with a cleft palate: the basis for a selective policy for ventilation tube insertion at time of palate repair. *Clin Otolaryngol Allied Sci* 2004; 29:10–17.

[49] Ahn JH, Kang WS, Kim JH, Koh KS, Yoon TH. Clinical manifestation and risk factors of children with cleft palate receiving repeated ventilating tube insertions for treatment of recurrent otitis media with effusion. *Acta Otolaryngol* 2012; 132:702–707.

[50] Klockars T, Rautio J. Early placement of ventilation tubes in cleft lip and palate patients: does palatal closure affect tube occlusion and short-term outcome? *Int J Pediatr Otorhinolaryngol* 2012; 76:1481–1484.

[51] Valtonen H, Dietz A, Qvarnberg Y. Long-term clinical, audiologic, and radiologic outcomes in palate cleft children treated with early tympanostomy for otitis media with effusion: a controlled prospective study. *Laryngoscope* 2005; 115:1512–1516.

[52] Ovesen T, Blegvad-Andersen O. Alterations in tympanic membrane appearance and middle ear function in 11-year-old children with complete unilateral cleft lip and palate compared with healthy age-matched subjects. *Clin Otolaryngol Allied Sci* 1992; 17:203–207.

[53] He Y, Xu H, Zhen Q, Liao X, Xu L, Zhen Y. The influence of palatoplasty and tympanotomy on middle ear function in cleft palate patients. *Hua Xi Kou Qiang Yi Xue Za Zhi* 2001; 19:243–245.

[54] Koempel JA, Kumar A. Long-term otologic status of older cleft palate patients. *Indian J Pediatr* 1997; 64:793–800.

[55] Fria TJ, Paradise JL, Sabo DL, Elster BA. Conductive hearing loss in infants and young children with cleft palate. *J Pediatr* 1987; 111:84–87.

[56] Frable MA, Brandon GT, Theogaraj SD. Velar closure and ear tubings as a primary procedure in the repair of cleft palates. *Laryngoscope* 1985; 95:1044–1046.

[57] Moller P. Hearing, middle ear pressure and otopathology in a cleft palate population. *Acta Otolaryngol* 1981; 92:521–528.

[58] Zheng Q, Xu H, He Y. Effects of tympanotomy and pressure equilibrium tube insertion during palatoplasty on prognoses of otitis media with effusion. *Hua Xi Kou Qiang Yi Xue Za Zhi* 2003; 21:28–30.

[59] Broen PA, Moller KT, Carlstrom J, Doyle SS, Devers M, Keenan KM. Comparison of the hearing histories of children with and without cleft palate. *Cleft Palate Craniofac J* 1996; 33:127–133.

[60] Hubbard TW, Paradise JL, McWilliams BJ, Elster BA, Taylor FH. Consequences of unremitting middle-ear disease in early life. Otologic, audiologic, and developmental findings in children with cleft palate. *N Engl J Med* 1985; 312:1529–1534.

[61] Kwan WM, Abdullah VJ, Liu K, van Hasselt CA, Tong MC. Otitis media with effusion and hearing loss in chinese children with cleft lip and palate. *Cleft Palate Craniofac J* 2011; 48:684–689.

[62] Hornigold R, Morley A, Glore RJ, Boorman J, Sergeant R. The long-term effect of unilateral t-tube insertion in patients undergoing cleft palate repair: 20-year follow-up of a randomised controlled trial. *Clin Otolaryngol* 2008; 33:265–268.

[63] Chen JL, Messner AH, Curtin G. Newborn hearing screening in infants with cleft palates. *Otol Neurotol* 2008; 29:812–815.

[64] Li W, Shang W, Yu AH, et al. Early treatment of middle ear disease in cleft palate infants. *Hua Xi Kou Qiang Yi Xue Za Zhi* 2007; 25:458–462.

[65] Liu L, Sun YG, Ma L, Zhao W, Wu R. Effect of ventilation tube insertion on otitis media with effusion in cleft palate children. *Zhonghua Er Bi Yan Hou Ke Za Zhi* 2004; 39:216–218.

[66] Maheshwar AA, Milling MA, Kumar M, Clayton MI, Thomas A. Use of hearing aids in the management of children with cleft palate. *Int J Pediatr Otorhinolaryngol* 2002; 66:55–62.

[67] Gordon AS, Jean-Louis F, Morton RP. Late ear sequelae in cleft palate patients. *Int J Pediatr Otorhinolaryngol* 1988; 15:149–156.

[68] Potsic WP, Cohen M, Randall P, Winchester R. A retrospective study of hearing impairment in three groups of cleft palate patients. *Cleft Palate J* 1979; 16:56–58.

[69] Merrick GD, Kunjur J, Watts R, Markus AF. The effect of early insertion of grommets on the development of speech in children with cleft palates. *Br J Oral Maxillofac Surg* 2007; 45:527–533.

[70] Kobayashi H, Sakuma T, Yamada N, Suzaki H. Clinical outcomes of ventilation tube placement in children with cleft palate. *Int J Pediatr Otorhinolaryngol* 2012; 76:718–721.

[71] Shaw R, Richardson D, McMahon S. Conservative management of otitis media in cleft palate. *J Craniomaxillofac Surg* 2003; 31:316–320.

[72] Freeland AP, Evans DM. Middle ear disease in the cleft palate infant: its effect on speech and language development. *Br J Plast Surg* 1981; 34:142–143.

[73] Spilsbury K, Ha JF, Semmens JB, Lannigan F. Cholesteatoma in cleft lip and palate: a population-based follow-up study of children after ventilation tubes. *Laryngoscope* 2013; 123:2024–2029.

[74] Kay DJ, Nelson M, Rosenfeld RM. Meta-analysis of tympanostomy tube sequelae. *Otolaryngol Head Neck Surg* 2001; 124:374–380.

[75] Golz A, Goldenberg D, Netzer A, et al. Cholesteatomas associated with ventilation tube insertion. *Arch Otolaryngol Head Neck Surg* 1999; 125:754–757.

[76] Herdman R, Wright JL. Grommets and cholesteatoma in children. *J Laryngol Otol* 1988; 102:1000–1002.

[77] Hellstrom S, Groth A, Jorgensen F, et al. Ventilation tube treatment: a systematic review of the literature. *Otolaryngol Head Neck Surg* 2011; 145:383–395.

[78] Moller P. Selective use of ventilating tubes in the treatment of secretory otitis media and retractions of the eardrum. *Acta Otolaryngol* 1982; 94(Suppl 386):158–160.

[79] Curtin G, Messner AH, Chang KW. Otorrhea in infants with tympanostomy tubes before and after surgical repair of a cleft palate. *Arch Otolaryngol Head Neck Surg* 2009; 135:748–751.

[80] Shapiro RS. Otologic findings in an Inuit population of cleft palate children. *J Otolaryngol* 1988; 17:101–102.

[81] Yamamoto Y, Takahashi K, Morita Y, Takahashi S. Clinical behavior and pathogenesis of secondary acquired cholesteatoma with a tympanic membrane perforation. *Acta Otolaryngol* 2013; 133:1035–1039.

[82] Kuo CL, Shiao AS, Yung M, et al. Updates and knowledge gaps in cholesteatoma research. *BioMed Res Int* 2015; 2015:854024.

[83] Kuo CL. Etiopathogenesis of acquired cholesteatoma: prominent theories and recent advances in biomolecular research. *Laryngoscope* 2015; 125:234–240.

[84] Kuo CL, Liao WH, Shiao AS. A review of current progress in acquired cholesteatoma management. *Eur Archives Oto-Rhino-Laryngol Off J Eur Fed Oto-Rhino-Laryngol Soc* 2015; 272:3601–3609.

[85] Kuo CL. *Chapter 12. Recent Advances in Understanding Pathogenesis of Acquired Cholesteatoma. Recent Advances in Otolaryngology Head and Neck Surgery*. India: Jaypee Brothers Medical Publishers. 2016, Vol. 5, pp. 167–190.

[86] Kuo CL. In reference to A new theory on the pathogenesis of acquired cholesteatoma: mucosal traction. *Laryngoscope* 2016; 126:E132.

[87] Vlastarakos PV, Nikolopoulos TP, Korres S, Tavoulari E, Tzagaroulakis A, Ferekidis E. Grommets in otitis media with effusion: the most frequent operation in children. But is it associated with significant complications? *Eur J Pediatr* 2007; 166:385–391.

[88] Caglar O, Bulbul F, Sennaroglu L. Incidence of otitis media with effusion and long-term clinical findings in children with cleft lip and palate types. *Kulak Burun Bogaz Ihtis Derg* 2013; 23:268–274.

[89] Kuscu O, Gunaydin RO, Icen M, et al. The effect of early routine grommet insertion on management of otitis media with effusion in children with cleft palate. *J Craniomaxillofac Surg* 2015; 43:2112–2115.

[90] Lithovius RH, Lehtonen V, Autio TJ, et al. The association of cleft severity and cleft palate repair technique on hearing outcomes in children in northern Finland. *J Craniomaxillofac Surg* 2015; 43:1863–1867.

[91] Huang CY, Wu CS, Tang CH, Wang MC, Kuo TY, Tu TY. Palatoplasty decreases the re-insertion rate of middle ear ventilation tube in cleft palate children – a population-based birth cohort study. *Acta Otolaryngol* 2016; 136:768–774.

[92] Kuo CL. A critical appraisal of ventilation tube insertion in children with cleft palate. *JAMA Otolaryngol Head Neck Sur* 2015; 141:189–190.

[93] Kuo CL, Tsao YH, Shiao AS. Critical reassessment of the probability of receiving additional ventilation tube insertion for recurrent otitis media with effusion in children with cleft palate. *Acta Otolaryngol* 2015; 135:519–520.

[94] Rosenfeld RM, Shin JJ, Schwartz SR, et al. Clinical practice guideline: otitis media with effusion executive summary (update). *Otolaryngol Head Neck Surg* 2016; 154:201–214.

[95] Browning GG, Rovers MM, Williamson I, Lous J, Burton MJ. Grommets (ventilation tubes) for hearing loss associated with otitis media with effusion in children. Cochrane Database of Systematic Reviews 2010, Issue 10. Art. No.: CD001801. DOI: 10.1002/14651858.CD001801.pub3

[96] Sheahan P, Blayney AW. Cleft palate and otitis media with effusion: a review. *Rev Laryngol Otol Rhinol (Bord)* 2003; 124:171–177.

[97] Paradise JL. Middle ear problems associated with cleft palate. An internationally-oriented review. *Cleft Palate J* 1975; 12:17–22.

[98] Yules RB. Current concepts of treatment of ear disease in cleft palate children and adults. *Cleft Palate J* 1975; 12:315–322.

[99] Rosenfeld RM, Schwartz SR, Pynnonen MA, et al. Clinical practice guideline: tympanostomy tubes in children. *Otolaryngol Head Neck Surg* 2013; 149:S1–S35.

[100] Wallace IF, Berkman ND, Lohr KN, Harrison MF, Kimple AJ, Steiner MJ. Surgical treatments for otitis media with effusion: a systematic review. *Pediatrics* 2014.

[101] Berkman ND, Wallace IF, Steiner MJ, et al. Otitis media with effusion: comparative effectiveness of treatments. *Comparative Effectiveness Review No. 101 (Prepared by the RTI-UNC Evidence-based Practice Center under Contract No. 290-2007-10056-1).* 2013.

[102] McDonald S, Langton Hewer CD, Nunez DA. Grommets (ventilation tubes) for recurrent acute otitis media in children. Cochrane Database of Systematic Reviews 2008, Issue 4. Art. No.: CD004741. DOI: 10.1002/14651858.CD004741.pub2.

[103] Perera R, Haynes J, Glasziou PP, Heneghan CJ. Autoinflation for hearing loss associated with otitis media with effusion. Cochrane Database of Systematic Reviews 2006, Issue 4. Art. No.: CD006285. DOI: 10.1002/14651858.CD006285.

[104] van den Aardweg MTA, Schilder AGM, Herkert E, Boonacker CWB, Rovers MM. Adenoidectomy for otitis media in children. Cochrane Database of Systematic Reviews 2010, Issue 1. Art. No.: CD007810. DOI: 10.1002/14651858.CD007810.pub2.

[105] van Zon A, van der Heijden GJ, van Dongen TMA, Burton MJ, Schilder AGM. Antibiotics for otitis media with effusion in children. Cochrane Database of Systematic Reviews 2012, Issue 9. Art. No.: CD009163. DOI: 10.1002/14651858.CD009163.pub2.

[106] Higgins JPT, Green S (eds). *Cochrane Handbook for Systematic Reviews of Interventions Version 5.1.0* [updated March 2011]. The Cochrane Collaboration, 2011. Available from http://handbook.cochrane.org.

[107] Liberati A, Altman DG, Tetzlaff J, et al. The PRISMA statement for reporting systematic reviews and meta-analyses of studies that evaluate health care interventions: explanation and elaboration. *PLoS Med* 2009; 6:e1000100.

[108] Moher D, Shamseer L, Clarke M, et al. Preferred reporting items for systematic review and meta-analysis protocols (PRISMA-P) 2015 statement. *Systematic Rev* 2015; 4:1.

[109] Kuo CL, Tsao YH, Cheng HM, et al. Grommets for otitis media with effusion in children with cleft palate: a systematic review. *Pediatrics* 2014; 134:983–994.

[110] Smallridge J, Hall AJ, Chorbachi R, et al. Functional outcomes in the Cleft Care UK study–Part 3: oral health and audiology. *Orthodontics Craniofacial Res* 2015; 18(Suppl 2):25–35.

10

Epidemiology of Cleft Lip and Palate

Mairaj K. Ahmed, Anthony H. Bui and
Emanuela Taioli

Abstract

Orofacial cleft (OFC) anomalies are amongst the most common congenital anomalies and the most common craniofacial anomalies. Despite their poorly characterized etiologies, cases of OFC are usually grouped by epidemiological studies as cleft lip, with or without cleft palate (CL/P), and cleft palate alone (CPO). Incidence of CL/P and CPO differs according to gender and ancestry and may vary widely across studies. Cases of OFC are characterized as either "syndromic" or "nonsyndromic," with further classification of nonsyndromic cases into isolated cases and cases that present with additional malformations. The genetic bases for many syndromic cases of OFC have been previously elucidated. Genetic associations have been described for nonsyndromic OFC as well. Importantly, etiology of OFC is known to involve interaction between genetic and environmental factors, including maternal nutrition and exposure to teratogenic agents. Furthermore, evidence points toward epigenetic as well as genetic factors influencing OFC etiology. Recent studies have begun to explore the association between CL/P and cancer. These studies report higher incidence of cancer among patients with CL/P and their family members as well as identification of common genetic markers mediating this increased risk, although much remains unknown about this link.

Keywords: cleft, epidemiology, etiology, genetics, epigenetics, environmental risk factors, cancer

1. Introduction

Orofacial cleft (OFC) anomalies may be unilateral or bilateral and involve the lip, the palate, or both. Due to similar phenotypic overlap and resulting health care needs of these patients, epidemiological studies usually group cleft lip, with or without cleft palate (CL/P), and cleft palate alone (CPO) even though the etiology of each may be unique. Whether or not CL/P and CPO have distinct etiology and should be combined in investigations is under debate.

It is often found in epidemiological studies that CL/P and CPO is considered underneath the umbrella of either "syndromic" or "nonsyndromic." Furthermore, "nonsyndromic" CL/P and CPO cases can be subgrouped into those that are isolated or those that have additional malformations that do not form a recognizable syndrome. Relatively, the etiology of non-syndromic cases of CL/P and CPO is lesser known compared to those found identified with a syndrome. Due to the poorly characterized etiology of CL/P and CPO, in general, there is still debate for the best method of grouping CL/P and CPO in epidemiological studies, but the most common current classifications are used to help determine associations and thus help the clinician with their diagnosis and subsequent treatment.

The genetic basis for many syndromic cases of CL/P and CPO are well-described. Evidence for genetic factors underlying nonsyndromic CL/P and CPO has begun to materialize as well. While less well-described, it is also known that epigenetic modifications can play a role in the development of CL/P and CPO. Recently, the association between OFC and cancer has been explored, with evidence suggesting existence of a link between the presence of OFC in patients and risk of cancer in these patients and/or their families.

2. Descriptive epidemiology

2.1. Prevalence

The overall prevalence of OFC is estimated to be approximately 1 in 700 live births, accounting for nearly one half of all craniofacial anomalies [1, 2]. As reported by the World Health Organization (WHO), the prevalence at birth of OFC varies worldwide, ranging 3.4–22.9 per 10,000 births for CL/P, and 1.3–25.3 per 10,000 births for CPO [3]. The incidence of CL/P and CPO can vary greatly between studies. The inclusion criteria, case definition, data sources, and selection bias contribute to the varying incidence estimates. Even though there are many different variables regarding the inclusion or exclusion criteria of in studies, the majority report a higher incidence of CL/P compared to CPO.

Prevalence has been found to vary based on ancestry, with the highest incidence rates observed amongst Asian populations (0.82–4.04 per 1000 live births), intermediate rates amongst Caucasians (0.9–2.69 per 1000 live births), and the lowest rates amongst African populations (0.18–1.67 per 1000 live births) [1, 4]. Prevalence has also been found to vary further by subgroup, for example, with one study reporting lower rates of OFC amongst Far East Asians compared to Filipinos [5].

2.2. Gender ratio

Prevalence of OFC additionally varies according to gender and cleft pattern. Male predominance has been consistently identified in CLP, with a male/female sex ratio of 1.81 (CI 95%:

1.75–1.86). For CP, the opposite has been shown, with a reported sex ratio of 0.93 (CI 95%: 0.89–0.96) [3]; however, this may be due in part to sampling bias, as one Danish study could not find a significant predominance of females in individuals with CP after combining both surgically treated and nonsurgically treated cases [6].

2.3. Laterality

OFC may be unilateral or bilateral. According to the International Perinatal Database of Typical Orofacial Clefts (IPDTOC) working group, the proportion of bilateral cases is 10.3% for cleft lip without palate (CL) and 30.2% for cleft lip with palate (CLP). Amongst unilateral cases, 36.9% of CL and 41.1% of CLP occur on the right side, suggesting that unilateral cases of CL/P occur more frequently on the left [7].

3. Classification

It is often found in epidemiological studies that CL/P and CPO are classified as either "syndromic" or "nonsyndromic." Cases of "nonsyndromic" CL/P and CPO are further categorized as isolated—those without an underlying syndrome or additional, nonsecondary malformations—or multiple—those that have additional malformations that do not form a recognizable syndrome. These distinctions are important epidemiologically, for identifying homogenous subgroups of cases, and clinically, for informing prognosis, recurrence risk, diagnosis, and treatment plan.

3.1. Syndromic

Individuals with "syndromic" CL/P or CP present with patterns of malformations and/or symptomatology that form a recognizable syndrome of known or unknown origin; hence, the CL/P or CP is part of a syndrome. Recognition of these syndromes is essential for assessing the risks faced by the child, providing the necessary treatment, and counseling the parents. Because the prevalence of associated anomalies varies across different populations of individuals with OFC, better understanding of the epidemiology of these anomalies could aid in the proper identification and characterization of the syndrome, leading to better care for the individual. Syndromes associated with OFC for which the underlying cause is known include chromosomal abnormalities, such as trisomy 13 or 18, Mendelian disorders such as Van der Woude Syndrome and teratogenic exposure.

A guideline for identifying syndromes in individuals with CL/P or CP is outlined by Venkatesh as follows [8]:

- Thorough clinical examination, preferably by geneticist or dysmorphologist.
- Comprehensive medical history: description of the cleft, antenatal history, birth history, developmental history, and family history.

- Physical examination: measurement of weight, length or height, and occipitofrontal circumference, identification of anomalies of eyes, ears, heart, extremities, and also to look for associated preauricular tags, lip pits, and epicanthal folds.
- Documentation by photographs of all affected individuals and first-degree relatives.
- Necessary laboratory and radiological evaluations.

3.2. Multiple

The multiple subset of CL/P and CPO includes those cases that are not a part of a recognizable syndrome and have major other malformations which may involve, but are not limited to, the eye, ear, head, neck, respiratory tract, gastrointestinal tract, and musculoskeletal system [5, 9]. Cases of "multiple nonsyndromic" CL/P and CPO may be classified as such simply by virtue of unrecognized syndromes or undocumented teratogenic exposures. Furthermore, wide variation exists in the classification of associated anomalies in cases of OFC [10].

3.3. Isolated

Cases of CL/P and CPO that are classified as "isolated" do not have an underlying syndrome or other secondary malformations. Most epidemiological studies of CL/P and CPO focus on those cases that are isolated in hopes to further gain insight into associations.

4. Etiology

Development of the head and face represents one of the most intricate events during embryonic development, synchronized by a network of transcription factors and signaling molecules together with proteins conferring cell polarity and cell-cell interactions. In mammals, the facial region develops from the facial primordia, which consists of the lateral and medial nasal prominences arising from the frontonasal process and the maxillary and mandibular processes arising from the first branchial arch. As demonstrated in **Figure 1**, fusion of medial nasal and maxillary prominences gives rise to the lip and primary palate, while fusion of separate palatal processes arising from the maxillary prominence gives rise to the secondary palate and occurs later during embryogenesis. These processes are known to be dependent, in part, on the migration and differentiation of neural crest cells from the neuroectoderm into the branchial arches [11].

Disturbance of this closely controlled cascade can result in a facial cleft where these facial primordia ultimately fail to meet and fuse or form the proper structures. Historically, OFCs have been classified as either CL/P or CPO [13, 14]. This broad subdivision is consistent with both the distinct developmental origins of the lip/primary palate and the secondary palate and the distinct cellular and genetic etiologies described for CL/P and CPO; cleft palate may occur secondary to or independently from cleft lip. However, there is some epidemiologic evidence suggesting that cleft lip only has distinct etiologic features from cleft lip with palate and should be classified accordingly [15, 16].

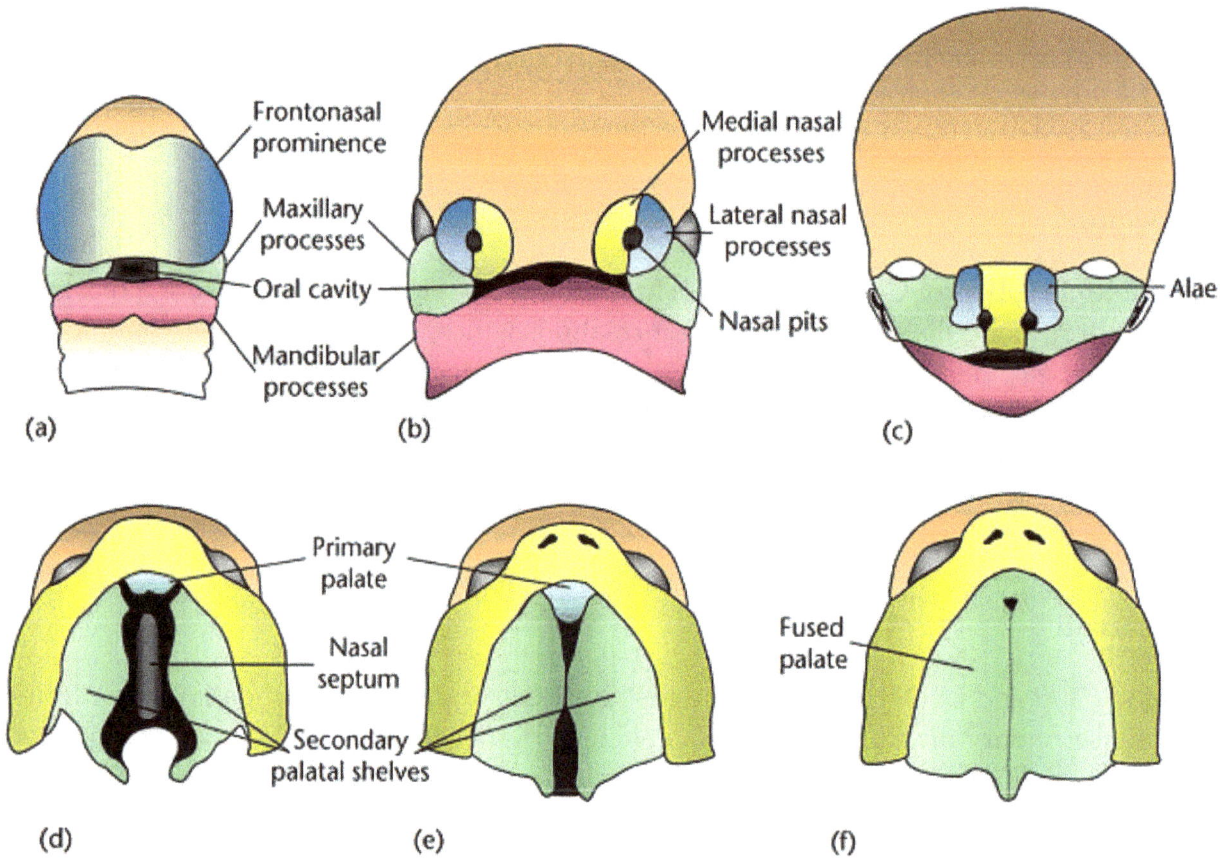

Figure 1. Schematic diagrams depicting human craniofacial development and formation of the secondary palate [12]. (a) By the fourth week of embryonic development, neural crest cells have migrated into the craniofacial region to form the frontonasal prominence, paired maxillary processes and the paired mandibular processes. (b) Formation of the nasal pits by the fifth week of embryogenesis divides the frontonasal prominence into paired medial and lateral nasal processes. (c) By the end of the sixth week of embryonic development, the medial nasal processes have merged with one another and with the maxillary processes to form the upper lip and primary palate, whereas the lateral nasal processes form the alae of the nose. The mandibular processes fuse together to form the lower jaw. (d) The secondary palate develops from the maxillary processes as bilateral outgrowths which grow vertically down the side of the tongue during the sixth week of embryogenesis. (e) During the seventh week of embryonic development, the palatal shelves elevate to a horizontal position above the tongue, make contact with one another and begin to fuse. (f) Fusion of the secondary palatal shelves with one another and with the primary palate and nasal septum is completed by the tenth week of embryogenesis. Figure is adapted from [12] © (2009) John Wiley and Sons Ltd.

5. Genetics

Both genetic and environmental factors have been shown to influence the risk of CL/P and CPO. Approximately 70% of all cases of CL/P and 50% of cases of CPO are designated as nonsyndromic [17], with the rest comprised of a wide range of malformation syndromes with known genetic and/or cellular etiologies. A summary of syndromic forms of CL/O and CPO in which the underlying genetic mutation has been elucidated is provided by Dixon et al. (**Table 1**; see original article for references) [18].

Cleft type	Syndrome	Gene
Cleft lip +/− cleft palate	Autosomal dominant developmental malformations, deafness, and dystonia	*ACTB*
	Familial gastric cancer and CLP	*CDH1*
	Craniofrontonasal	*EFNB1*
	Roberts	*ESCO2*
	Holoprosencephaly	*GLI2*
	"Oro-facial-digital"	*GLI3*
	Hydrolethalus	*HYLS1*
	Van der Woude/popliteal pterygium	*IRF6*
	X-linked mental retardation and CL/P	*PHF8*
	Gorlin	*PTCH1*
	CLP—ectodermal dysplasia	*PVRL1*
	Holoprosencephaly	*SHH*
	Holoprosencephaly	*SIX3*
	Branchio-oculo-facial	*TFAP2A*
	Holoprosencephaly	*TGIF*
	Ectrodactyly-ectodermal dysplasia-clefting	*TP73L*
	Ankyloblepharon-ectodermal dysplasia-clefting	*TP73L*
	Tetra-amelia with CLP	*WNT3*
Cleft palate only	Oculofaciocardiodental	*BCOR*
	CHARGE	*CHD7*
	Lethal and Escobar multiple pterygium	*CHRNG*
	Stickler type 1	*COL2A1*
	Stickler type 2	*COL11A1*
	Stickler type 3	*COL11A2*
	Desmosterolosis	*DHCR24*
	Smith-Lemli-Opitz	*DHCR7*
	Miller	*DHODH*
	Craniofrontonasal	*EFNB1*
	Kallmann	*FGFR1*
	Crouzon	*FGFR2*
	Apert	*FGFR2*
	Otopalatodigital types 1 and 2	*FLNA*
	Larsen syndrome; atelosteogenesis	*FLNB*
	Hereditary lymphedema-distichiasis	*FOXC2*

Cleft type	Syndrome	Gene
	Bamforth-Lazarus	*FOXE1*
	"Oro-facial-digital"	*GLI3*
	Van der Woude/popliteal pterygium	*IRF6*
	Andersen	*KCNJ2*
	Kabuki	*MLL2*
	Cornelia de Lange	*NIPBL*
	X-linked mental retardation	*PQBP1*
	Isolated cleft palate	*SATB2*
	Diastrophic dysplasia	*SLC26A2*
	Campomelic dysplasia	*SOX9*
	Pierre Robin	*SOX9*
	DiGeorge	*TBX1*
	X-linked cleft palate and ankyloglossia	*TBX22*
	Treacher Collins	*TCOF1*
	Loeys-Dietz	*TGFBR1*
	Loeys-Dietz	*TGFBR2*
	Saethre-Chotzen	*TWIST1*
Midline cleft lip	Opitz G/BBB	*MID1*
	Oro-facial-digital type I	*OFD1*

Table 1. Clefting syndromes in which the mutated gene has been identified. Adapted from Ref. [18].

In contrast, nonsyndromic CL/P is complex and multifactorial in origin. Both genetic and environmental risk factors have been shown to influence the probability of occurrence. Furthermore, there is evidence that the presence of environmental factors—in particular, maternal smoking—modulates the risk conferred by genetic factors and vice-versa, complicating the genetic analysis of nonsyndromic forms of CLP [19]. As such, multifactorial models of inheritance which allow for the evaluation of these risk factors both independently and in interaction with each other are preferred.

Association studies such as candidate gene studies, which test correlation between a phenotype and prespecified genes of interest, and genome-wide association studies (GWAS), which identify genetic variations across entire genomes that are associated with a phenotype, have been used to evaluate a variety of genetic polymorphisms associated with nonsyndromic OFC. Genes that have been examined through these studies for associations with nonsyndromic OFC exhibit a range of functions, including growth, DNA transcription, nutrient metabolism, immunity, and oncogenesis. A few such genes are described here.

5.1. Growth factors

Transforming growth factor alpha (TGF-α) is a growth factor encoded by the *TGFA* gene that serves as a ligand for the epidermal growth factor receptor, which is involved in cell proliferation, differentiation, and development [20]. The first association study of genes associated with CL/P found an association with *TFGA* [21]; however, evidence of this linkage since then has been mixed [22, 23]. *TGFA* is currently viewed as a modifier, rather than a necessary or sufficient determinant, of risk for OFC.

Proteins in the transforming growth factor beta (TGF-β) family bind various TGF-β receptors leading to recruitment and activation of the SMAD family of transcription factors. TGF-β is involved in processes including apoptosis, modulation of immune cell function, and wound healing; disruption of TGF-β has been implicated in cancer, Loeys-Dietz syndrome, and other conditions [20]. Knockout experiences in mice have shown the *TGFB3* gene to be associated with OFC [24, 25], and subsequent association studies have identified these results in humans [26].

5.2. Transcription factors

The *MSX1* gene, which is a part of the homeobox gene family, codes for a protein that is involved in transcriptional regulation during embryogenesis as well as limb pattern formation, craniofacial development (in particular odontogenesis), and tumor growth inhibition [20]. This gene has been implicated in the development of cleft in several candidate gene studies, and may even account for 1–2% of all isolated cases of OFC [27].

Interferon regulatory factor 6 (IRF6) is a transcription factor protein that is involved in early development, especially of tissue in the head and face [20]. Mutations of the *IRF6* gene at 1q32 causes Van der Woude syndrome, a Mendelian-inherited disorder which induces CL/P or CPO and accounts for about 2% of all CL/P cases [28, 29]. The overlap between phenotypic presentation of Van der Woude syndrome and isolated CL/P motivated further study into the role of *IRF6* in development of OFC. Variation at *IRF6* has been found to be strongly associated with CL/P and may account for up to 12% of the genetic contribution to CL/P at the population level [30–32]. Furthermore, the discovery of *ILF6* as a risk factor for CL/P served as an important example of elucidating genetic variants associated with cases of nonsyndromic OFC, which are often excluded from genetic analyses [33].

5.3. Nutrient metabolism

Deficient maternal folate intake has long been implicated in risk of OFC in children, leading to suggestions that mutations of the enzyme 5,10-methyltetranhydrofolate reductase (MTHFR), which catalyzes the synthesis of 5-methylenetetrahydrofolate, play a role in the etiology of cases of nonsyndromic CL/P [34]. However, results from several association studies evaluating the role of *MTHFR* mutations in CL/P have been conflicting [35–37].

Retinoic acid plays an important role during development. Its functions, mediated by retinoic acid receptor alpha (RAR-α), include regulation of development, differentiation, apoptosis, granulopoeisis, as well as transcription of genes involved in the circadian rhythm [20]. Transgenic and knockout mice studies have additionally proposed a role in facial development [38]. Mutations of the *RARA* gene have been associated with development of OFC [39].

6. Epigenetics

Due to the relative lack of success in identifying causal genetic factors involved in OFC despite the numerous association studies that have been performed, recent attention has been directed toward the role of epigenetic programming, or modifications that do not involve DNA sequencing. Commonly studied epigenetic events include histone modification, chromatin remodeling, posttranscriptional gene alteration via noncoding MicroRNAs, and DNA methylation. MicroRNAs and DNA methylation, in particular, have begun to demonstrate distinct roles in etiologies of OFC.

6.1. MicroRNAs

While protein-coding genes make up only about 1.2% of the human genome, recent estimates suggest that up to 93% of the human genome codes for RNA transcripts. MicroRNAs (miRNAs) represent the largest family of such noncoding RNAs in the human genome. They are involved in gene silencing and play important roles in cell and tissue differentiation, including development of the secondary palate [40–43]. miRNAs have been shown to orchestrate many of the processes that are central to palatal morphogenesis, including epithelial-mesenchymal transformation, platelet-derived growth factor (PDGF) and TGF-β signaling, cell migration and proliferation, and collagen synthesis [44–48]. As such, further analysis of miRNA expression and gene networks will be key to elucidating mechanisms of palatal development as well as etiologies of OFC.

6.2. DNA methylation

DNA methylation, one of the most important epigenetic modifications in mammalian cells, is a process by which methyl groups are added to DNA in order to regulate gene expression. Methylation generally occurs at cytosines within the context of symmetrical CpG dinucleotide sequences, which are often concentrated in regions known as *CpG islands* and found in both gene bodies and promoter regions [49, 50]. Classically, methylation of *CpG islands* at gene promoters is thought to induce silencing of gene transcription; however, *positive* correlation between gene body methylation and gene expression has been observed [51, 52].

DNA methylation was first identified as a potential mediator of palatal development after a series of studies in which DNA demethylating agents were used to induce cleft palate in mice [53–55]. Since then, failures in DNA methylation demonstrated involvement in craniofacial malformations including cleft palate [56, 57]. Despite the current lack of knowledge regarding the epigenetic mechanisms mediating palatal development, evidence strongly indicates that DNA methylation plays a central role in regulating this process, and may perhaps serve as future risk assessment and therapeutic targets for patients with OFC.

7. Risk factors

The role of environmental factors in the etiology of OFC has been extensively studied. Known and suspected risk factors for CL/P and CP include family history, maternal nutrition, and exposure to teratogenic agents. The upper lip and palate are developed by 7 and 9 weeks after conception, respectively. Therefore, risk factors must be present before these times to influence the risk of CL/P and CPO.

7.1. Heredity

Family history is one of the strongest risk factors for both CL/P and CP. The risk of CL/P and CP has been reported to be increased in the first-, second-, and third-degree relatives and the identical twins of individuals with CL/P and CP, with even nonsyndromic cases of CL/P exhibiting evidence of genetic components [58–61]. However, few cases demonstrate true Mendelian inheritance patterns [62]. Moreover, CL/P and CP are known to be influenced by environmental risk factors. Specifically, there is growing evidence of gene-environment interactions that may influence the risk of these conditions.

7.2. Maternal drug use

Maternal drug use seems to play only a small role for the origin of orofacial clefts, but studies have shown that maternal use of folate antagonists (valproic acid and carbamazepine), dihydrofolate reductase inhibitors (trimethoprim, triamterene, and sulfasalazine), benzodiazepines, nonsteroidal anti-inflammatory drugs, retinoids, and corticosteroids is associated with a marked increase of cleft lip and palate [63–67].

7.3. Maternal diseases

The increased risk of having a child with CL/P or CP in women with nongestational diabetes or maternal hyperthermia is well-characterized [68, 69]. Additionally, a study conducted in Hungary found an increased risk of CL/P for children born to mothers with influenza, common cold, orofacial herpes, and gastroenteritis during pregnancy, posterior CP in mothers with influenza, sinusitis, and bronchitis, and OFC in mothers with epilepsy or angina pectoris [70].

7.4. Nutrition

The role of maternal nutrient intake in the development of congenital malformations in the child has long been studied with the aim of elucidating the etiologies of specific birth defects and informing effective prevention strategies. Evidence indicates that maternal nutrient intake affects the risk of giving birth to a child with CL/P or CP. In particular, a lack of vitamin B9, more commonly known as folate (or its synthetic form, folic acid), in the mother's diet has long been linked to the risk of congenital malformations. An association between maternal folate intake and reduced risk of having a child with CL/P or CP has previously been demonstrated [71]. However, studies have not consistently linked folic acid with OFC as they have with neural tube defects [72, 73].

Previous reports have shown maternal intake of vitamins other than folate, such as other B vitamins (e.g. riboflavin), iron, zinc, and the amino acids choline, methionine, and cysteine, to be associated with reduced risk of having a child with CL/P or CP [72, 74, 75].

Vitamin A is known to play a crucial role in fetal development. Deficient and excessive intakes of vitamin A increase the risk of birth defects, including OFC, in animals as well as humans [76–79], but exact daily intake numbers have not been established [80].

7.5. Maternal exogenous exposures

Most of the CL/P and CPO epidemiologic studies support a role for environmental factors in the etiology of clefting. The most common risk factors reported were maternal exposure to tobacco products [81, 82], alcohols [83], some viral infections [70], pesticides [84], and teratogens in the workplace or at home in early pregnancy [85–87]. Recognized teratogens included rare exposures such as phenytoin, valproic acid, thalidomide, and herbicides such as dioxin. As mentioned previously, risk of CL/P or CPO conferred by these exposures—in particular tobacco—may be modulated by the presence or absence of certain genetic factors [19, 88, 89].

8. Cleft palate and cancer

Several studies from different countries (USA, Latvia, Denmark, and Brazil) have identified an association between cleft palate and cancer [90–95]. The first epidemiological studies addressed the presence of cancer in cleft lip/palate subjects and their families. Parents of kids with sporadic CL/P have a higher risk of developing cancer than control families [96], and increased risk of cancer in adulthood can be seen in a Danish population-based cohort of CL/P subjects [97]. Such studies suggested that the association was most frequent for breast cancer but also colorectal, gastric, prostate, and uterus cancers. In a large study, 313 families segregating cases of isolated CL/P, including information of 13,879 individuals, were analyzed by Vieira [93]. The study brings further evidence that individuals born with CL/P and their family members have a higher prevalence of cancer than the general population. This risk is three times higher in first- and second-degree relatives and decreases to 1.5 times in third-degree relatives.

A possible genetic link was identified in two families with mutations in the E-cadherin gene CDH1 with CL/P and hereditary diffuse gastric cancer [98]. CDH1 is highly expressed in the palate. Vogelaar et al. also identified germline mutations multiple families with gastric cancer and orofacial clefts [99]. One concern in interpreting these studies is that cleft lip/palate patients tend to have a higher prevalence of behavioral risk factors, such as smoking and drinking because of their limited social interactions as adolescents, thus are at higher risk of tobacco and alcohol-related cancers independently from their initial malformation.

What is lacking is a study of cancer cases and the risk of cleft palate in their family members. Such studies are limited by the fact that the genetic defect is still a rare event, and the number of cancer cases necessary to address the problem would be extremely large. A study conducted on family members of cancer patients (Taioli et al. [95]) involved an epidemiological questionnaire including family history of cancer and congenital oral cleft malformations that was administered to 168 cancer survivors and a population-based sample of 170 healthy subjects. In the control group, 1.2% reported a family member with CL/P; among cancer survivors, the figure was 4.2% (odds ratio: 3.7; 95% confidence interval: 0.75–17.8; $p = .07$). Among cancer survivors with a family member with CL/P, there was an apparent excess of testicular cancer and melanoma in comparison with the cancer survivors with no family history of CL/P. These preliminary results suggest a common etiologic background for cancer and CL/P.

Taken all together, the data suggest that there are shared environmental and genetic factors in families that predispose to both cleft palate and cancer.

9. Conclusion

OFCs are the most common craniofacial anomalies, and one of the most common congenital anomalies worldwide. OFCs have historically been grouped as CL/P or CPO. However, existing evidence suggests that separate etiologies may exist for cleft lip alone versus cleft lip with palate. CL/P and CPO are classified as syndromic or nonsyndromic; nonsyndromic cases are further subclassified as multiple or isolated.

Both genetic and environmental factors have been implicated in the etiology of OFC. The genes underlying a number of known syndromes associated with OFC have been identified. Furthermore, environmental factors such as alcohol and tobacco have been shown to modulate the risk of OFC conferred by certain genetic factors.

Although nonsyndromic OFCs are not traditionally the subject of genetic analysis, a number of genomic association studies have evaluated the link between genetic variants and nonsyndromic OFC. Examples of genes that have been examined in such studies include those that code for growth factors, transcription factors, and nutrient metabolism proteins. In addition to genetic factors, studies have recently begun to explore the role of epigenetic modifications in palatal ontogeny and etiology of OFC.

A number of environmental and maternal factors that influence the risk of having a child with OFC are well-described. In particular, family history, maternal drug use, nutrition, and exogenous exposures demonstrate strong links with development of OFC in the child.

Several studies have shown a higher incidence of cancer amongst patients with CL/P and their families. Additionally, studies have begun to identify higher rates of CL/P in the families of patients with cancer, although less is known about this. Combined, these suggest that CL/P and cancer may be mediated by shared environmental and genetic etiologies.

Author details

Mairaj K. Ahmed[1*], Anthony H. Bui[2] and Emanuela Taioli[3]

*Address all correspondence to: mairaj.ahmed@mountsinai.org

1 Cleft/Craniofacial Center, Icahn School of Medicine at Mount Sinai, NY, NY, USA

2 Icahn School of Medicine at Mount Sinai, NY, NY, USA

3 Institute for Translational Epidemiology, Icahn School of Medicine at Mount Sinai, NY, NY, USA

References

[1] Mossey PA, Modell B. Epidemiology of oral clefts 2012: an international perspective. Front Oral Biol 2012;16:1–18. doi:10.1159/000337464

[2] Gorlin RJ, Cohen MM, Hennekam RCM. Syndromes of the Head and Neck. New York: Oxford University Press; 2001.

[3] Mossey PA, Castilla EE. Global Registry and Database on Craniofacial Anomalies: Report of a WHO Registry Meeting on Craniofacial Anomalies. Geneva, Switzerland: World Health Organization; 2001.

[4] Allam E, Windsor L, Stone C. Cleft lip and palate: etiology, epidemiology, preventive and intervention strategies. Anat Physiol 2014;4:940–2161. doi:10.4172/2161-0940.1000150

[5] Forrester MB, Merz RD. Descriptive epidemiology of oral clefts in a multiethnic population, Hawaii, 1986–2000. Cleft Palate-Craniofacial J 2004;41:622–8. doi:10.1597/03-089.1

[6] Christensen K, Holm NV, Olsen J, Kock K, Fogh-Andersen P. Selection bias in genetic-epidemiological studies of cleft lip and palate. Am J Hum Genet 1992;51:654–9.

[7] Mastroiacovo P, Maraschini A, Leoncini E, Mossey P, Bower C, Castilla EE, et al. Prevalence at birth of cleft lip with or without cleft palate: data from the International Perinatal Database of Typical Oral Clefts (IPDTOC). Cleft Palate-Craniofacial J 2011;48:66–81. doi:10.1597/09-217

[8] Venkatesh R Syndromes and anomalies associated with cleft. Indian J Plast Surg 2009;42 Suppl:S51–5. doi:10.4103/0970-0358.57187

[9] Shaw GM, Carmichael SL, Yang W, Harris JA, Lammer EJ. Congenital malformations in births with orofacial clefts among 3.6 million California births, 1983–1997. Am J Med Genet A 2004;125A:250–6. doi:10.1002/ajmg.a.20508

[10] Wyszynski DF, Sarkozi A, Czeizel AE. Oral clefts with associated anomalies: methodological issues. Cleft Palate-Craniofacial J 2006;43:1–6. doi:10.1597/04-085R2.1

[11] Bronner ME, LeDouarin NM. Development and evolution of the neural crest: an overview. Dev Biol 2012;366:2–9. doi:10.1016/j.ydbio.2011.12.042

[12] Thomason HA, Dixon MJ, Thomason HA, Dixon MJ. Craniofacial defects and cleft lip and palate. Encycl Life Sci Chichester, UK: John Wiley & Sons, Ltd.; 2009. doi:10.1002/9780470015902.a0020915

[13] Fogh-Andersen P Inheritance of harelip and cleft palate: contribution to the elucidation of the etiology of the congenital clefts of the face. J Am Med Assoc 1947;133:276. doi:10.1001/jama.1947.02880040062031

[14] Fraser FC. Thoughts on the etiology of clefts of the palate and lip. Acta Genet Stat Med 1955;5:358–69.

[15] Harville EW, Wilcox AJ, Lie RT, Vindenes H, Åbyholm F. Cleft lip and palate versus cleft lip only: are they distinct defects? Am J Epidemiol 2005;162:448–53. doi:10.1093/aje/kwi214

[16] Weinberg SM, Brandon CA, McHenry TH, Neiswanger K, Deleyiannis FWB, De Salamanca JE, et al. Rethinking isolated cleft palate: evidence of occult lip defects in a subset of cases. Am J Med Genet Part A 2008;146:1670–5. doi:10.1002/ajmg.a.32291

[17] Jones MC. Etiology of facial clefts: prospective evaluation of 428 patients. Cleft Palate J 1988;25:16–20.

[18] Dixon MJ, Marazita ML, Beaty TH, Murray JC. Cleft lip and palate. Synthesizing genetic and environmental influences. Natl Inst Heal 2011;12:167–78. doi:10.1038/nrg2933.Cleft

[19] Beaty TH, Ruczinski I, Murray JC, Marazita ML, Munger RG, Hetmanski JB, et al. Evidence for gene-environment interaction in a genome wide study of isolated, non-syndromic cleft palate. Genet Epidemiol 2011;35:469–78. doi:10.1002/gepi.20595.Evidence

[20] The NCBI handbook [Internet]. Bethesda (MD): National Library of Medicine (US), National Center for Biotechnology Information; 2002 Oct. Chapter 18, The Reference Sequence (RefSeq) Project. Available from http://www.ncbi.nlm.nih.gov/books/NBK21091.

[21] Ardinger HH, Buetow KH, Bell GI, Bardach J, VanDemark DR, Murray JC. Association of genetic variation of the transforming growth factor-alpha gene with cleft lip and palate. Am J Hum Genet 1989;45:348–53.

[22] Jugessur A, Lie RT, Wilcox AJ, Murray JC, Taylor JA, Saugstad OD, et al. Variants of developmental genes (TGFA, TGFB3, and MSX1) and their associations with orofacial clefts: a case-parent triad analysis. Genet Epidemiol 2003;24:230–9. doi:10.1002/gepi.10223

[23] Mitchell LE. Transforming growth factor alpha locus and nonsyndromic cleft lip with or without cleft palate: a reappraisal. Genet Epidemiol 1997;14:231–40. doi:10.1002/(SICI)1098-2272(1997)14:3<231::AID-GEPI2>3.0.CO;2-8

[24] Proetzel G, Pawlowski SA, Wiles MV, Yin M, Boivin GP, Howles PN, et al. Transforming growth factor-beta 3 is required for secondary palate fusion. Nat Genet 1995;11:409–14. doi:10.1038/ng1295-409

[25] Kaartinen V, Voncken JW, Shuler C, Warburton D, Bu D, Heisterkamp N, et al. Abnormal lung development and cleft palate in mice lacking TGF-beta 3 indicates defects of epithelial-mesenchymal interaction. Nat Genet 1995;11:415–21. doi:10.1038/ng1295-415

[26] Marazita ML, Murray JC, Lidral AC, Arcos-Burgos M, Cooper ME, Goldstein T, et al. Meta-analysis of 13 genome scans reveals multiple cleft lip/palate genes with novel loci on 9q21 and 2q32–35. Am J Hum Genet 2004;75:161–73. doi:10.1086/422475

[27] Jezewski PA, Vieira AR, Nishimura C, Ludwig B, Johnson M, O'Brien SE, et al. Complete sequencing shows a role for MSX1 in non-syndromic cleft lip and palate. J Med Genet 2003;40:399–407. doi:10.1136/jmg.40.6.399

[28] Rintala AE, Ranta R. Lower lip sinuses: I. Epidemiology, microforms and transverse sulci. Br J Plast Surg 1981;34:26–30.

[29] Ferrero GB, Baldassarre G, Panza E, Valenzise M, Pippucci T, Mussa A, et al. A heritable cause of cleft lip and palate-Van der Woude syndrome caused by a novel IRF6 mutation. Review of the literature and of the differential diagnosis. Eur J Pediatr 2010;169:223–8. doi:10.1007/s00431-009-1011-3

[30] Zucchero TM, Cooper ME, Maher BS, Daack-Hirsch S, Nepomuceno B, Ribeiro L, et al. Interferon regulatory factor 6 (IRF6) gene variants and the risk of isolated cleft lip or palate. N Engl J Med 2004;351:769–80. doi:10.1056/NEJMoa032909

[31] Houdayer C, Bonaïti-Pellié C, Erguy C, Soupre V, Dondon MG, Bürglen L, et al. Possible relationship between the van der Woude syndrome (vWS) locus and nonsyndromic cleft lip with or without cleft palate (NSCL/P). Am J Med Genet 2001;104:86–92.

[32] Lidral AC, Moreno LM. Progress toward discerning the genetics of cleft lip. Curr Opin Pediatr 2005;17:731–9. doi:10.1097/01.mop.0000185138.65820.7f

[33] Stanier P, Moore GE. Genetics of cleft lip and palate: syndromic genes contribute to the incidence of non-syndromic clefts. Hum Mol Genet 2004;13Spec No:R73–81. doi:10.1093/hmg/ddh052

[34] Martinelli M, Scapoli L, Pezzetti F, Carinci F, Carinci P, Stabellini G, et al. C677T variant form at the MTHFR gene and CL/P: a risk factor for mothers? Am J Med Genet 2001;98:357–60. doi:10.1002/1096-8628(20010201)98:4<357::AID-AJMG1108>3.0.CO;2-F

[35] Shaw GM, Rozen R, Finnell RH, Todoroff K, Lammer EJ. Infant C677T mutation in MTHFR, maternal periconceptional vitamin use, and cleft lip. Am J Med Genet 1998;80:196–8. doi:10.1002/(SICI)1096-8628(19981116)80:3<196::AID-AJMG2>3.0.CO;2-V

[36] Blanton SH, Patel S, Hecht JT, Mulliken JB. MTHFR is not a risk factor in the development of isolated nonsyndromic cleft lip and palate. Am J Med Genet 2002;110:404–5. doi:10.1002/ajmg.10496

[37] Jugessur A, Wilcox AJ, Lie RT, Murray JC, Taylor JA, Ulvik A, et al. Exploring the effects of methylenetetrahydrofolate reductase gene variants C677T and A1298C on the risk of orofacial clefts in 261 Norwegian case-parent triads. Am J Epidemiol 2003;157:1083–91.

[38] Lohnes D, Mark M, Mendelsohn C, Dollé P, Dierich A, Gorry P, et al. Function of the retinoic acid receptors (RARs) during development (I). Craniofacial and skeletal abnormalities in RAR double mutants. Development 1994;120:2723–48.

[39] Shaw D, Ray A, Marazita M, Field L. Further evidence of a relationship between the retinoic acid receptor alpha locus and nonsyndromic cleft lip with or without cleft palate (CL+/−P). Am J Hum Genet 1993;53:1156–7.

[40] Conrad R, Barrier M, Ford LP. Role of miRNA and miRNA processing factors in development and disease. Birth Defects Res Part C—Embryo Today Rev 2006;78:107–17. doi:10.1002/bdrc.20068

[41] Hinton A, Hunter S, Reyes G, Fogel GB, King CC. From pluripotency to islets. miRNAs as critical regulators of human cellular differentiation. Adv Genet. 2012;79:1–34. doi:10.1016/B978-0-12-394395-8.00001-3

[42] Pasquinelli AE, Ruvkun G. Control of developmental timing by microRNAs and their targets. Annu Rev Cell Dev Biol 2002;18:495–513. doi:10.1146/annurev.cellbio.18.012502.105832

[43] Mukhopadhyay P, Brock G, Pihur V, Webb C, Pisano MM, Greene RM. Developmental microRNA expression profiling of murine embryonic orofacial tissue. Birth Defects Res A Clin Mol Teratol 2010;88:511–34. doi:10.1002/bdra.20684

[44] Gregory PA, Bracken CP, Bert AG, Goodall GJ. MicroRNAs as regulators of epithelial-mesenchymal transition. Cell Cycle 2008;7:3112–7. doi:10.4161/cc.7.20.6851

[45] Eberhart JK, He X, Swartz ME, Yan Y-L, Song H, Boling TC, et al. MicroRNA mirn140 modulates PDGF signaling during palatogenesis. Nat Genet 2008;40:290–8. doi:10.1038/ng.82

[46] Shin J-O, Lee J-M, Cho K-W, Kwak S, Kwon H-J, Lee M-J, et al. MiR-200b is involved in TGF-β signaling to regulate mammalian palate development. Histochem Cell Biol 2012;137:67–78. doi:10.1007/s00418-011-0876-1

[47] Shin J-O, Nakagawa E, Kim E-J, Cho K-W, Lee J-M, Cho S-W, et al. miR-200b regulates cell migration via Zeb family during mouse palate development. Histochem Cell Biol 2012;137:459–70. doi:10.1007/s00418-012-0915-6

[48] Li L, Shi JY, Zhu GQ, Shi B. MiR-17-92 cluster regulates cell proliferation and collagen synthesis by targeting TGFB pathway in mouse palatal mesenchymal cells. J Cell Biochem 2012;113:1235–44. doi:10.1002/jcb.23457

[49] Bonasio R, Tu S, Reinberg D. Molecular signals of epigenetic states. Science 2010;330:612–6. doi:10.1126/science.1191078

[50] Jones PA, Takai D. The role of DNA methylation in mammalian epigenetics. Science 2001;293:1068–70. doi:10.1126/science.1063852

[51] Ndlovu MN, Denis H, Fuks F. Exposing the DNA methylome iceberg. Trends Biochem Sci 2011;36:381–7. doi:10.1016/j.tibs.2011.03.002

[52] Jjingo D, Conley AB, Yi S V, Lunyak V V, Jordan IK. On the presence and role of human gene-body DNA methylation. Oncotarget 2012;3:462–74. doi:10.18632/oncotarget.497

[53] Rogers JM, Francis BM, Sulik KK, Alles AJ, Massaro EJ, Zucker RM, et al. Cell death and cell cycle perturbation in the developmental toxicity of the demethylating agent, 5-aza-2′-deoxycytidine. Teratology 1994;50:332–9. doi:10.1002/tera.1420500504

[54] Branch S, Chernoff N, Brownie C, Magnus FB. 5-AZA-2′-deoxycytidine-induced dysmorphogenesis in the rat. Teratog Carcinog Mutagen 1999;19:329–38. doi:10.1002/(SICI)1520-6866(1999)19:5<329::AID-TCM3>3.0.CO;2-S

[55] Bulut HE, Ozdemir O, Başimoglu-Koca Y, Korkmaz M, Atalay A. Effects of a DNA demethylating agent—5-azacytidine—on testicular morphology during mouse embryo development. Okajimas Folia Anat Jpn 1999;76:47–53.

[56] Kuriyama M, Udagawa A, Yoshimoto S, Ichinose M, Sato K, Yamazaki K, et al. DNA methylation changes during cleft palate formation induced by retinoic acid in mice. Cleft Palate-Craniofacial J 2008;45:545–51. doi:10.1597/07-134.1

[57] Seelan RS, Appana SN, Mukhopadhyay P, Warner DR, Brock GN, Pisano MM, et al. Developmental profiles of the murine palatal methylome. Birth Defects Res A Clin Mol Teratol 2013;97:171–86. doi:10.1002/bdra.23126

[58] Mitchell LE, Christensen K. Analysis of the recurrence patterns for nonsyndromic cleft lip with or without cleft palate in the families of 3,073 Danish probands. Am J Med Genet 1996;61:371–6.doi:10.1002/(SICI)1096-8628(19960202)61:4<371::AID-AJMG12>3.0.CO;2-P

[59] Grosen D, Chevrier C, Skytthe A, Bille C, Mølsted K, Sivertsen A, et al. A cohort study of recurrence patterns among more than 54,000 relatives of oral cleft cases in Denmark: support for the multifactorial threshold model of inheritance. J Med Genet 2010;47:162–8. doi:10.1136/jmg.2009.069385

[60] Grosen D, Bille C, Petersen I, Skytthe A, Hjelmborg JvB, Pedersen JK, et al. Risk of oral clefts in twins. Epidemiology 2011;22:313–9. doi:10.1097/EDE.0b013e3182125f9c

[61] Christensen K, Mitchell LE. Familial recurrence-pattern analysis of nonsyndromic isolated cleft palate—a Danish Registry study. Am J Hum Genet 1996;58:182–90.

[62] Jugessur A, Shi M, Gjessing HK, Lie RT, Wilcox AJ, Weinberg CR, et al. Genetic determinants of facial clefting: analysis of 357 candidate genes using two national cleft studies from Scandinavia. PLoS One 2009;4:e5385. doi:10.1371/journal.pone.0005385

[63] Hernández-Díaz S, Werler MM, Walker AM, Mitchell AA. Folic acid antagonists during pregnancy and the risk of birth defects. N Engl J Med 2000;343:1608–14. doi:10.1056/NEJM200011303432204

[64] Dolovich LR, Addis A, Vaillancourt JM, Power JD, Koren G, Einarson TR. Benzodiazepine use in pregnancy and major malformations or oral cleft: meta-analysis of cohort and case-control studies. BMJ 1998;317:839–43.

[65] Lammer EJ, Chen DT, Hoar RM, Agnish ND, Benke PJ, Braun JT, et al. Retinoic acid embryopathy. N Engl J Med 1985;313:837–41. doi:10.1056/NEJM198510033131401

[66] Hernandez RK, Werler MM, Romitti P, Sun L, Anderka M, National Birth Defects Prevention Study. Nonsteroidal antiinflammatory drug use among women and the risk of birth defects. Am J Obstet Gynecol 2012;206:228.e1–8. doi:10.1016/j.ajog.2011.11.019

[67] Carmichael SL, Shaw GM, Ma C, Werler MM, Rasmussen SA, Lammer EJ, et al. Maternal corticosteroid use and orofacial clefts. Am J Obstet Gynecol 2007;197:585.e1–7; discussion 683–4, e1–7. doi:10.1016/j.ajog.2007.05.046

[68] Aberg A, Westbom L, Källén B. Congenital malformations among infants whose mothers had gestational diabetes or preexisting diabetes. Early Hum Dev 2001;61:85–95.

[69] Hashmi SS, Gallaway MS, Waller DK, Langlois PH, Hecht JT. Maternal fever during early pregnancy and the risk of oral clefts. Birth Defects Res Part A—Clin Mol Teratol 2010;88:186–94. doi:10.1002/bdra.20646

[70] Métneki J, Puhó E, Czeizel AE. Maternal diseases and isolated orofacial clefts in Hungary. Birth Defects Res A Clin Mol Teratol 2005;73:617–23. doi:10.1002/bdra.20177

[71] Wilcox AJ, Lie RT, Solvoll K, Taylor J, McConnaughey DR, Abyholm F, et al. Folic acid supplements and risk of facial clefts: national population based case-control study. BMJ 2007;334:464. doi:10.1136/bmj.39079.618287.0B

[72] Goh YI, Bollano E, Einarson TR, Koren G. Prenatal multivitamin supplementation and rates of congenital anomalies: a meta-analysis. J Obstet Gynaecol Canada JOGC = J D'obstétrique Gynécologie Du Canada JOGC 2006;28:680–9.

[73] Ray JG, Meier C, Vermeulen MJ, Boss S, Wyatt PR, Cole DEC. Association of neural tube defects and folic acid food fortification in Canada. Lancet (London, England) 2002;360:2047–8. doi:10.1016/S0140-6736(02)11994-5

[74] Shaw GM, Carmichael SL, Laurent C, Rasmussen SA. Maternal nutrient intakes and risk of orofacial clefts. Epidemiology 2006;17:285–91. doi:10.1097/01.ede.0000208348.30012.35

[75] Carmichael SL, Yang W, Feldkamp ML, Munger RG, Siega-Riz AM, Botto LD, et al. Reduced risks of neural tube defects and orofacial clefts with higher diet quality. Arch Pediatr Adolesc Med 2012;166:121–6. doi:10.1001/archpediatrics.2011.185

[76] Rothman KJ, Moore LL, Singer MR, Nguyen US, Mannino S, Milunsky A. Teratogenicity of high vitamin A intake. N Engl J Med 1995;333:1369–73. doi:10.1097/00006254-199605000-00007

[77] Shaw GM, Wasserman CR, Block G, Lammer EJ. High maternal vitamin A intake and risk of anomalies of structures with a cranial neural crest cell contribution. Lancet (London, England) 1996;347:899–900.

[78] Mills JL, Simpson JL, Cunningham GC, Conley MR, Rhoads GG. Vitamin A and birth defects. Am J Obstet Gynecol 1997;177:31–6. doi:10.1016/S0002-9378(97)70434-4

[79] Mastroiacovo P, Mazzone T, Addis A, Elephant E, Carlier P, Vial T, et al. High vitamin A intake in early pregnancy and major malformations: a multicenter prospective controlled study. Teratology 1999;59:7–11. doi:10.1002/(SICI)1096-9926(199901)59:1<7::AID-TERA4>3.0.CO;2-6

[80] Johansen AMW, Lie RT, Wilcox AJ, Andersen LF, Drevon CA. Maternal dietary intake of vitamin A and risk of orofacial clefts: a population-based case-control study in Norway. Am J Epidemiol 2008;167:1164–70. doi:10.1093/aje/kwn035

[81] Chevrier C, Bahuau M, Perret C, Iovannisci DM, Nelva A, Herman C, et al. Genetic susceptibilities in the association between maternal exposure to tobacco smoke and the risk of nonsyndromic oral cleft. Am J Med Genet Part A 2008;146:2396–406. doi:10.1002/ajmg.a.32505

[82] Li Z, Liu J, Ye R, Zhang L, Zheng X, Ren A. Maternal passive smoking and risk of cleft lip with or without cleft palate. Epidemiology 2010;21:240–2. doi:10.1097/EDE.0b013e3181c9f941

[83] Boyles AL, Deroo LA, Lie RT, Taylor JA, Jugessur A, Murray JC, et al. Maternal alcohol consumption, alcohol metabolism genes, and the risk of oral clefts: a population-based case-control study in Norway, 1996–2001. Am J Epidemiol 2010;172:924–31. doi:10.1093/aje/kwq226

[84] Romitti PA, Herring AM, Dennis LK, Wong-Gibbons DL. Meta-analysis: pesticides and orofacial clefts. Cleft Palate-Craniofacial J 2007;44:358–65. doi:10.1597/06-100.1

[85] Lin S, Herdt-Losavio ML, Chapman BR, Munsie J-P, Olshan AF, Druschel CM. Maternal occupation and the risk of major birth defects: a follow-up analysis from the National Birth Defects Prevention Study. Int J Hyg Environ Health 2013;216:317–23. doi:10.1016/j.ijheh.2012.05.006

[86] Desrosiers TA, Lawson CC, Meyer RE, Richardson DB, Daniels JL, Waters MA, et al. Maternal occupational exposure to organic solvents during early pregnancy and risks of neural tube defects and orofacial clefts. Occup Env Med 2013;69:493–9. doi:10.1136/oemed-2011-100245.Maternal

[87] Cordier S, Garlantézec R, Labat L, Rouget F, Monfort C, Bonvallot N, et al. Exposure during pregnancy to glycol ethers and chlorinated solvents and the risk of congenital malformations. Epidemiology 2012;23:806–12. doi:10.1097/EDE.0b013e31826c2bd8

[88] Li L, Zhu G, Meng T, Shi J, Wu J, Xu X, et al. Biological and epidemiological evidence of interaction of infant genotypes at Rs7205289 and maternal passive smoking in cleft palate. Am J Med Genet Part A 2011;155:2940–8. doi:10.1002/ajmg.a.34254

[89] Wu T, Fallin MD, Shi M, Ruczinski I, Liang KY, Hetmanski JB, et al. Evidence of gene-environment interaction for the RUNX2 gene and environmental tobacco smoke in controlling the risk of cleft lip with/without cleft palate. Birth Defects Res A Clin Mol Teratol 2012;94:76–83. doi:10.1002/bdra.22885

[90] Dietz A, Pedersen DA, Jacobsen R, Wehby GL, Murray JC, Christensen K. Risk of breast cancer in families with cleft lip and palate. Ann Epidemiol 2012;22:37–42. doi:10.1016/j.annepidem.2011.09.003

[91] Steinwachs EF, Amos C, Johnston D, Mulliken J, Stal S, Hecht JT. Nonsyndromic cleft lip and palate is not associated with cancer or other birth defects. Am J Med Genet 2000;90:17–24.

[92] Menezes R, Marazita ML, Goldstein McHenry T, Cooper ME, Bardi K, Brandon C, et al. AXIS inhibition protein 2, orofacial clefts and a family history of cancer. J Am Dent Assoc 2009;140:80–4.

[93] Vieira AR, Khaliq S, Lace B. Risk of cancer in relatives of children born with isolated cleft lip and palate. Am J Med Genet A 2012;158A:1503–4. doi:10.1002/ajmg.a.35359

[94] Lima LS, Silvério MO, Swerts MSO, Aquino SN, Martelli DRB, Martelli-Júnior H. Frequency of cancer in first-degree relatives of patients with cleft lip and/or palate in the Brazilian population. Braz Dent J 2013;24:200–3. doi:10.1590/0103-6440201302191

[95] Taioli E, Ragin C, Robertson L, Linkov F, Thurman NE, Vieira AR. Cleft lip and palate in family members of cancer survivors. Cancer Invest 2010;28:958–62. doi:10.3109/07357907.2010.483510

[96] Zhu JL, Basso O, Hasle H, Winther JF, Olsen JH, Olsen J. Do parents of children with congenital malformations have a higher cancer risk? A nationwide study in Denmark. Br J Cancer 2002;87:524–8. doi:10.1038/sj.bjc.6600488

[97] Bille C, Winther JF, Bautz A, Murray JC, Olsen J, Christensen K. Cancer risk in persons with oral cleft—a population-based study of 8,093 cases. Am J Epidemiol 2005;161:1047–55. doi:10.1093/aje/kwi132

[98] Frebourg T, Oliveira C, Hochain P, Karam R, Manouvrier S, Graziadio C, et al. Cleft lip/palate and CDH1/E-cadherin mutations in families with hereditary diffuse gastric cancer. J Med Genet 2006;43:138–42. doi:10.1136/jmg.2005.031385

[99] Vogelaar IP, Figueiredo J, van Rooij IALM, Simões-Correia J, van der Post RS, Melo S, et al. Identification of germline mutations in the cancer predisposing gene CDH1 in patients with orofacial clefts. Hum Mol Genet 2013;22:919–26. doi:10.1093/hmg/dds497

11

Surgical Strategy of Cleft Palate Repair and Nasometric Results

Norifumi Nakamura and Masahiro Tezuka

Abstract

The goal of cleft palate (CP) repair is to achieve normal speech. Despite the recent development of surgical repair of cleft palate, there is no standard procedure that ensures patients' speech to the same level as that in noncleft children. In this chapter, we describe our surgical strategy of cleft palate repair that approaches each anatomical and pathological abnormality of cleft palate and the postoperative speech outcomes using the subjective and objective manners. After palate repair based on our surgical strategy, patients' speech was significantly improved, and the nasalance scores were recovered to almost the same levels as those of Japanese children without cleft palate.

Keywords: cleft palate, palatal repair, nasometry, speech

1. Introduction

The surgical goals of primary repair for cleft palate (CP) include closure of the defect of the hard and soft palate and achievement of normal speech based on favorable velopharyngeal (VP) closure. Patients and family members always desire their speech in the same level as that of healthy children. However, it is said that approximately 40% of patients have a persistent, often lifelong, speech impairment in connected to CP [1]. Despite the recent development of surgical repair of cleft palate, there has been no standard procedure that can ensure complete VP closure (VPC) in patients with CP to date.

The Department of Oral and Maxillofacial Surgery, Kagoshima University Hospital, worked on cleft lip and palate repair for 30 years. We assessed their speech from 2000 to 2005 and revealed that more than 30% of patients had a moderate or poor VPC, and only 40% had achieved normal articulation. Therefore, to improve our speech results, the following countermeasures were carried out: First, we tried to standardize the surgical procedures for palatal repair. Second, postoperative speech results were assessed objectively by speech language therapists (SLT). Third, these objective data were shared with all surgeons to provide feedback for the next operation.

In this chapter, we described our surgical strategy of cleft palate repair that approaches each anatomical and pathological abnormality of cleft palate and evaluated postoperative speech outcomes including presence/severity of hypernasality, nasal emission, and nasalance scores after standardize palatal repair. We then compared speech outcomes to ones using our previous palatal repair protocol without following surgical strategy. Furthermore, we also compared them to the nasalance scores of Japanese noncleft children.

2. Surgical strategy of palate repair approaching each anatomical and pathological abnormality

The concept of our strategy for CP repair was to approach each anatomical and pathological abnormality that may cause postoperative velopharyngeal incompetence (VPI): short palate, asymmetric palate, insufficient velar elevation, and a midline defect of the velum, to establish CP repair that can ensure VP closure (**Table 1**) [2]. The above factors were identified based on our experiences during the treatment of persistent VPI after CP repair. Therefore, our CP repair consisted of (1) presurgical orthopedics using Hotz's plate as much as possible to minimize the cleft space, (2) modified V-Y palatoplasty, allowing conservation of the periosteum in the anterior part of the maxilla, minimizing maxillary growth disturbance, (3) lengthening of the nasal mucosa using a large Z-plasty and a free mucosal graft, (4) muscular reconstruction producing a symmetrical levator sling and pharyngeal arch, and (5) two-layered suture of the palatal muscles.

Possible causes of VPI	Anatomical pathological abnormalities	Surgical procedures in palatal repair
Short palate	• Wide cleft palate. • Growth deficiency of the soft palate. • Insufficient retropositioning of the palatal muscles.	• Presurgical orthopedics for narrowing the cleft space using Hotz's plate, as much as possible. • Sufficient retropositioning of the palatal muscle.
Asymmetric velopharynx	• Antero-posterior discrepancy between the maxillary segments. • Discrepancy of the velar length between the segments. • Malpositioning of the palatal muscles.	• Presurgical orthopedics improving the positional gap using Hotz's plate, as much as possible. • Extension of the nasal mucosa by large Z-plasty with a free mucosal graft. • Symmetrical reconstruction of the palatal muscle referencing the anatomical landmarks.

Possible causes of VPI	Anatomical pathological abnormalities	Surgical procedures in palatal repair
Insufficient velar elevation	• Insufficient releasing of the palatal muscles from the palatal bone. • Muscular pooling in the soft palate. • Wide scar in the soft palate.	• Freeing the palatal muscle in a single layer on the tensor aponeurosis. • Sufficient retropositioning of the palatal muscle. • Sufficient extension of the oral and nasal mucosa.
Midline defect of the velum	• Unsatisfactory repair or defect of musculus uvulae.	• Two-layer suture of the palatal muscles in the midline of the velum.

Table 1. Our surgical strategy for palatal repair approaching each anatomical and pathological abnormality and possible causes of VPI [2].

3. Surgical procedures for cleft palate repair

We adopt a modified V-Y palatoplasty for cleft palatal repair, although a large number of surgeons have developed surgical procedures for palatal repair [3–10]. The reason why we adopt a modified V-Y palatoplasty for cleft palatal repair is due to the following previous reports. Brothers et al. observed that the success rates for VP closure after Furlow palatoplasty and the modified Wardill-Kilner procedure were 64.0 and 70.0%, respectively, using pressure-flow testing, and they concluded that there was no difference between the two procedures [11]. Van Lierde et al. also compared Furlow palatoplasty and the Wardill-Kilner procedure using the nasometry and observed significantly better results in those treated with the Wardill-Kilner procedure [12].

The surgical procedures of a modified V-Y palatoplasty are shown in **Figure 1**. On designing the incision line, anatomical landmarks at the velopharynx were marked carefully (**Figure 1a**). The palatal flaps were elevated while preserving the periosteum in the anterior and lateral parts of the hard palate, and the palatal muscles were bluntly dissected along the surface of the tensor aponeurosis and nasal mucosa in a single layer. For extension of the nasal mucosa of the soft palate, large Z-plasty was performed in the nasal surface of the soft palate (**Figure 1b**). Mucosal incision for the large Z-plasty was extended until the surgeon could confirm contact between the soft palate and posterior pharyngeal wall without any tension. When the velar length became shorter on complete closure of the Z-plasty, the mucosal defect that remained on the nasal side was filled using a free mucosal graft donated from the buccal area (**Figure 1c**). Palatal muscles were then sutured in the midline of the soft palate by the two-layered suture (**Figure 1d**).

Palatal muscle was sutured carefully on producing a symmetrical levator sling and also the symmetrical palatopharyngeal and palatoglossal arches and uvula, while referencing five anatomical landmarks, as described above.

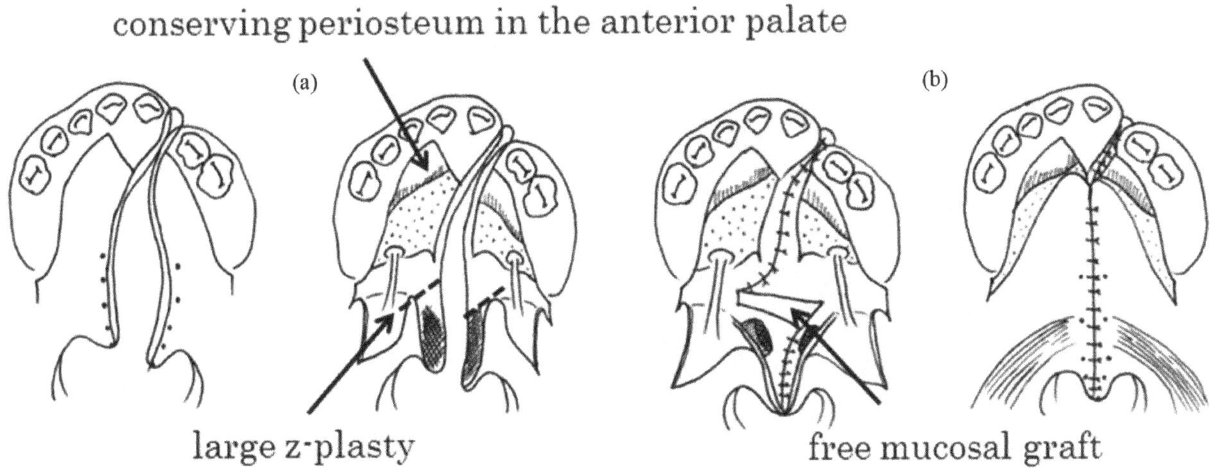

Figure 1. Surgical steps in palate repair for UCLP.

On designing the incision line, anatomical landmarks at the velopharynx were marked using 0.05% Toluidine blue solution (**Figure 2**). The marked points included the tip and base of the uvula (nos. 1 and 2), point in which the extension line of the palatoglossal arch crossed the cleft edge (no. 3), posterior edge of the hard palate (no. 4), and midpoint between nos. 3 and 4 (no. 5).

The palatal flaps were elevated while preserving the periosteum in the anterior and lateral parts of the hard palate, and the palatal muscles including the levator veli palatini muscle, palatopharyngeal muscle, and musculus uvulae, although these muscles were not clearly identified, were bluntly dissected along the surface of the tensor aponeurosis and nasal mucosa in a single layer. Muscles were sufficiently retropositioned as the direction was turned sideways. The hamular process was not fractured.

For extension of the nasal mucosa of the soft palate, a large Z-plasty was made in the nasal mucosa of the soft palate (**Figure 3a**). Mucosal incision for the large Z-plasty was extended until the soft palate contact to the posterior pharyngeal wall without any tension. The mucosal defect produced by a large Z-plasty was closed. However, when the velar length became shorter on complete closure of the Z-plasty, the mucosal defect that remained on the nasal side was filled using a free mucosal graft donated from the buccal area (**Figure 3b**). Because the shortened velar length due to complete closure of a Z-plasty might cause an asymmetric VP form and asymmetric closure motion.

Palatal muscles were then sutured in the midline of the soft palate by the two-layered suture (nasal and oral sides) using a nonabsorbable thread (5-0 Nylon; **Figure 3c**). Palatal muscle was sutured carefully on producing a symmetrical levator sling and also the symmetrical palatopharyngeal and palatoglossal arches and uvula, while referencing five anatomical landmarks, as described above. The raw area of the hard palate was dressed using a collagen-based artificial dermis and covered using an acrylic plate for 1 week.

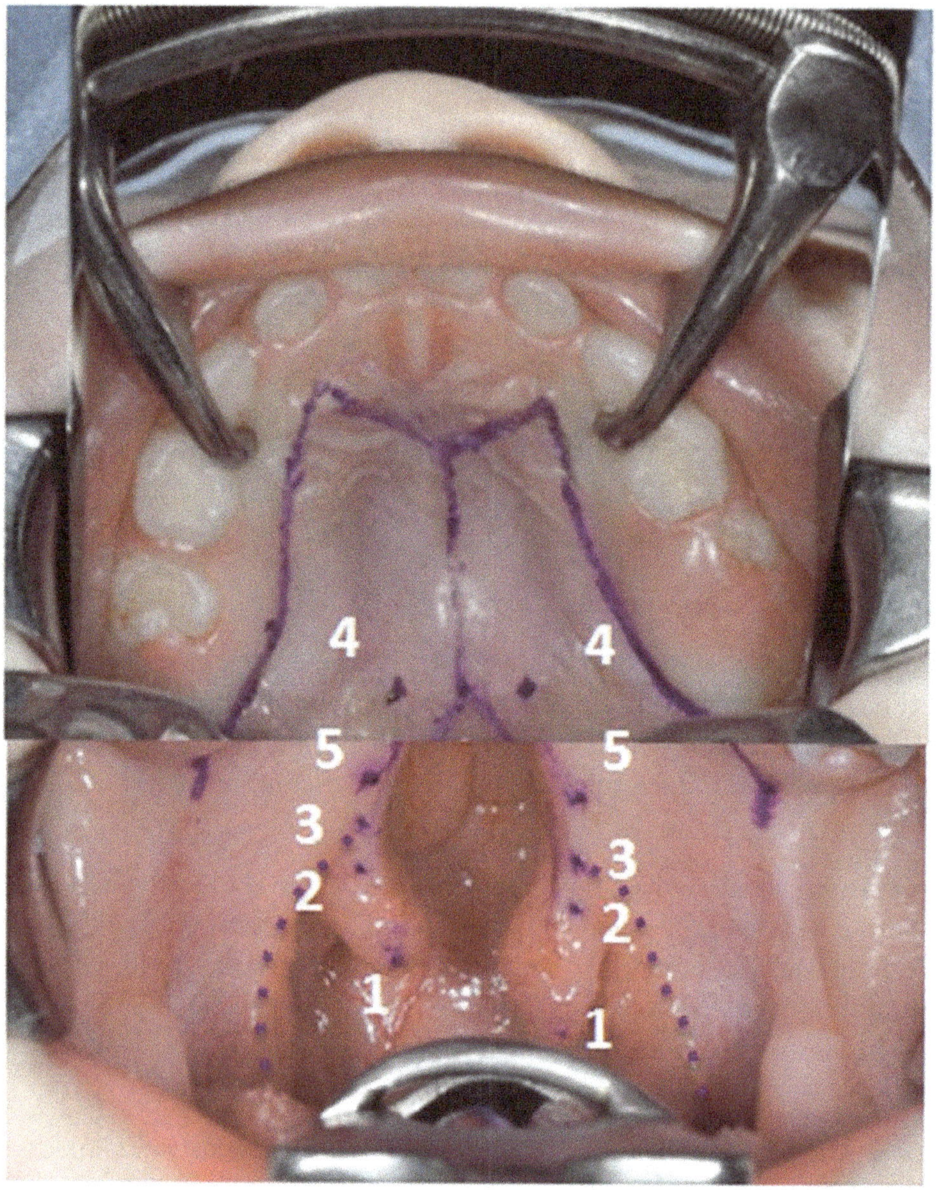

Figure 2. Surgical steps in palatal repair. The figure demonstrates anatomical landmarks and the incision line.

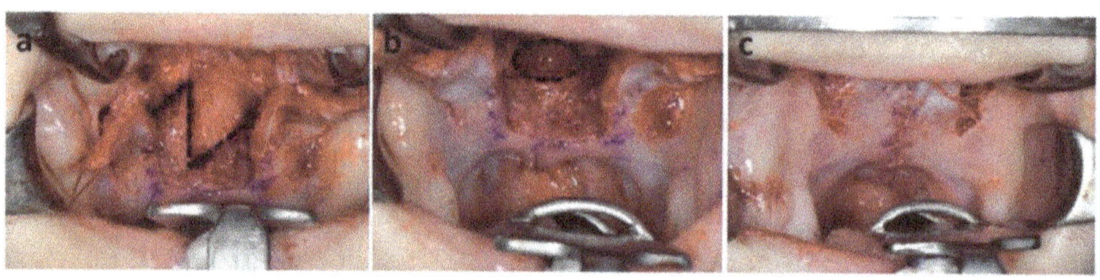

Figure 3. Surgical steps in palatal repair. The figure demonstrates elevation of the palatal flaps conserving the periosteum in the anterior and lateral parts of the hard palate and a large Z-plasty on the nasal side (dotted line) (a), a free mucosal graft on the nasal side (b), and symmetrical muscular reconstruction producing a levator sling while referring to the anatomical landmarks (c).

4. Speech assessment

Figure 4 shows our treatment schedule for speech in cleft palate patients. Speech management by a speech therapist starts just after birth, and the patient's motor development is facilitated. A check by an ENT doctor for the presence of otitis media is performed every 6 months. Palatal repair is then performed at 1.5 years. And after palatal repair, exercise facilitating VP closure is performed by a speech therapist. When the patient reaches the age of 4 years, VP closure (VPC) function is evaluated more precisely. If VPI remains, speech therapist starts training facilitating VPC. Our goal is to achieve a normal speech before entering elementary school.

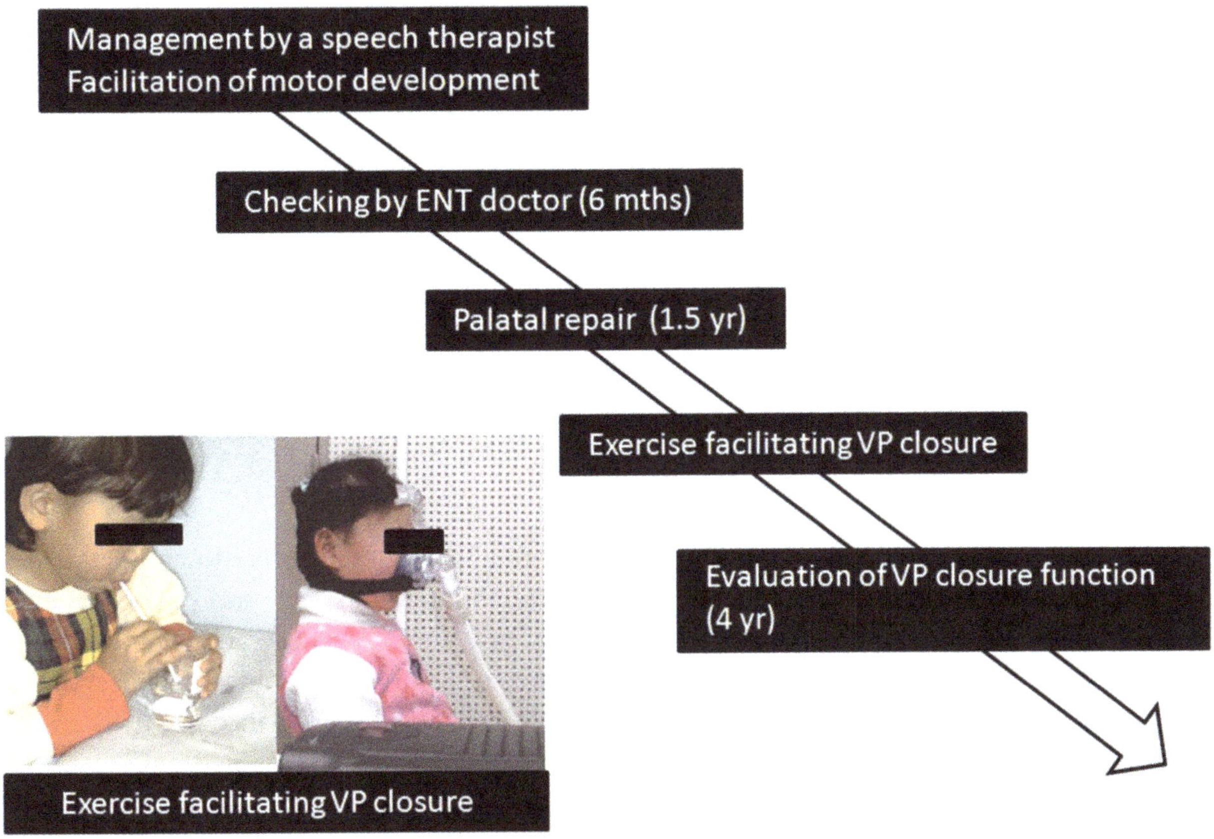

Figure 4. Treatment schedule for speech in cleft palate patients in Kagoshima University Hospital.

Postoperatively, patients were followed by 2 SLTs every 3 months until around 4 years. In this study, perceptual rating of hypernasality and nasal emission was carried out for all participants using the preserved sound sources by SLTs. In perceptual rating, hypernasality and nasal emission were classified into four categories: none, slight/mild, moderate, and severe. Articulation was also evaluated using the articulation test of the Japan Society of Logopedics and Phoniatrics and then converted to IPA 2005 phonetic symbols so that all abnormalities could be diagnosed and transcribed in IPA.

Nasometry scores were obtained for all patients using the Kay 6200 Nasometer II (Kay Elemetics, Lincoln Park, NJ, USA). For speech stimuli, the low-pressure vowel /i:/ and low-pressure sentence /yooi wa ooi/ and the high-pressure consonant-vowel syllable /tsu/ and high-pressure sentence /kitsutsuki ga kiwotsutsuku/ were used [13]. The reason, why we selected /i:/ extending the verbalization of /i/ among the all low-pressured vowels, was based on our previous study on the relationship between nasalance score and the perceptual rating of resonance in Japanese cleft and noncleft subjects [14]. In the previous study, we found that nasalance score during phonation of /i:/ was correlated with perceptual rating of resonance and cleft and noncelft subjects with normal resonance demonstrated the mean nasalance score less than 20% during phonation of /i:/.

5. Postoperative speech results comparing to the previously operated patients and noncleft controls

Postoperative speech results of 94 patients who underwent palate repair based on our surgical strategy during 2006–2012 (strategy group) and those of 109 patients who previously underwent palate repair without following strategy during 2000–2005 (previous group) were compared. As control group, speech data on 37 Japanese noncleft controls were used. For speech assessment, perceptual rating of hypernasality and nasal emission was classified into four categories: none, slight/mild, moderate, and severe, by one experienced speech language therapist for all participants. Articulation was also evaluated using the articulation test. For objective assessment, Nasometer test was performed for all patients. This study was approved by the Clinical Research Ethical Review Boards of Kagoshima University Hospital.

Comparison of the rate of achieving normal resonance in each cleft type is shown in **Figure 5**. Normal resonance was achieved in 35/37 (94.6%) in Unilateral cleft lip and palate (UCLP), 15/18 (83.3%) in Bilateral cleft lip and palate (BCLP), 24/27 (88.9%) in CP, and 8/12 (66.7%) in Submucous cleft palate (SMCP) in the strategy group. Severe hypernasality was observed in each one patient with BCLP and SMCP. On the other hand, normal resonance was achieved in 40/57 (70.2%) in UCLP, 16/25 (64.0%) in BCLP, and 19/27 (70.3%) in CP in the previous group. Successful achievement of normal resonance was obtained more reliably in all types of CP following palate repair based on our surgical strategy.

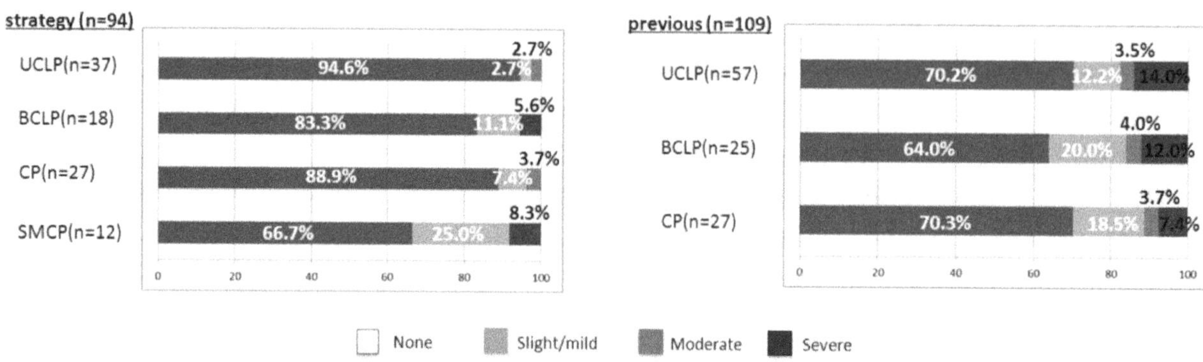

Figure 5. Postoperative hypernasality of each cleft type in the strategy and previous group.

The mean and SD of the nasalance scores of the strategy and previous groups and controls are shown in **Table 2**. The mean nasalance scores in the strategy group were less than 20% and were significantly lower than those of the previous group. When comparing the nasalance scores of control groups, those in the previous group were significantly higher on phonating /i:/ and the low-pressure sentence than in controls. On the other hand, there was no significant difference between the strategy and control groups. In other words, the nasalance scores representing hypernasality in the subjects of the strategy group recovered to almost the same levels as those of Japanese children without cleft palate.

Regarding articulation at 4 years of age, normal articulation was obtained in 68.4% in the strategy group, and this was better than that of the previous group (**Figure 6**).

	Nasalance score (%)				
	Strategy (*n* = 94)		**Previous** (*n* = 109)		**Controls** (*n* = 37)
/i/	20.3 ± 13.5	<0.01	33.6 ± 23.9	<0.01	22.7 ± 14.4
/tsu/	16.8 ± 13.5	<0.05	22.6 ± 19.3	<0.05	15.2 ± 8.5
/youihaooi/	19.7 ± 13.6	NS	24.2 ± 17.0	<0.01	13.0 ± 9.7
/kitsutsuki ga kiwo tsutsuku/	19.2 ± 12.7	NS	23.6 ± 18.3	NS	17.5 ± 9.8

Table 2. Mean ± SD of the nasalance score in the strategy, previous, and control groups.

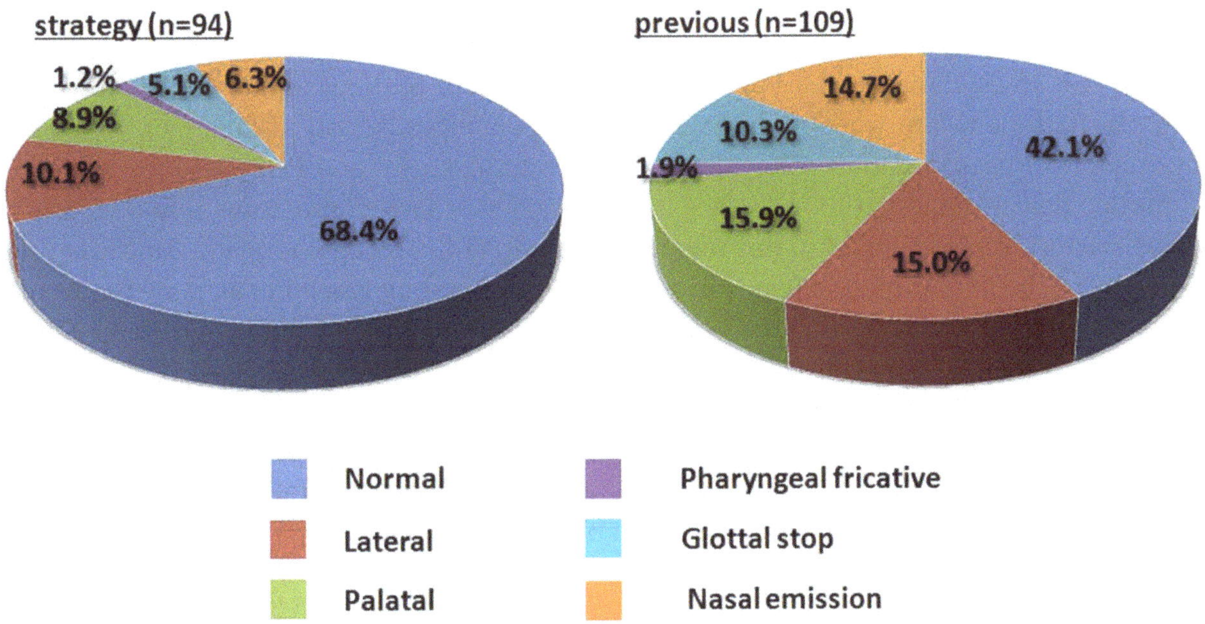

Figure 6. Postoperative articulation in the strategy and previous groups.

6. Discussion

When considering the postoperative VPI following CP repair, there are several main causes, including a wide cleft, short palate, deep pharynx, and unsatisfactory muscle reconstruction, when syndromic conditions, hearing loss, and mental retardation are excluded (**Figure 7a, b**). The preoperative portion between the velar length and pharyngeal depth bilaterally often differed, especially in subject with UCLP whose major and minor segments dislocated antero-posteriorly. During palatal repair, Z-plasty was usually used for adjusting the velar length; however, complete closure of the mucosal defect by large Z-plasty sometimes moved the uvula forward remaining asymmetry of the uvula position and pharyngeal arches (**Figure 7c**). The authors thought that these asymmetries in the velopharyngeal form may disturb the symmetrical muscular approximation and cause different sizes of the velopharyngeal orifice, resulting in persistent VPI following palatal repair [15, 16]. Therefore, it is thought to be useful to add a mucosal graft on the nasal side to fill the mucosal defect and to avoid an asymmetric VP form that may facilitate symmetrical velar motion in the VP closure mechanism.

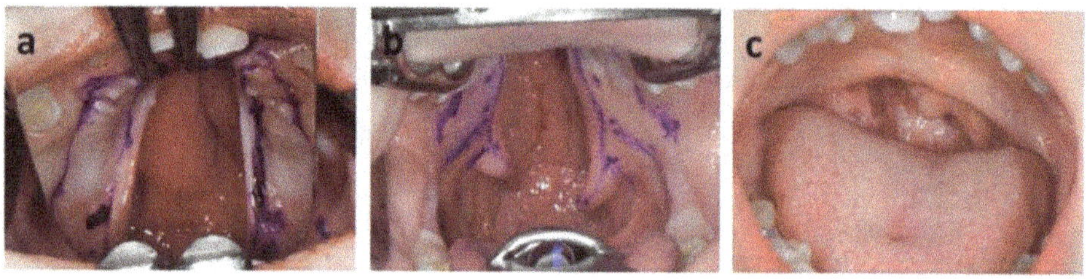

Figure 7. The reasons for postoperative VPI following CP repair: (a) the wide cleft, (b) short palate, (c) asymmetry of the uvula position and pharyngeal arch.

Furthermore, in the authors' experience during endoscopic examination of patients with persistent VPI, an asymmetric pharyngeal form or movement of the velopharynx and the midline defect of the velum were often observed, and they might be critical causes of VP closure dysfunction. Regarding the midline defect of the velum, Kuehn and Perry also reported that a midline defect suggested the presence of a deficiency or lack of musculus uvulae tissue or unsatisfactory surgical repair of this muscle (**Figure 8**) [17]. The anatomy and functional significance of the uvular muscle for VP closure was described by Kuehn et al. [18]. The uvular muscle courses posteriorly from its origin along the midline of the velum near the nasal surface of the velum. It is in its most cohesive form in the area overlying, and cradled by, the levator sling. The uvular muscle adds bulk to the dorsal aspect of the velum, thereby helping to fill the area between the velum and posterior pharyngeal wall. Without such bulk, the dorsal region would be concave, rather than convex, demonstrating a midline defect in the velum. In these cases, complete VP closure would not be achieved [17].

Considering the above, to ensure complete VP closure on CP repair, it is important to construct a symmetrical and functional velopharynx. Therefore, the authors have established a surgical strategy for palatal repair focusing on sufficient lengthening of the nasal mucosa, retropositioning the palatal muscles to produce a symmetrical levator sling, and unionizing the palatal muscles with a certain width in the midline of the velum. In the result, the surgical strategy for palatal repair facilitates successful speech outcomes in almost the same levels as those of Japanese children without cleft palate. There was no description about speech results of the CP patients based on the successful achievement of postoperative Velopharyngeal closure function equal to normal children.

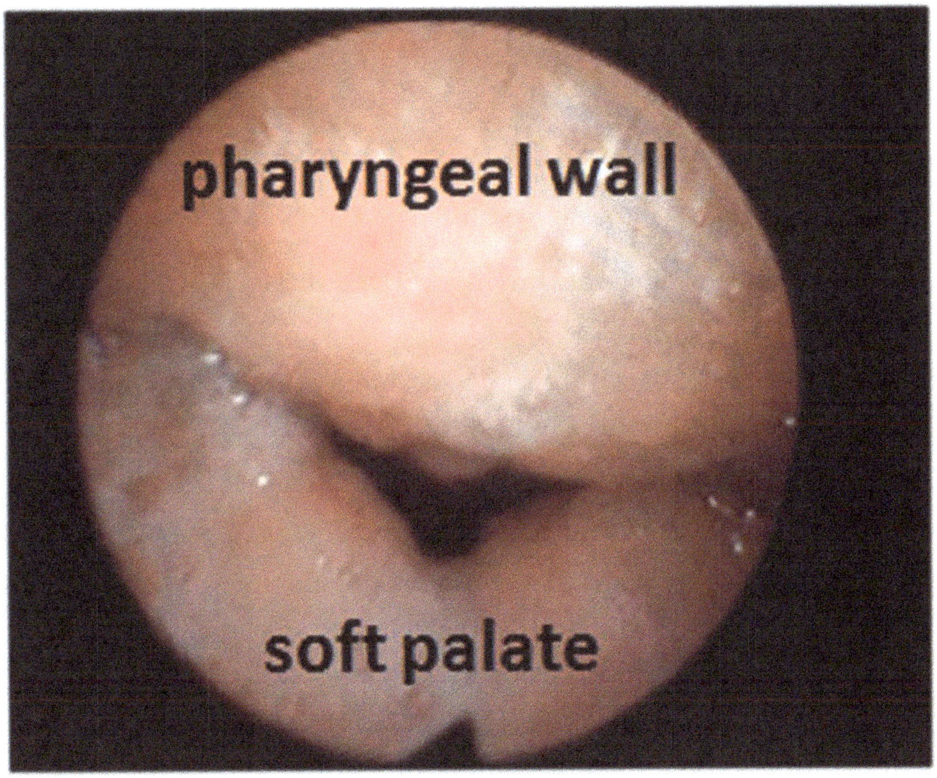

Figure 8. The midline defect of the velum of endoscopic examination might be a critical cause of VP closure dysfunction.

7. Conclusions

Cleft palate repair using a modified V-Y palatoplasty combining with a large Z-plasty and a mucosal graft on the nasal side of the velum for symmetrical muscular reconstruction based on the surgical strategy that approaches each anatomical and pathological abnormalities of cleft palate. Following palate repair based on our surgical strategy, patients' speech was significantly improved, and the nasalance scores were recovered to almost the same levels as those of Japanese children without cleft palate.

Author details

Norifumi Nakamura* and Masahiro Tezuka

*Address all correspondence to: nakamura@dent.kagoshima-u.ac.jp

Department of Oral and Maxillofacial Surgery, Field of Maxillofacial Rehabilitation, Kagoshima University Graduate School of Medical and Dental Sciences, Kagoshima, Japan

References

[1] Stengelhofen J: The nature and causes of communication problems in cleft palate. In: Sengelhofen J, editors. Cleft Palate: The Nature and Remediation of Communication Problems. Edinburg: Churchill Livingstone; 1989:1-30.

[2] Oyama K, Nishihara K, Matsunaga K, Miura N, Kibe T, Nakamura N: Perceptual-speech, nasometric, and cephalometric results after modified V-Y palatoplasties with or without mucosal graft. Cleft Palate Craniofac J. 2016;53:469-480.

[3] Dorrance GM, Bransfield JW: Cleft palate. Ann Surg. 1943;117:1-27.

[4] Ruding R: Cleft palate. Plast Reconstr Surg. 1964;33:132-147.

[5] Kreins OB: Fundamental anatomic findings for and intravelar veloplasty. Cleft Palate J. 1970;7:27-36.

[6] Edgerton MT, Dellon L: Surgical retrodisplacement of the levator veli palatine muscle. Preliminary report. Plast Reconstr Surg. 1971;47:154-167.

[7] Kaplan EN: Soft palate repair by levator muscle reconstruction and a buccal mucosal flap. Plast Reconstr Surg. 1975;56:129-136.

[8] Millard DR Jr: Refining the V-Y palate retropositioning. In: Millard DR Jr, editors. Cleft Craft. The Evolution of Its Surgery III. Alveolar and Palatal Deformities. Boston: Little Brown and Co.; 1980:419-448.

[9] Jackson IT, Moreira-Gonzales AA, Rogers A, Beal BJ: The buccal flap – a useful techniqque in cleft palate repair? Cleft Palate-Craniofac J. 2004;41:144-151.

[10] Nishio J, Yamanishi T, Kohara H, Hirano Y, Sako M, Adachi T, Mukai T, Miya S: Early two-stage palatoplasty using modified Furlow's veloplasty. Cleft Palate-Craniofac J. 2010;47:73-81.

[11] Brothers DB, Dalston RW, Peterson HD: Comparison of the Furlow double-opposing z-plasty with the Wardill-Kilner procedure for isolated cleft of the soft palate. Plast Reconstr Surg. 1995;95:969-977.

[12] van Lierde KM, Monstrey S, Bonte K, Van Cauwenberg P, Vinck B: The long-term speech outcome in Flemish young adults after two different types of palatoplasty. Int J Pediatr Otorhinolaryngol. 2004;68:865-875.

[13] Ogata Y, Tezuka M, Matsunaga K, Nakamura N: A trial for characterizing the behaviors of velopharyngeal closure insufficiency under various oral pressure conditions in cleft palate. In: Jaso N, Maria D'Cruz A, editors. Cleft Lip and Palate: Etiology, Surgery & Repair and Sociopsychological Consequences. New York: Nova Science Publishers Inc.; 2013:145-158.

[14] Ogata Y, Nakamura N, Kubota Y, Sasaguri M, Kikuta R, Shirasuna K, Ohishi M: Nasometer test for analysis on velopharyngeal function of patients with cleft palate (in Japanese with English Abstract). Jpn J Cleft Palate Assoc. 2003:28;9-19.

[15] Nakamura N, Ogata Y, Sasaguri M, Suzuki A, Kikuta R, Ohishi M: Aerodynamic and cephalometric analyses of velopharyngeal structure and function following re-pushback surgery for secondary correction in cleft palate. Cleft Palate-Craniofac J. 2003:40(1):46-53.

[16] Nakamura N, Ogata Y, Kunimitsu K, Suzuki A, Sasaguri M, Ohishi M: Velopharyngeal morphology of patients with persistent velopharyngeal incompetence following repushback surgery for cleft palate. Cleft Palate-Craniofac J. 2003:40(6):612-617.

[17] Kuehn DP, Perry JL: Anatomy and physiology of the velopharynx. Part V Cleft palate speech and management of velopharyngeal dysfunction. In: Losee JE, Kirshner RE, editors. Comprehensive Cleft Care. New York: The McGraw-Hill Companies Inc.; 2009:557-567.

[18] Kuehn DP, Folkins JW, Cutting CB: Relationships between muscle activity and velar position. Cleft Palate J. 1982;19:25-35.

12

Structural Analysis of Calderas by Semiautomatic Interpretation of the Gravity Gradient Tensor: A Case Study in Central Kyushu, Japan

Shigekazu Kusumoto

Abstract

In order to understand the formation history and mechanism of volcanoes and their related structures, including calderas, their subsurface structures play an important role. In recent years, gravity gradiometry survey has been introduced, and new analyses techniques for gravity gradient tensors obtained by the survey have been developed. In this chapter, we first describe the gravity gradient tensor and its characteristics, and the method for obtaining the tensor from the gravity anomaly. Next, we review the semiautomatic interpretation methods for extracting information on subsurface structures, and apply some of the techniques to the volcanic zone of central Kyushu, Japan. The results showed that the horizontal and vertical gravity gradient methods, and the *CLP* method were useful for extracting outlines of important volcanic and tectonic structures in this region. Using the maximum eigenvector of the gravity gradient tensor, the caldera wall dip of the Aso caldera was successfully estimated to be in the range of 50–70°, and the dip of the Median Tectonic Line which was the largest tectonic line in the southwest Japan was consistent with seismic reflection surveys. In addition, a large circular structure surrounding the Shishimuta caldera with a diameter of 35 km was distinguished in some analyses.

Keywords: caldera, gravity gradient tensor, subsurface structure, semi-automatic interpretation method, edge emphasis, dip estimation, curvature of the potential field, Hohi Volcanic Zone, Shishimuta caldera, Aso caldera

1. Introduction

Subsurface structures reveal the current form of the static basement and crust and may also indicate the result of past crustal deformation. Consequently, subsurface structures are essentially fossil evidence of crustal movement, such as faulting, dyke emplacement, and/or volcanic activity, and the restoration of these subsurface structures provides important information on the tectonic and/or volcanic history of a region.

In volcanic areas, large eruptions produce widespread volcanic ejecta at the Earth's surface, such as ash and lava flows, as well as volcanic depressions in the Earth's crust. And, there are fossil magma chambers, that is, plutons. These are frequently recorded as gravity and magnetic anomalies, and especially collapse calderas formed by partial or total collapse of a magma chamber roof (e.g., [1–3]) have low gravity anomalies and it is a roughly concentric circular shape. Large eruption forming calderas occur with a very low frequency, however, since much smaller calderas such as the Miyake-jima caldera (e.g., [4]) form more frequently (e.g., [5]), understanding the mechanisms behind caldera formation is very important not only for advancing scientific knowledge but also for social purposes such as the construction of hazard maps.

Thus, studies on caldera formation have been conducted not only by geological surveys in the field but with analogue experiments, numerical simulations, and theoretical approaches (e.g., [6–21]). Although results obtained by these experiments have been compared with surface topography and ring-fault distributions, they have not been compared with subsurface structures or gravity anomalies reflecting subsurface structures. This is a result of the difficulty inherent in estimating caldera subsurface structures and in transforming analogue experiment results into gravity anomalies. Nevertheless, many researchers have recognized the importance of caldera subsurface structures and observed significant relationships between the dip of the caldera wall, the radius of the magma chamber, processes of caldera formation, and the type of caldera (e.g., [14, 19–21]).

Geoelectromagnetic and gravity surveys are popular geophysical techniques used in volcanic areas and have been employed frequently to estimate shallow to medium depth subsurface structures. In recent years, gravity gradiometry has been introduced. This measures the gravity gradient tensor generated by a source body, which consists of six components of three-dimensional (3D) gravity gradients. Gravity gradiometry survey has higher sensitivity than gravity surveys. Various analysis techniques for gravity gradient tensors have been developed and have given excellent results in subsurface structure estimation and edge detection, for example (e.g., [22–25]).

In this chapter, we first describe the gravity gradient tensor and its characteristics. Generally, the gravity gradient tensor is obtained by gravity gradiometry. However, surveys of this type have been made in only a few areas, so that tensor data are rarely available. Therefore, in Section 2.2, we present a method based on the work of Mickus and Hinojosa [26] that is used to obtain the tensor from the gravity anomaly. We then review the semiautomatic interpretation methods used to extract information on subsurface structures without additional geological and geophysical information, and apply some of these techniques to the volcanic zone of central Kyushu in Japan.

2. Gravity gradient tensor

2.1. Characteristics of gravity gradient tensor

The gravity gradient tensor Γ is defined by the differential coefficients of the gravitational potential W (e.g., [27, 28]), as follows:

$$\Gamma = \begin{bmatrix} \frac{\partial^2 W}{\partial x^2} & \frac{\partial^2 W}{\partial x \partial y} & \frac{\partial^2 W}{\partial x \partial z} \\ \frac{\partial^2 W}{\partial y \partial x} & \frac{\partial^2 W}{\partial y^2} & \frac{\partial^2 W}{\partial y \partial z} \\ \frac{\partial^2 W}{\partial z \partial x} & \frac{\partial^2 W}{\partial z \partial y} & \frac{\partial^2 W}{\partial z^2} \end{bmatrix} \tag{1}$$

Defining g_x, g_y, and g_z, as the first derivative of W along the x, y, and z directions, we can rewrite Eq. (1) as follows:

$$\Gamma = \begin{bmatrix} \frac{\partial g_x}{\partial x} & \frac{\partial g_x}{\partial y} & \frac{\partial g_x}{\partial z} \\ \frac{\partial g_y}{\partial x} & \frac{\partial g_y}{\partial y} & \frac{\partial g_y}{\partial z} \\ \frac{\partial g_z}{\partial x} & \frac{\partial g_z}{\partial y} & \frac{\partial g_z}{\partial z} \end{bmatrix} = \begin{bmatrix} g_{xx} & g_{xy} & g_{xz} \\ g_{yx} & g_{yy} & g_{yz} \\ g_{zx} & g_{zy} & g_{zz} \end{bmatrix} \tag{2}$$

Here, g_z is the well-known gravity anomaly and g_{zz} is the vertical gradient of the gravity anomaly. The gravity gradient tensor is symmetric (e.g., [27]) and the sum of its diagonal components is zero since the gravitational potential satisfies Laplace's equation ($\Delta W = 0$).

Here, we set a point mass model under the surface (**Figure 1**). In this case, the gravitational potential W is:

$$W = -\frac{GM}{r} \tag{3}$$

where

$$r = \sqrt{(x-x')^2 + (y-y')^2 + (z-z')^2} \tag{4}$$

G is the gravitational constant and M is the mass. Taking the first derivative along the x-, y-, and z-directions gives

$$g_x = W_x = \frac{\partial W}{\partial x} = GM\frac{x-x'}{r^3} \tag{5}$$

$$g_y = W_y = \frac{\partial W}{\partial y} = GM\frac{y-y'}{r^3} \tag{6}$$

and

$$g_z = W_z = \frac{\partial W}{\partial z} = GM\frac{z-z'}{r^3} \tag{7}$$

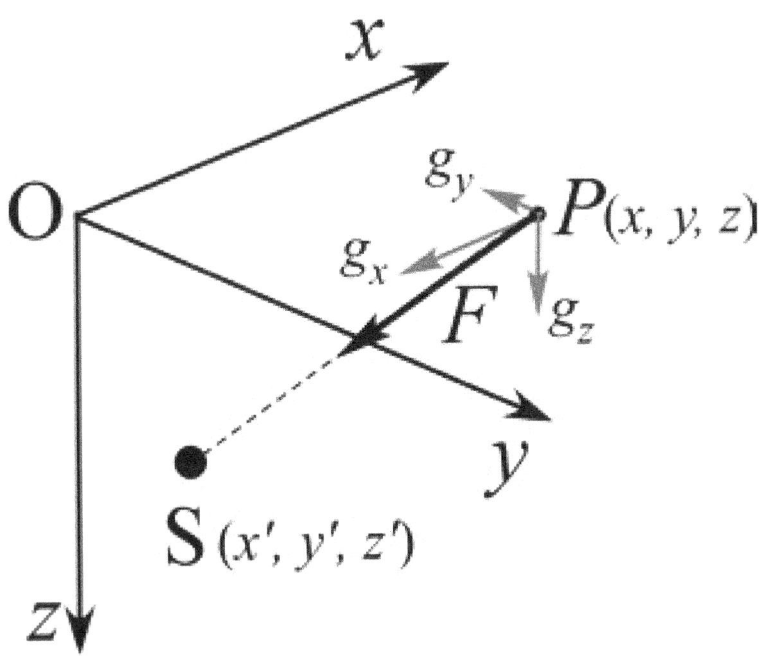

Figure 1. Point mass model. Schematic illustration of the gravitational vector due to a positive mass anomaly.

These are xyz components of the gravitation vector, F, due to the mass anomaly M.

Taking the second derivatives of the potential W along x, y, and z directions, six of the nine second derivatives are given by

$$g_{xx} = W_{xx} = \frac{\partial^2 W}{\partial x^2} = GM \frac{-3(x-x')^2 + r^2}{r^5} \tag{8}$$

$$g_{xy} = W_{xy} = \frac{\partial^2 W}{\partial x \partial y} = GM \frac{-3(x-x')(y-y')}{r^5} \tag{9}$$

$$g_{xz} = W_{xz} = \frac{\partial^2 W}{\partial x \partial z} = GM \frac{-3(x-x')(z-z')}{r^5} \tag{10}$$

$$g_{yy} = W_{yy} = \frac{\partial^2 W}{\partial y^2} = GM \frac{-3(y-y')^2 + r^2}{r^5} \tag{11}$$

$$g_{yz} = W_{yz} = \frac{\partial^2 W}{\partial y \partial z} = GM \frac{-3(y-y')(z-z')}{r^5} \tag{12}$$

and

$$g_{zz} = W_{zz} = \frac{\partial^2 W}{\partial z^2} = GM \frac{-3(z-z')^2 + r^2}{r^5} \tag{13}$$

These are six independent components of the gravity gradient tensor. The other three second derivatives can be obtained using the symmetry characteristics of the second derivative. And, since the sum of Eqs. (8), (11), and (13) is zero, namely

$$\begin{aligned} g_{xx} + g_{yy} + g_{zz} &= GM\left[\frac{-3(x-x')^2 + r^2}{r^5} + \frac{-3(y-y')^2 + r^2}{r^5} + \frac{-3(z-z')^2 + r^2}{r^5}\right] \\ &= GM\left\{\frac{-3\left[(x-x')^2 + (y-y')^2 + (z-z')^2\right] + 3r^2}{r^5}\right\} = 0 \end{aligned}$$

diagonal components satisfy Laplace's equation ($\Delta W = 0$).

We show a numerical example for the point mass model in **Figure 2**. In the numerical example, we set the point mass model with a depth of 4 km and a mass anomaly of -5.7×10^4 kg. Here, negative mass anomaly means lack of mass caused by negative density contrast such as hole in the crust, and the mass anomaly of -5.7×10^4 kg is equivalent to a sphere having radius of 3 km and density contrast of -500 kg/m^3. The vertical component, g_z, of the gravitational vector is negative because of a negative mass anomaly (**Figure 2(i)**). The horizontal components of the gravitational vector, g_x (**Figure 2(a)**) and g_y (**Figure 2(e)**), are positive in the area where the terms $(x - x')$ or $(y - y')$ in Eqs. (5) and (6) are positive, and negative in the area where the terms are negative, because material surrounding the point mass is denser and gravitation vectors point to dense area, that is, the outside of the point mass.

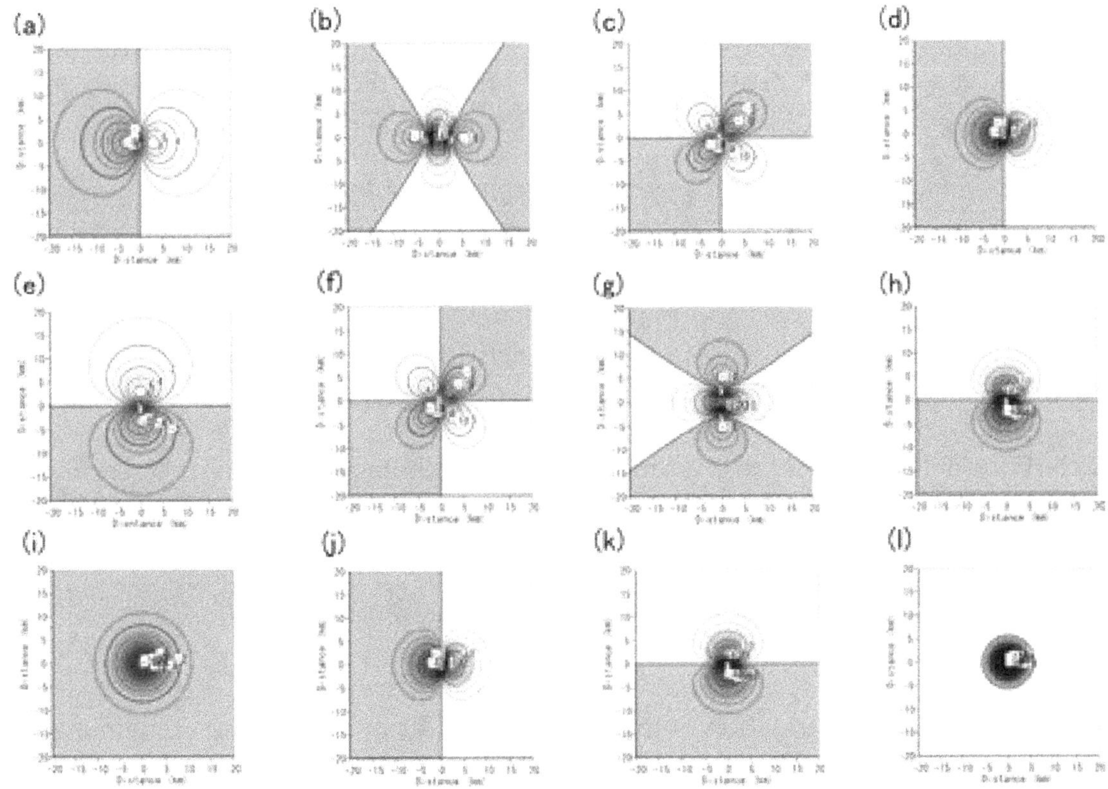

Figure 2. Components of the gravitational vector and gravity gradient tensor caused by a point mass with a depth of 4 km and a mass anomaly of -5.7×10^4 kg. Negative mass anomaly means lack of mass caused by negative density contrast such as hole in the crust. Negative areas are colored gray. The gravitational vector unit is given in mGal, and mGal = 10^{-5} m/s^2. The unit of the gravity gradient tensor is given in E (Eötvös), and 1 E = 0.1 mGal/km. (a) g_x component of gravitational vector, (b) g_{xx} component of gravity gradient tensor, (c) g_{xy} component, (d) g_{xz} component, (e) g_y component, (f) g_{yx} component, which is equal to g_{xy}, (g) g_{yy} component, (h) g_{yz} component, (i) $g_z$component; gravity anomaly, (j) g_{zx} component, which is equal to g_{xz}, (k) g_{zy} component, which is equal to g_{yz}, and (l) g_{zz} component.

In the gravity gradient tensor, Γ, we first find the triplet pattern, negative-positive-negative, in the g_{xx} component (**Figure 2(b)**). This pattern can be understood by examining the slopes of the anomalies of g_x as we proceed from left to right along the x-axis. We notice that the steepest slope is at the center of the map of g_x and it is positive; the zero slopes are at the trough and peak of g_x, and the gentle negative slopes are to the left and right of the trough and peak, respectively. In a similar manner, we can explain the triplet pattern of the g_{yy} component (**Figure 2(g)**). In the g_{xy} component (**Figure 2(c)**), we find the quadruplet pattern, negative-positive-negative-positive. This pattern can be understood by examining the slopes of the anomalies of g_y as we proceed from left to right along the x-axis, or by examining the slopes of the anomalies of g_x as we proceed from left to right along the y-axis. The components g_{xz} (**Figure 2(d)**), g_{yz} (**Figure 2(h)**), and g_{zz} (**Figure 2(l)**) are differential coefficients of g_x, g_y, and g_z in the z direction and emphasize the high frequencies of each gravitational component without any changes in the location or shape of the anomalies.

2.2. Derivation of gravity gradient tensor from gravity anomaly

In general, the gravity gradient tensor is measured with gravity gradiometry (e.g., [29–31]). However, we can obtain the tensor from gravity anomaly data using calculations shown in [26], even if the gravity gradiometry surveys have not yet been undertaken.

As a technique for calculating the gravity gradient tensor from the gravity anomaly data, Mickus and Hinojosa [26] used the following procedure: (1) application of a Fourier transformation to the gravity anomaly, (2) estimation of the gravitational potential by integration of the gravity anomaly in the Fourier domain, (3) calculation of the gravity gradient components from second-order derivatives of the potential in each direction, and (4) application of a Fourier inverse transformation to finally obtain all components of the tensor in the spatial domain.

When the Fourier transformation of a function $f(x, y)$ is denoted by the shorthand notation $\mathscr{F}[f]$, that is,

$$\mathscr{F}[f] = F(k_x, k_y) = \int_{-\infty}^{\infty}\int_{-\infty}^{\infty} f(x, y) e^{-i(k_x x + k_y y)} dx dy, \tag{14}$$

The Fourier inverse transformation of the function $F(k_x, k_y)$ in the Fourier domain is denoted by the shorthand notation $\mathscr{F}^{-1}[F]$ (e.g., [32]), that is,

$$\mathscr{F}^{-1}[F] = f(x, y) = \frac{1}{4\pi^2}\int_{-\infty}^{\infty}\int_{-\infty}^{\infty} F(k_x, k_y) e^{i(k_x x + k_y y)} dk_x dk_y, \tag{15}$$

where k_x and k_y are wave numbers and are inversely related to wavelengths λ_x and λ_y in the x and y directions, respectively: $k_x = 2\pi/\lambda_x$ and $k_y = 2\pi/\lambda_y$. If G_z is the Fourier transform of the gravity anomaly g_z, the relationships between g_z and G_z are as follows:

$$G_z = \mathscr{F}[g_z] \tag{16}$$

$$g_z = \mathscr{F}^{-1}[G_z] \tag{17}$$

and we use the notation $g_z \leftrightarrow G_z$ for this relationship. Differentiation of a function in the space domain is equivalent to multiplication by a power of the wavenumber in the Fourier domain (e.g., [32]). If $f(x, y) \leftrightarrow F(k_x, k_y)$, then,

$$\frac{\partial^m}{\partial x^m}\frac{\partial^n}{\partial y^n}f(x,y)\leftrightarrow(ik_x)^m(ik_y)^n F(k_x,k_y) \quad (18)$$

Integration of the function in the Fourier domain is given by division of the wavenumber. From these and relationships between gravity and gravitational potential, we derive the following equations on gravitational vector components:

$$G_x = ik_x U \quad (19)$$

$$G_y = ik_y U \quad (20)$$

$$G_z = |\mathbf{k}|U \quad (21)$$

where U is the Fourier transform of the gravitational potential, W, and $|\mathbf{k}| = (k_x^2 + k_y^2)^{1/2}$. From Eq. (21), we can obtain the gravitational potential U from the gravity anomaly by

$$U = \frac{G_z}{|\mathbf{k}|} \quad (22)$$

and Eqs. (19) and (20) are rewritten as follows:

$$G_x = \frac{ik_x}{|\mathbf{k}|}G_z \quad (23)$$

$$G_y = \frac{ik_y}{|\mathbf{k}|}G_z \quad (24)$$

Therefore, we can obtain g_x and g_y from g_z by the Fourier inverse transformation of G_x and G_y.

In a similar manner, we derive equations to obtain each component of the gravity gradient tensor:

$$G_{xx} = -k_x^2 U = \frac{-k_x^2}{|\mathbf{k}|}G_z \quad (25)$$

$$G_{yy} = -k_y^2 U = \frac{-k_y^2}{|\mathbf{k}|} G_z \tag{26}$$

$$G_{zz} = |\mathbf{k}| G_z \tag{27}$$

$$G_{xy} = ik_x ik_y U = \frac{-k_x k_y}{|\mathbf{k}|} G_z \tag{28}$$

$$G_{zx} = ik_x G_z \tag{29}$$

and

$$G_{zy} = ik_y G_z \tag{30}$$

From these equations, as summarized in [26], we can obtain all components of the gravity gradient tensor from the gravity anomaly as follows:

$$\begin{bmatrix} g_{xx} & g_{xy} & g_{xz} \\ g_{yx} & g_{yy} & g_{yz} \\ g_{zx} & g_{zy} & g_{zz} \end{bmatrix} = \mathscr{F}^{-1} \left\{ \begin{bmatrix} \frac{-k_x^2}{|\mathbf{k}|} & \frac{-k_x k_y}{|\mathbf{k}|} & ik_x \\ \frac{-k_x k_y}{|\mathbf{k}|} & \frac{-k_y^2}{|\mathbf{k}|} & ik_y \\ ik_x & ik_y & |\mathbf{k}| \end{bmatrix} G_z(\mathbf{k}) \right\}. \tag{31}$$

3. Semiautomatic interpretation techniques

3.1. Edge emphasis

Edge emphasis techniques are extraction techniques used to find locations (namely, edge) where the gravity anomaly changes abruptly due to density variations, and these techniques play an important role in interpretation of potential field data (e.g., [33–35]).

In these techniques, the horizontal and vertical gravity gradient methods have frequently been employed to find structural boundaries such as faults or contacts between different materials (e.g., [36–39]). The vertical gravity gradient (*VG*) is the g_{zz} component of the gravity gradient tensor, and the horizontal gravity gradient (*HG*) is given using the components of the gravity gradient tensor shown in Eq. (2) as follows:

$$HG = \sqrt{g_{zx}^2 + g_{zy}^2} \tag{32}$$

In addition to these gravity gradients, the second vertical derivative, $\partial^2 g_z/\partial z^2$, is well known and is a classical edge emphasis technique for edge detection (e.g., [40–43]).

Miller and Singh [44] proposed the *TDR* (tilt derivative), defined by the arctangent of the ratio of the vertical gravity gradient to the *HG*:

$$TDR = \arctan\left(\frac{g_{zz}}{\sqrt{g_{zx}^2 + g_{zy}^2}}\right) \tag{33}$$

This emphasis technique does not extract extremely large amplitude signals in the short wavelength range and is known as a balanced method. However, it is noted that the *TDR* extracts a phantom boundary at the zero line if positive and negative anomalies exist side by side (e.g., [45, 46]).

Wijns et al. [47] proposed the *THETA* map that could be used to obtain the structural boundaries,

$$THETA = \arccos\left(\frac{\sqrt{g_{zx}^2 + g_{zy}^2}}{\sqrt{g_{zx}^2 + g_{zy}^2 + g_{zz}^2}}\right) \tag{34}$$

and Cooper and Cowan [44] proposed the *TDX* defined by the following equation:

$$TDX = \arctan\left(\frac{\sqrt{g_{zx}^2 + g_{zy}^2}}{|g_{zz}|}\right) \tag{35}$$

Li et al. [48] conducted a numerical test of these emphasis techniques for structural boundary extraction. As a result, they found that (1) the *HG* method can determine structural boundaries of the causative body but its ability decreases with depth, (2) the *TDR* and *THETA* methods are also able to retrieve the structural boundaries but their extracted shapes are not clear and, as mentioned above, these methods introduce a phantom boundary at the zero line in case of side by side positive and negative anomalies, and (3) the *TDX* has the same phantom boundary limitation but the method can give clearer boundary location than both *TDR* and *THETA*.

Based on these discussions, Li et al. [48] suggested the *CLP* method, which extracts the outlines of subsurface structures without the phantom boundary. The *CLP* is defined as follows:

$$CLP = \arctan\left[\frac{\sqrt{\left(\frac{\partial g_z}{\partial x}\right)^2 + \left(\frac{\partial g_z}{\partial y}\right)^2}}{p + k \times \left|\frac{\partial g_z}{\partial z}\right|}\right] \tag{36}$$

where p is a previously determined constant, typically 1/10 of the maximum value of the horizontal gravity gradient. And k is defined as follows:

$$k = \frac{mean\left|\frac{\partial g_z}{\partial z}\right|}{mean\left|\frac{\partial^2 g_z}{\partial z^2}\right|} \tag{37}$$

In recent years, specialized edge emphasis techniques have been developed to find the edges of potential field data related to multi subsurface structures. For example, Ma [46] suggested the Improved Local Phase method (*ILP*):

$$ILP = \arcsin\left[\frac{\sqrt{\left(\frac{\partial g_z}{\partial x}\right)^2 + \left(\frac{\partial g_z}{\partial y}\right)^2}}{\sqrt{\left(\frac{\partial g_z}{\partial x}\right)^2 + \left(\frac{\partial g_z}{\partial y}\right)^2 + \left(\frac{\partial^2 g_z}{\partial x^2} + \frac{\partial^2 g_z}{\partial y^2}\right)^2}}\right] \tag{38}$$

And, Ferreira et al. [49] have suggested the *TAHG*:

$$TAHG = \arctan\left[\frac{\frac{\partial HG}{\partial z}}{\sqrt{\left(\frac{\partial HG}{\partial x}\right)^2 + \left(\frac{\partial HG}{\partial y}\right)^2}}\right] \tag{39}$$

Using numerical tests, Zhang et al. [50] showed that the *ILP* and the *TAHG* successfully extract the edges of potential field data relating to multi subsurface structures, and they also suggested a more sensitive edge detection method, *THVH*. The *THVH* is defined as follows:

$$THVH = \arctan\left[\frac{\dfrac{\partial^2 HG}{\partial z^2}}{\sqrt{\left(\dfrac{\partial}{\partial x}\dfrac{\partial HG}{\partial z}\right)^2 + \left(\dfrac{\partial}{\partial y}\dfrac{\partial HG}{\partial z}\right)^2}}\right] \tag{40}$$

Kusumoto [51] pointed out that because the *CLP, ILP, TAHG,* and *THVH* are all very sensitive high pass filters, which respond to very small signals (perhaps also including noise), other geological or geophysical data of the region would be required in order to fully understand the results obtained by these techniques.

3.2. Curvature of the potential field

Curvatures of potential field data vary in response to density changes in the subsurface structure, and these curvatures are described by the g_{xx}, g_{yy}, and g_{xy} components (e.g., [27, 28]).

Pedersen and Rasmussen [52] defined the invariant ratio, *I*, of the gravity gradient tensor as follows:

$$I = \frac{-27 I_2^2}{4 I_1^3} \tag{41}$$

Here, I_1 and I_2 are invariants of the tensor. Each invariant is given by three eigenvalues (λ_1, λ_2, λ_3) of the gravity gradient tensors, as follows:

$$\begin{aligned} I_1 &= \lambda_1\lambda_2 + \lambda_2\lambda_3 + \lambda_1\lambda_3 \\ I_2 &= \lambda_1\lambda_2\lambda_3 \end{aligned} \tag{42}$$

The invariant ratio *I* varies between 0 and +1. If the body causing a gravity anomaly is a 2D structure, *I* is 0. If the causative body is 3D, *I* is +1. Beiki and Pedersen [53] named this ratio the dimensionality index and suggested $I = 0.5$ as the threshold between a 2D and 3D causative structure. In addition, for the case of a 2D causative structure such as a dike, the maximum eigenvector of the gravity gradient tensor points to the causative body and the minimum eigenvector is parallel to the strike direction of the structure.

Cevallos et al. [54] and Cevallos [55] pointed out that the shape index (e.g., [56, 57]) is useful for determining the characteristics of potential fields and is defined by

$$Si = \frac{2}{\pi}\arctan\left[\frac{g_{zz}}{\sqrt{\left(g_{xx} - g_{yy}\right)^2 + 4g_{xy}^2}}\right] \tag{43}$$

The shape index, Si, varies from –1 to +1, and it is suggested that values of –1, –0.5, 0, +0.5, and +1 correspond to bowl, valley, flat, ridge, and dome structures, respectively. Cevallos [55] found that a map of the shape index at depth was consistent with deep structures integrated by geophysical and geological data in the King Sound area of the Canning Basin, Western Australia.

Studies on the curvature of the potential field have recently been developed as new interpretation techniques because they use a lot of the characteristics of the gravity gradient tensor (e.g., [58–62]). However, some problems relating to its practical usage remain unsolved. In fact, Li [63] conducted numerical tests for 13 well-known semiautomatic interpretation methods based on the curvature of the potential field and concluded that the shape of the potential does not always correspond to the subsurface structure, and therefore care should be taken when interpreting these results.

3.3. Euler deconvolution

Euler deconvolution is a semiautomatic interpretation method based on Euler's homogeneity equation and is often employed to estimate locations and/or outlines of causative bodies. Because the Euler deconvolution technique can provide rapid interpretations of any potential field data in terms of depth and geological structures, it has been used by several researchers for analyzing both magnetic anomalies (e.g., [64–66]) and gravity anomalies (e.g., [67]).

The Euler deconvolution based on the three orthogonal gradient components of the potential field is simply called Euler deconvolution or conventional Euler deconvolution. For the gravity anomaly g_z, it uses the following equation:

$$(x - x_0)g_{zx} + (y - y_0)g_{zy} + (z - z_0)g_{zz} = N(B_z - g_z) \tag{44}$$

In Eq. (44), x_0, y_0, and z_0 are unknown location parameters of the causative body center or edge that have to be estimated, and x, y, and z are known location parameters of the observation point of the gravity and its gradients. N is the structural index and B_z is the regional component of the gravity anomaly that has to be estimated.

Rewriting Eq. (44), we obtain the following equation in which we can separate unknown parameters from known parameters:

$$x_0 g_{zx} + y_0 g_{zy} + z_0 g_{zz} + NB_z = xg_{zx} + yg_{zy} + zg_{zz} + Ng_z \tag{45}$$

There are four unknown parameters in Eq. (45). If we have enough data, namely $n \geq 4$, to solve for these unknowns within a selected window, we can estimate these four parameters using the least-squares method.

Zhang et al. [68] suggested the Tensor Euler deconvolution, designed to consider the full gravity gradient tensor (Eq. (2)) and all components (g_x, g_y, g_z) of the gravitational vector. The Tensor Euler deconvolution is defined by the following simultaneous equations:

$$\begin{aligned}(x - x_0) g_{xx} + (y - y_0) g_{xy} + (z - z_0) g_{xz} &= N(B_x - g_x) \\ (x - x_0) g_{yx} + (y - y_0) g_{yy} + (z - z_0) g_{yz} &= N(B_y - g_y) \\ (x - x_0) g_{zx} + (y - y_0) g_{zy} + (z - z_0) g_{zz} &= N(B_z - g_z)\end{aligned} \tag{46}$$

Here, B_x and B_y are the regional components of the gravity anomaly that have to be estimated. Thus, there are six unknown parameters in this equation, and if we have enough data to solve for these six unknowns within a selected window, namely $n \geq 6$, these parameters can be estimated using the least squares method. Using a numerical study and applying it to field data, Zhang et al. [68] showed that the Tensor Euler deconvolution produces a significantly improved resolution compared to the conventional Euler deconvolution.

3.4. Dip estimation of a fault or structural boundary

In recent years, a technique estimating the dip of structures such as dikes, faults, or other geological structure boundaries has been developed and produced good results as a semiautomatic interpretation method using the gravity gradient tensor.

Beiki [69] suggested that the dip, α, of the causative body could be estimated from the three components (x, y, z) of the maximum eigenvector (v_1) of the gradient tensor of the potential field (**Figure 3**) as follows:

$$\alpha = \arctan\left(\frac{v_{1z}}{\sqrt{(v_{1x})^2 + (v_{1y})^2}}\right) \tag{47}$$

where v_{1x}, v_{1y}, and v_{1z} are the x, y, and z components of the maximum eigenvector, v_1. Beiki [69] applied this method to an aeromagnetic data set of the Åsele area in Sweden, and provided useful information on the dip of dike swarms. Kusumoto [70] applied this technique to estimate the dip of the Median Tectonic Line located in southwest Japan, and obtained a dip distribution compatible with results from other geophysical surveys, including a reflection survey. Since gravity gradient tensor consists of differential coefficients of gravitation caused by causative body the tensor has higher accuracy than gravity anomaly. In addition, since analysis using eigenvalues and eigenvectors of the tensor considers all components of the tensor, this technique would give good results. In this technique, we do not need to know or assume density contrast between layers or structures.

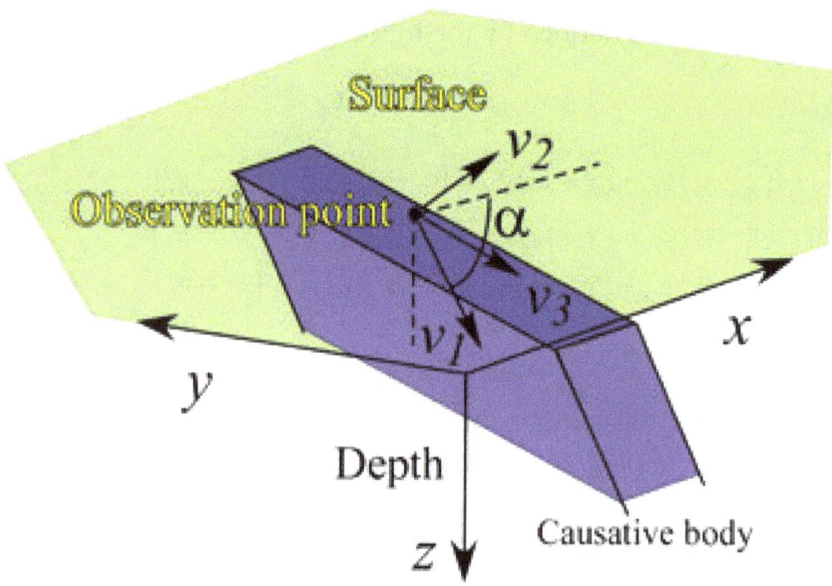

Figure 3. Schematic illustration of the eigenvectors for a 2D structure such as dike. In this figure, v_1, v_2, and v_3 are the maximum, intermediate, and minimum eigenvectors of the gravity gradient tensor, respectively. The maximum eigenvector points to the causative body and the minimum eigenvector is parallel to the strike direction of the body. The angle α between the surface and maximum eigenvector is the angle of the structural boundary and/or fault.

4. Application of semiautomatic interpretation method

Here, we apply the semiautomatic interpretation methods shown in the previous section to a volcanic area located in central Kyushu, Japan. This area consists of the Aso caldera and the Hohi Volcanic Zone containing a buried caldera, the Shishimuta caldera, where many previous geological and geophysical studies have been conducted. In addition, a database of the Bouguer gravity anomaly is available for use (e.g., [71]), although a gravity gradiometory survey covering this area has not yet been carried out. Since this gravity anomaly database employed in this study gives users 1 km × 1 km mesh data, we discussed structures larger than several kilometers in this study. If we would like to discuss fine structures, it would be possible by employing denser mesh data.

4.1. Background of Hohi Volcanic Zone and Aso caldera

4.1.1. Hohi Volcanic Zone and Shishimuta caldera

The Hohi Volcanic Zone (e.g., [73]) is located in the eastern part of central Kyushu (**Figure 4**) and is characterized by a wedge-shaped low gravity anomaly area, which becomes narrow toward the east (**Figure 5**). In the Hohi Volcanic Zone, there are four conspicuous low anomaly areas toward the west-southwest from Beppu Bay, which correspond to the Beppu Bay, Shonai Basin, Shishimuta caldera, and Kuju basin, respectively. The Beppu Bay has the lowest gravity anomaly, which reaches –50 mGal.

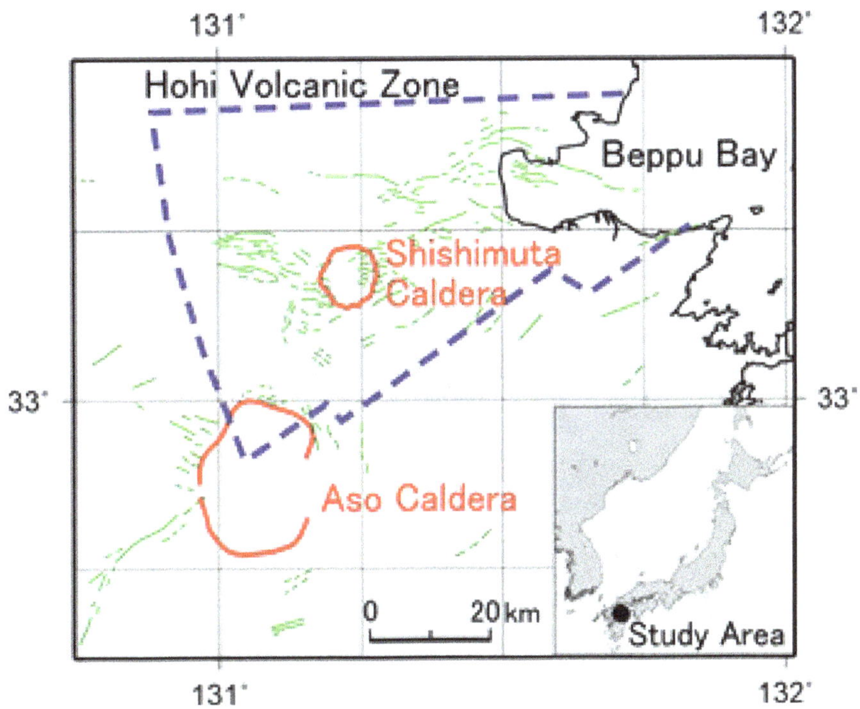

Figure 4. Location map of study area. Blue dashed line indicates the outline of the Hohi volcanic zone. Red lines indicate the caldera. Green lines are active faults (e.g., [72]).

Subsurface structures in this region have been estimated by gravity anomaly data, drill core data, reflection survey, and surface geology data (e.g., [74, 75]). Kusumoto et al. [75] showed that, although the average depth of the basement was estimated to be approximately 1.2 km in the Hohi Volcanic Zone, the small basins (the Shonai basin and the Kuju basin) along the Oita-Kumamoto Tectonic Line (the tectonic line suggested by a steep gravity gradient (e.g., [76])) are deeper than 2 km. In addition, it was shown that the basement depth in Beppu Bay reaches to approximately 4 km. Detailed geological surveys have shown that this volcanic zone consists of half-grabens detailing volcanic activity that began 6 Ma (e.g., [73]) and pull-apart basins that formed after the half-graben formation (e.g., [77]).

During formation of the Hohi Volcanic Zone, it is known that eruption of more than 5000 km^3 of material occurred in the last six million years, and that eruption rate gradually decreased. The volcanic zone erupted 2900 km^3/Ma in its initial stage of activity from 5 to 4 Ma. After that, the zone erupted approximately 1300, 900, 400, and 200 km^3 between 4–3, 3–2, 2–1, and 1–0 Ma, respectively [73]. The formation of the pull-apart basin began 1.5 Ma; this tectonic change occurred due to a counter-clockwise shift of the subducting Philippine Sea Plate (e.g., [77]).

Kusumoto et al. [78] attempted to restore the tectonic structures by numerical simulations based on the dislocation theory (e.g., [79]). They showed that tectonic structures such as half-grabens and pull-apart basins can be restored by obeying the tectonics suggested by Itoh et al. [77]. Kusumoto et al. [80] assumed a simple two-layer structure model, which consisted of the basement and the sediment, and estimated the gravity anomaly field from the vertical displacement field of the basement obtained by tectonic modeling [78]. As a result, it was shown that a gravity anomaly of volcanic origin cannot be restored. In this model, the unrestored gravity anomaly was that relating to the Shishimuta caldera.

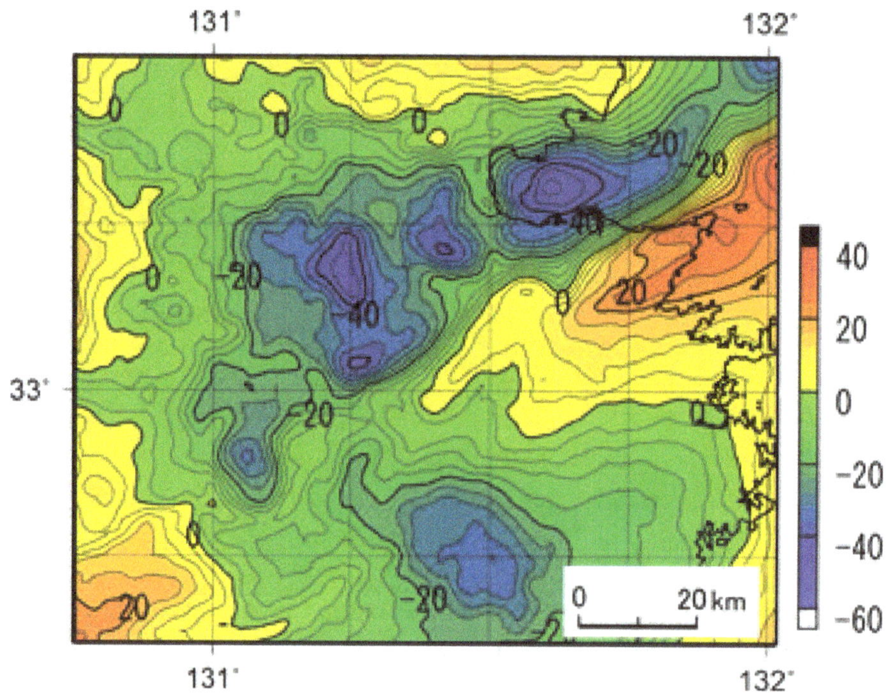

Figure 5. Residual Bouguer gravity anomaly map of the study area and surroundings. The contour interval is 4 mGal. In the residual Bouguer gravity anomaly map, the regional linear trend of the Bouguer gravity anomalies, such as the effect of the subducting plate, is estimated and removed by the least squares method from the Bouguer gravity anomalies. The Bouguer gravity anomaly used here is based on the gravity anomaly database (1 km × 1 km mesh data) by Komazawa [71], and a Bouguer density of 2670 kg/m^3 is employed.

The Shishimuta caldera is a buried caldera and is the origin of the Yabakei and Imaichi pyroclastic flows that are widely distributed throughout central Kyushu (e.g., [81, 82]). The volumes of these flows have been estimated as 40 km^3 (e.g., [81]) and 90 km^3 (e.g., [82]), respectively, based on detailed surface geological surveys. The red circle shown in **Figure 4** indicates the caldera wall at 1 km depth with a diameter of approximately 8–10 km, estimated from drilling core data and gravity anomalies (e.g., [81]). Density contrast between basement and sedimentary layers is estimated to be in the range of 300–700 kg/m^3 by Kusumoto et al. [75]. As shown in **Figure 5**, this Shishimuta caldera does not have the concentrically circular low gravity anomaly found in many calderas; rather, this caldera has a triangular low gravity anomaly.

The subsurface structure of the Shishimuta caldera was estimated from a geological perspective, and the structure shallower than 3 km depth was revealed by drill core data and gravity anomalies. On the basis of drill core data, gravity anomalies, active fault distribution, microearthquake activity, and geological surveys in and near the Shishimuta caldera, Kamata [81] estimated that the shape of this caldera is a funnel type. In addition, Kamata [81] estimated a magma chamber depth of the Shishimuta caldera would be 7–12 km depth. This was estimated by assuming that the original depth of the Yabakei pyroclastic flow is equal to the source depth of the Ito pyroclastic flow of Aira caldera, Kagoshima (e.g., [83]).

4.1.2. Aso caldera

The Aso caldera, like the Shishimuta caldera, is located in central Kyushu (**Figure 4**). However, it extends approximately 25 km in the south-north direction and about 18 km in the east-west direction and is thus elliptical in plan view, and is one of the largest calderas in the world.

It is known that the Aso caldera was formed by four eruptions with large-scale pyroclastic flows. The first large pyroclastic flow is called Aso-1 and flowed out from the present Aso caldera prior to 0.27 Ma. The second is called Aso-2 and was erupted before 0.14 Ma. The Aso-2 was the smallest pyroclastic flow and its volume is estimated at approximately 25 km^3. The third pyroclastic flow is called Aso-3 and is dated at 0.12 Ma. The fourth pyroclastic flow is called Aso-4 and is the largest pyroclastic flow with a volume of more than 80 km^3. From detailed geological surveys, it has been found that Aso-4 would have flown over the sea (the Seto inland sea and Tachibana Bay) and reached Yamaguchi Prefecture and Shimabara Peninsula. In the Aso caldera, there is also a central group of volcanic cones, which are currently active (e.g., [84]).

Gravity surveys of this region have been initiated by Tsuboi et al. [76] and Kubotera et al. [85]. Yokoyama [86] estimated that the subterranean caldera structure is similar to a funnel-shape. Komazawa [87] accumulated gravity data and conducted high accuracy, high-resolution analyses for the compiled gravity data. As a result, they found that the Aso caldera has a piston-cylinder type structure rather than a funnel-shaped structure with a single low anomaly. In addition, five minor local gravity lows exist in the caldera, which make up the major low gravity zone of the Aso caldera. The major gravity low has a steep gradient inside the caldera rim, and the central area of the minor gravity anomalies has a relatively flat bottom.

4.2. Gravity gradient tensor in central Kyushu

In **Figure 6**, we show all components of the gravitation vector and gravity gradient tensor. Since the gravity gradiometry survey covering this region has not been conducted, the gravitation vector and gravity gradient tensor were calculated from the Bouguer gravity anomaly data shown in **Figure 5**.

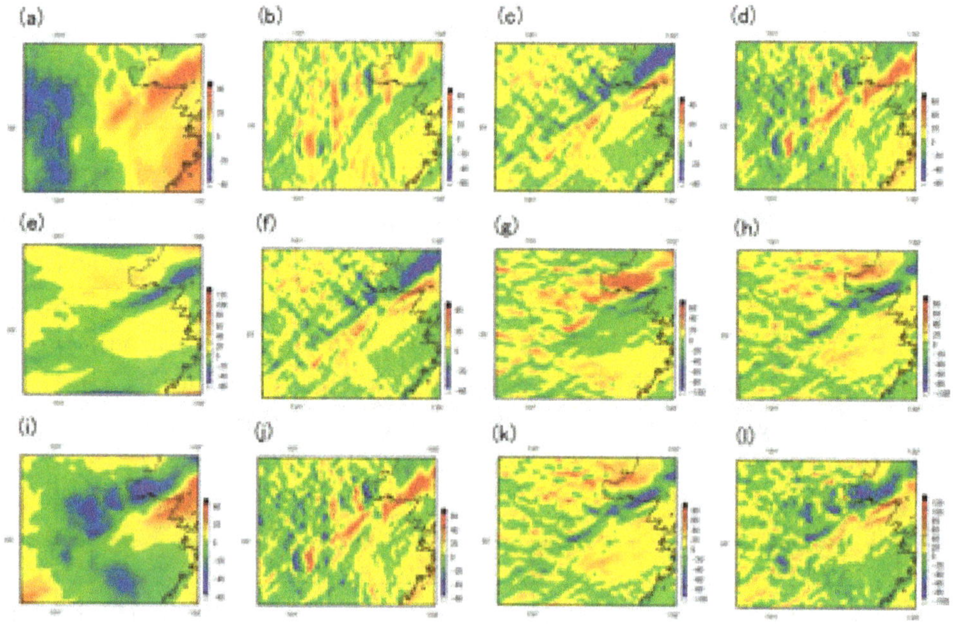

Figure 6. Components of gravitational vector and gravity gradient tensor calculated from g_z data shown in **Figure 5**, using the method of Mickus and Hinojosa [24]. The gravitational vector unit is given in mGal, and mGal = 10^{-5} m/s^2. The unit of the gravity gradient tensor is given in E (Eötvös), and 1 E = 0.1 mGal/km. (a) g_x component of gravitational vector, (b) g_{xx} component of gravity gradient tensor, (c) g_{xy} component, (d) g_{xz} component, (e) g_y component, (f) g_{yx} component, which is equal to g_{xy}, (g) g_{yy} component, (h) g_{yz} component, (i) $g_z$component; gravity anomaly, (j) g_{zx} component, which is equal to g_{xz}, (k) g_{zy} component, which is equal to g_{yz}, and (l) g_{zz} component.

Although all components of the gravity gradient tensor were theoretically estimated by the method of Mickus and Hinojosa [26], we also obtained components of the gravity gradient tensor by numerical differentiation of g_x, g_y, and g_z in the space domain, since short wavelength noise due to differentiation in the Fourier domain can sometimes be generated. The gravitation vector was, however, calculated using the method of Mickus and Hinojosa [26].

5. Results and discussion

5.1. Edge emphasis

In this section, we applied the 10 edge emphasis techniques shown in Section 3.1 to the field data. The results obtained by each method are shown in **Figures 7–16**.

The maps of the horizontal gravity gradient (*HG*: Eq. (32)), the vertical gravity gradient (*VG:* g_{zz}), and the second vertical derivative ($\partial^2 g_z/\partial z^2$, or g_{zzz}) are shown in **Figures 7–9**, respectively. The horizontal gravity gradient map extracts the outlines of the Hohi Volcanic Zone, the Shishimuta caldera, and the Aso caldera. In addition to these caldera or volcanic depressions, tectonic lines such as the Median Tectonic Line and Oita-Kumamoto Tectonic Line, which are important structures in this region, are also extracted (**Figure 7**). These lineaments were extracted as a high gravity gradient belt with an NE-SW trend crossing the Aso caldera. The land area of the belt corresponds to the Oita-Kumamoto Tectonic Line, and the sea area of the belt corresponds to the Median Tectonic Line. The Median Tectonic Line is the largest tectonic line in the southwest Japan, and it is known that the tectonic line has moved as a right lateral fault with normal faulting in the Quaternary. Furthermore, we also detect a large circular belt with a high gravity gradient outside of the high gradient belt that represents the Shishimuta caldera.

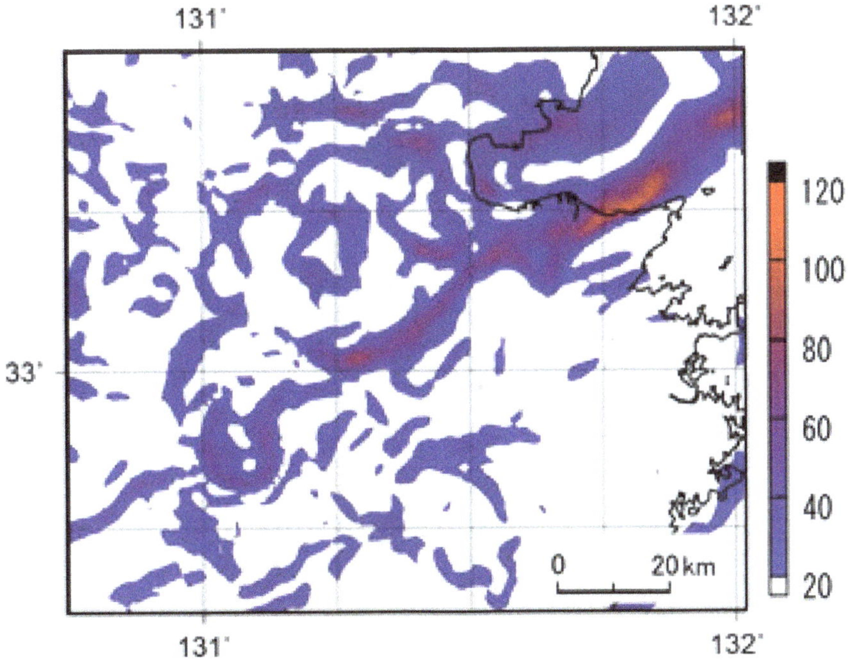

Figure 7. Horizontal gravity gradient map for values over 20 E. Units are given in E (Eötvös). Colored areas indicate locations of structural boundaries such as faults or contacts between different materials.

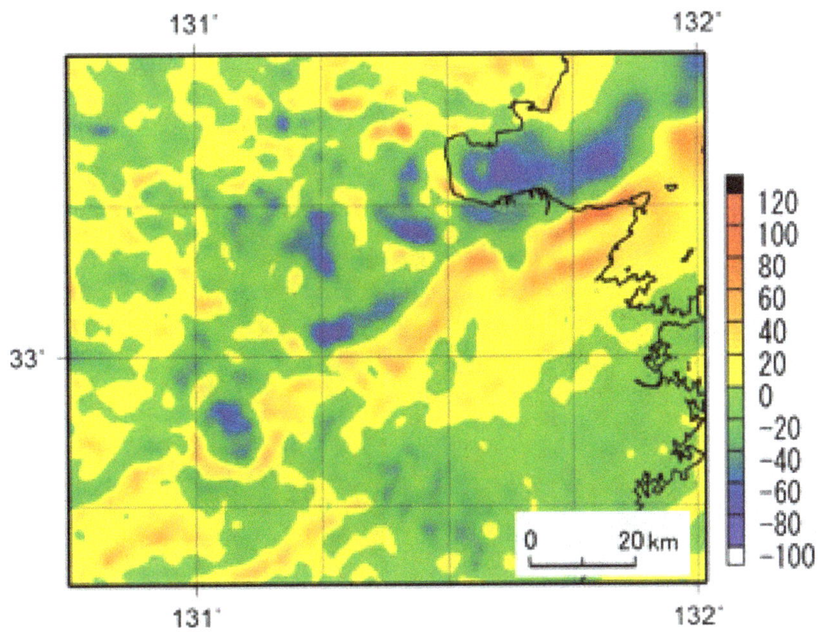

Figure 8. Vertical gravity gradient (g_{zz}) map. Units are given in E (Eötvös). Vertical gravity gradient evaluates vertical gradient of the Bouguer gravity anomaly, and estimates geological or structure boundary by line $g_{zz} = 0$.

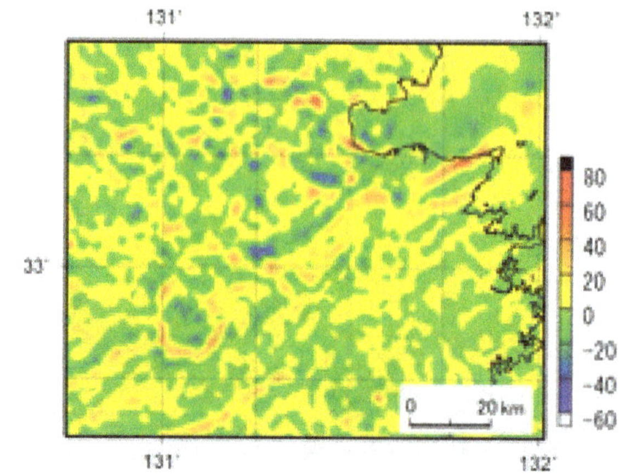

Figure 9. Vertical gravity gradient (second differential coefficient: $\partial^2 g_z/\partial z^2$, g_{zzz}) map. Units are given in E/km. E (Eötvös) is unit of the gravity gradient tensor, and 1 E = 0.1 mGal/km. This map indicates geological or structure boundary more sharply than g_{zz}.

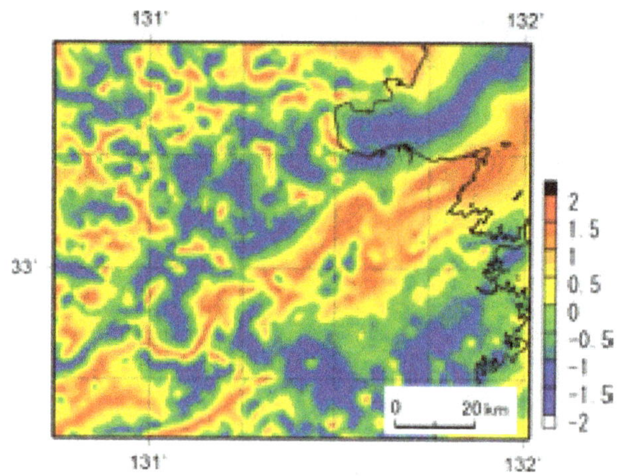

Figure 10. *TDR* map. Units are radians. This map indicates geological or structure boundary by line *TDR* = 0.

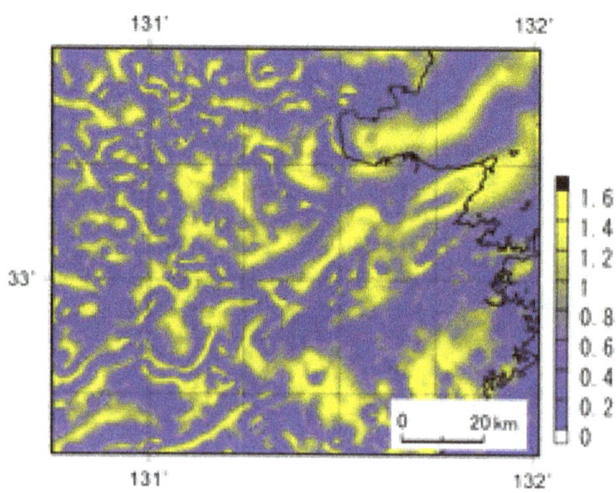

Figure 11. *THETA* map. Units are radians. This map indicates geological or structure boundary by line *THETA* = 0.

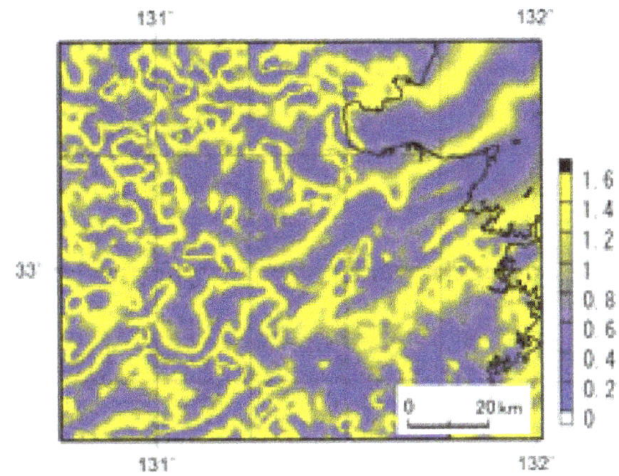

Figure 12. *TDX* map. Units are radians. This map indicates geological or structure boundary by line *TDX* = max (here, *TDX* = 1.6).

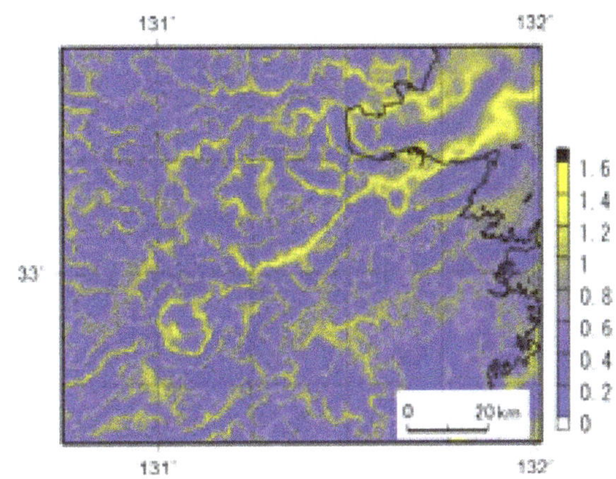

Figure 13. *CLP* map. Units are radians. This map indicates geological or structure boundary by line *CLP* = max (here, *CLP* = 1.6).

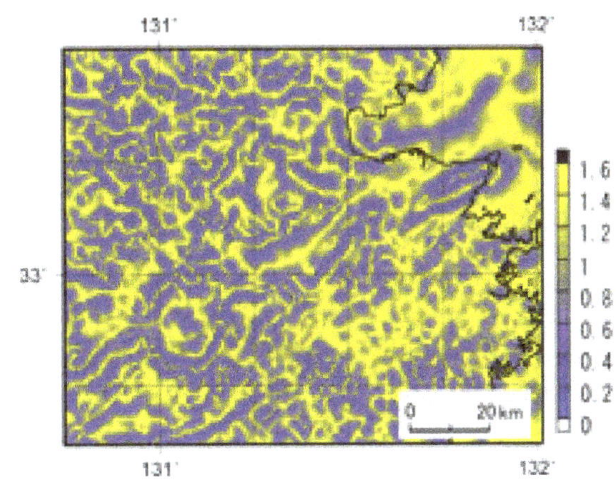

Figure 14. *ILP* map. Units are radians. This map extracts the edge of the gravity anomaly related to multi subsurface structures.

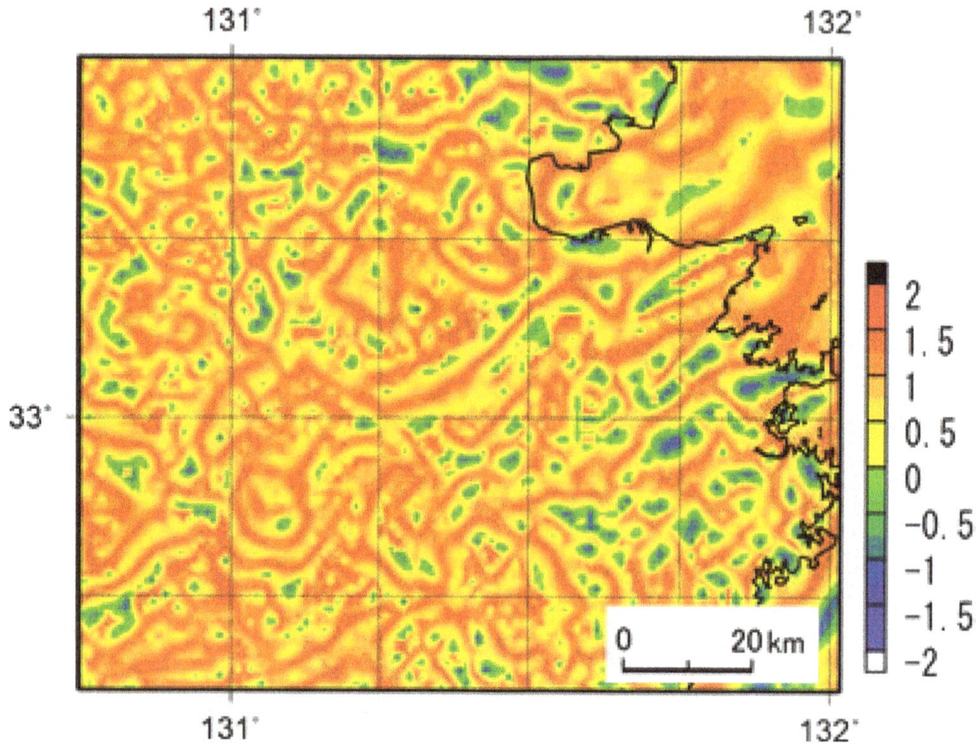

Figure 15. *TAHG* map. Units are radians. This map extracts the edge of the gravity anomaly related to multi subsurface structures.

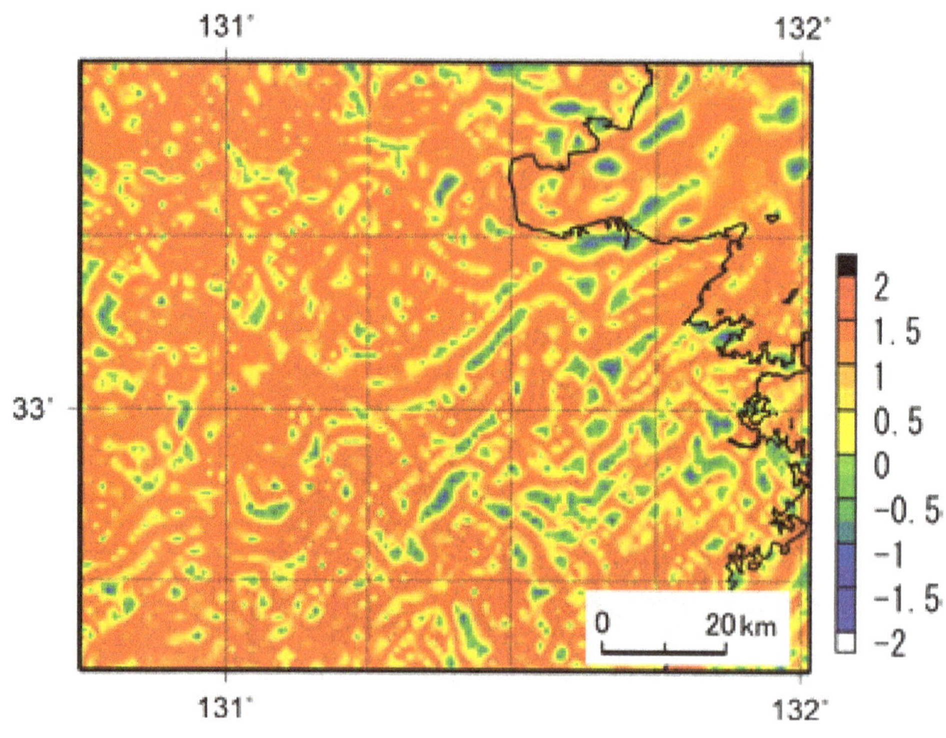

Figure 16. *THVH* map. Units are radians. This map extracts the edge of the gravity anomaly related to multi subsurface structures.

The vertical gravity gradient extracts the boundaries of the low gravity and high gravity areas, and emphasizes areas of low density (**Figure 8**). In particular, the caldera rim of the Aso caldera and boundaries of the tectonic lines and sedimentary basins are clearly extracted. In addition, areas of low-density material such as ash, pyroclastic flows, and sediments are accurately predicted and emphasized, and correspond to the inner areas of the Aso caldera, Shishimuta caldera, Kuju basin, Shonai basin, and Beppu Bay. The g_{zzz} map (**Figure 9**) shows each rim of the Aso caldera and Shishimuta caldera more clearly and emphasizes shorter wavelength signals. However, it seems that this technique does not highlight the density structures as effectively as the vertical gravity gradient, g_{zz}.

The maps of the *TDR* (Eq. (33)), the *THETA* (Eq. (34)), the *TDX* (Eq. (35)), and the *CLP* (Eq. (36)) are shown in **Figures 10–13**, respectively. The *TDR* shows the original structural boundaries at zero lines [44]. If we obeyed this judgment criterion, the boundaries of the green and yellow areas would be the structural boundaries such as lineaments, faults, and caldera rims. And, if we did not persist in the criterion, from this *TDR* we can derive information on both the structural boundaries and the density structures extracted by *HG* and *VG*. In fact, the *TDR* shows local low gravity areas more clearly or in greater detail than the vertical gravity gradient map.

The *THETA* map, the *TDX* map, and the *CLP* map extract structural boundaries by lines. In particular, it appears that the *CLP* technique is an excellent boundary extraction technique as it extracts very distinctly the caldera rims of the Aso caldera and the Shishimuta caldera, as well as locations of the Median Tectonic Line and the Oita-Kumamoto Tectonic Line (**Figure 13**). In addition, we also observe the larger circular lines outside the yellow lines indicating the Shishimuta caldera rim and the Aso caldera rim. The larger circular line outside of the Shishimuta caldera was also shown in the horizontal gravity gradient (*HG*) map (**Figure 7**).

The maps of the *ILP* (Eq. (38)), *TAHG* (Eq. (39)), and *THVH* (Eq. (40)) are shown in **Figures 14–16**, respectively. These techniques have been developed for finding the edges of the potential field related to multi subsurface structures, and generally they emphasize very small signals caused by the deep structures. The *ILP* map extracts the Aso caldera rim, but it is difficult to interpret what the other strong short wavelength lines represent. The *TAHG* and *THVH* maps are similar to the *ILP* map and have similar interpretation difficulties.

5.2. Curvature analysis

Figures 17 and **18** are the dimensionality index map and the shape index map. The dimensionality index map indicates whether the subsurface structure in the region is 2D, such as a vertical or subvertical dike or fault, or 3D, such as a dome structure. If the subsurface structure is 2D, the dimensionality index, $I < 0.5$. Since areas of $I \leq 0.5$ are widely distributed in **Figure 17**, we can conclude that the subsurface structures in the study area predominantly consist of 2D structures. However, in the inner area of the Shishimuta caldera rim, the dimensionality index is more than 0.7, and 3D structures are therefore predicted (**Figure 17**). In addition, the dimensionality index is also more than 0.7 in part of the inner area of the Aso caldera rim. This area corresponds to the volcanic cone group in the Aso caldera.

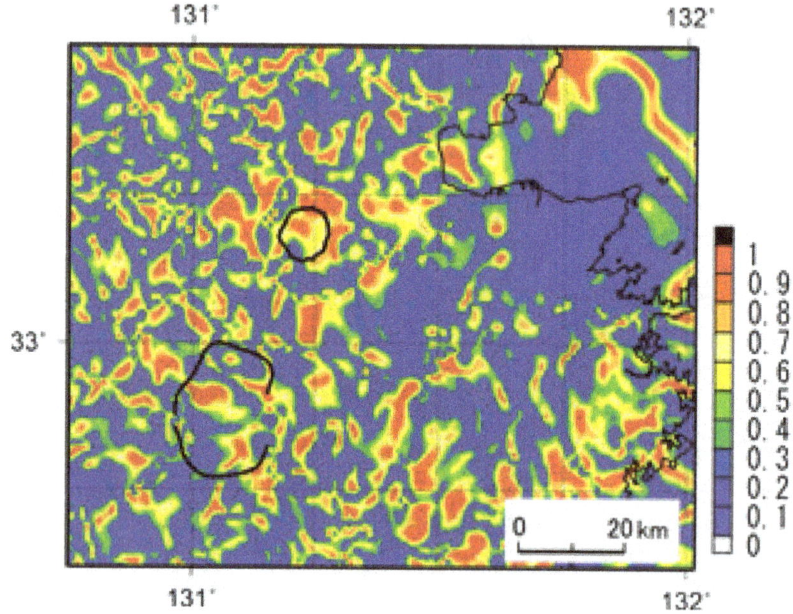

Figure 17. Map of dimensionality index, *I*. 2D structures are predicted in areas where $I < 0.5$. Locations of the caldera rim are shown by black lines. The northern small caldera is the Shishimuta caldera and its diameter is 8–10 km. The southern large caldera is the Aso caldera and its diameter is approximately 25 km in the south-north direction and about 18 km in the east-west direction.

The shape index in the Shishimuta caldera rim reaches –1 (**Figure 18**). This indicates that the potential shape of the low-density material is either bowl-like, a downward convex structure, or both. In fact, since Kamata [81] predicted that the Shishimuta caldera would be a funnel type caldera, the obtained results are considered suitable. Furthermore, these results are compatible with the result shown in **Figure 17**; the inner structure of the Shishimuta caldera would be 3D. In addition, locally low shape index areas are distributed around the Shishimuta caldera.

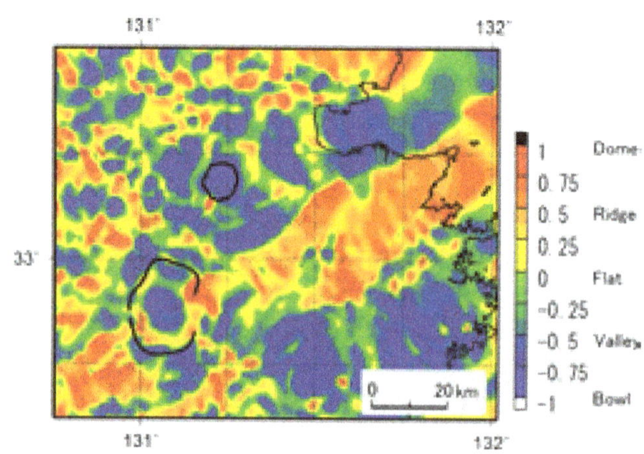

Figure 18. Shape index map. Values of –1, –0.5, 0, +0.5, and +1 indicate bowl, valley, flat, ridge, and dome structures, respectively. Locations of the caldera rim are shown by black lines. The northern small caldera is the Shishimuta caldera and its diameter is 8–10 km. The southern large caldera is the Aso caldera and its diameter is approximately 25 km in the south-north direction and about 18 km in the east-west direction.

In the Aso caldera, the shape index is in the range of –1 to +1. This indicates that the subsurface structures would be complex since the Aso caldera has experienced four caldera formations. Moreover, areas of locally low shape index less than –0.75 correspond to the five local minor gravity lows found by Komazawa [87].

5.3. Euler deconvolution

We employed here the Tensor Euler deconvolution [68] to obtain information on the subsurface structures. In the calculation, we set a 24 km width window (the required amount of data to solve Eq. (9) is 576) with a structure index of 0.001. Generally, a structure index of 0 is employed for sills, dikes, and faults (e.g., [88]), but calculations with this value did not give solutions in our study field. The value of 0.001 was obtained through trail and error.

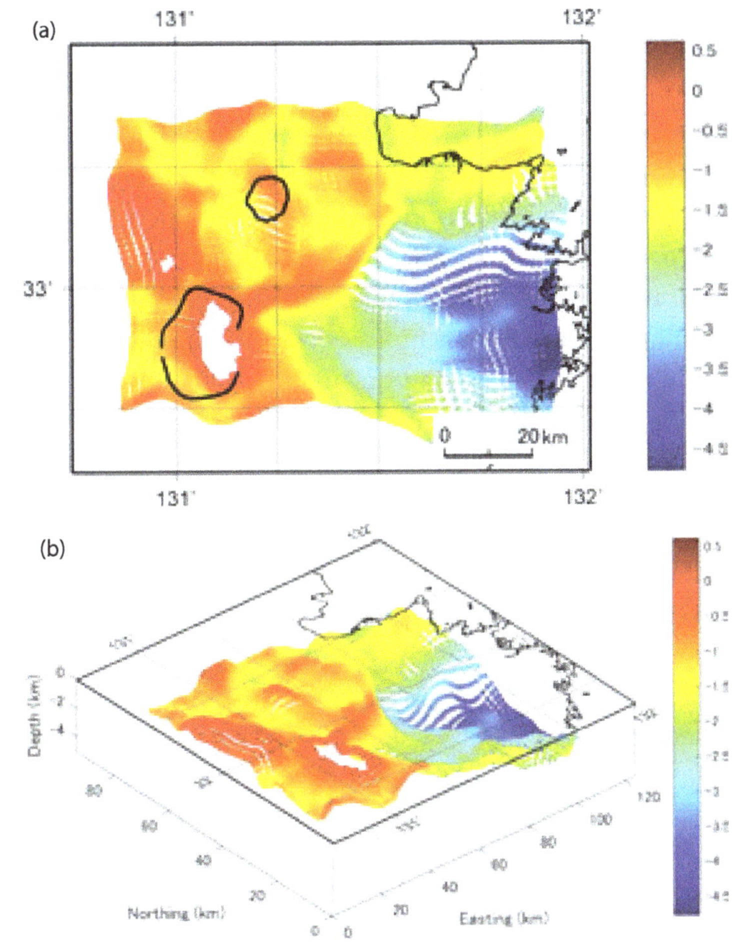

Figure 19. Solution clouds given by the Tensor Euler deconvolution. In the calculation, a 14km width window and a structure index of 0.5 are assumed. (a) Distribution of the solutions in map view. Units are km. Locations of the caldera rim are shown by black lines. The northern small caldera is the Shishimuta caldera and its diameter is 8–10 km. The southern large caldera is the Aso caldera and its diameter is approximately 25 km in the south-north direction and about 18 km in the east-west direction. (b) Distribution of the solutions in bird's-eye view. Units are km.

In **Figure 19**, we show the solution clouds given by the Tensor Euler deconvolution. We identify a deep and flat structure like a sedimentary basin at the east of the Aso caldera. There are large structural gaps between this structure and the Hohi Volcanic Zone, and the gaps appear to resemble a cliff (**Figure 19b**). In the Aso caldera, structural boundaries within the caldera are extracted as a void area of the solutions. However, these inner boundaries were not extracted in the Shishimuta caldera. In addition, we detect a large circular wall structure surrounding the Shishimuta caldera. Although partially observable in map view (**Figure 19a**), the structure is more clearly distinguished in bird's-eye view (**Figure 19b**).

5.4. Dip estimation

Dips of faults and/or structural boundaries were estimated in the areas that satisfied the conditions I (dimensionality index) < 0.5 and HG (horizontal gravity gradient) ≥ 20 E (**Figure 20**). From **Figure 20**, we found that dip of the Median Tectonic Line and Oita-Kumamoto Tectonic Line are in the range of 40–70°, and are interpreted as high angle faults. In part of the Median Tectonic Line, the dip is very high, exceeding 70°. Since it is known that the Median Tectonic Line moved as a right lateral fault with normal faulting in the Quaternary, it is reasonable that this tectonic line has a high dip reaching 70° or 80°. The dip of the Median Tectonic Line becomes gradually lower to the north, toward Beppu Bay area. Seismic reflection surveys (e.g., [89]) confirm that dip of normal faults distributed in the Beppu Bay are <45°. Consequently, the obtained dip distribution is consistent with the observed data, suggesting that this technique is a useful semiautomatic interpretation method. In our results, the dip of the Oita-Kumamoto Tectonic Line is estimated to be approximately 60°, but its actual dip is unknown. Since, for many numerical simulations evaluating deformation fields by fault motions, the dip of the fault plays an important role, this technique will give us useful information on fault shape even if the result is a first approximation solution.

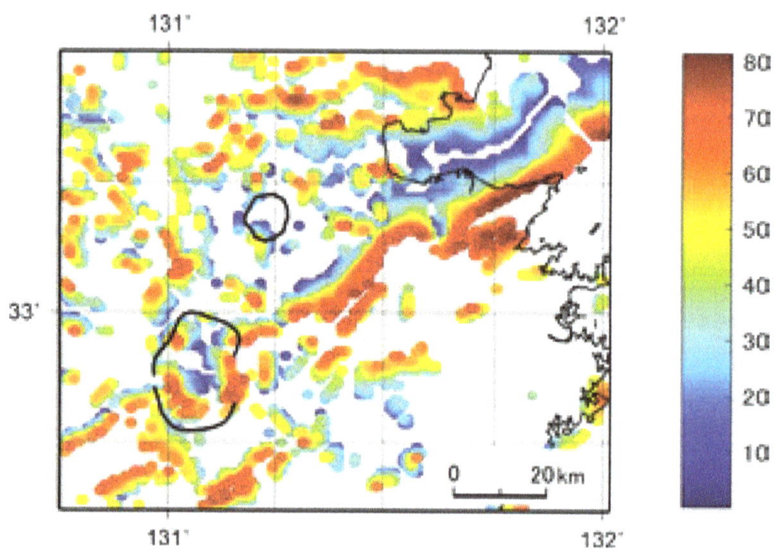

Figure 20. Distribution of estimated dip of faults and/or structural boundaries. Locations of the caldera rim are shown by black lines. The northern small caldera is the Shishimuta caldera and its diameter is 8–10 km. The southern large caldera is the Aso caldera and its diameter is approximately 25 km in the south-north direction and about 18 km in the east-west direction. Dip estimation was conducted for the areas that satisfied the conditions I < 0.5 and HG (horizontal gravity gradient) ≥ 20 E.

In the Aso caldera, dip of its caldera wall are in the range of 50–70° (inward dipping), as shown in **Figure 20**. Dips become gradually lower toward the caldera center, which is almost flat. These subsurface structural characteristics in the inner area of the Aso caldera have already been observed by detailed gravity analysis [87], and our results and Komazawa's results support to each other. However, this is the first time that caldera wall dips have been explicitly determined. In the Shishimuta caldera, because the condition of the dimensionality index was not satisfied, the distribution of caldera wall dips could not be estimated. Since the dip of the caldera wall leads to a discussion of the radius of the magma chamber, the process of caldera formation, and the type of caldera (e.g., [9, 14, 19–20]), the dip of the wall is thought to be as important as the fault dip.

The dips of the large circular wall structure surrounding the Shishimuta caldera are in the range of approximately 45–60° (inward dipping). This large structure appears in *HG* (**Figure 7**), *VG* (**Figure 8**), *TDR* (**Figure 10**), *CLP* (**Figure 13**), shape index (**Figure 18**), and Tensor Euler deconvolution (**Figure 19**) data, and it has a diameter of approximately 35 km. Since the Hohi Volcanic Zone was formed by eruption of more than 5000 km^3 or material during six million years (e.g., [73]), it is suggested that this structure represents a depression or group of depressions resulting from these eruptions. However, because the obvious sedimentary basins such as the Kuju basin and the Shonai basin are included within this area, more detailed surveys and studies would be required to discuss this large structure surrounding the Shishimuta caldera.

6. Conclusions

By obtaining the gravity gradient tensor from the gravity anomaly, we can use a variety of techniques to extract subsurface structures. In this study, we reviewed semiautomatic interpretation methods using the gravity gradient tensor, and applied some of the techniques to the volcanic zone of central Kyushu, Japan. This area consists of the Aso caldera and the Hohi Volcanic Zone containing a buried caldera, the Shishimuta caldera, and has large tectonic lines such as the Median Tectonic Line and the Oita-Kumamoto Tectonic Line, and tectonic sedimentary basins such as the Beppu Bay, the Kuju basin, and the Shonai basin.

Most edge detection methods extracted the outlines of these structures, and some of them indicated density structures. In spite of classical methods, the horizontal gravity gradient method and the vertical gravity gradient method were excellent edge detection methods. As for recent methods, the *CLP* method clearly extracted structural boundaries such as the caldera rim and tectonic lines as lines.

In the curvature analysis, we obtained useful information from the shape index and the dimensionality index that indicated caldera shape. In the estimation of the dip of structural boundaries using the eigenvector of the gravity gradient tensor, we obtained the fault dip of the Median Tectonic Line, which is consistent with seismic reflection surveys, and estimated the caldera wall dip of the Aso caldera, which corresponds to that obtained by detailed gravity analysis.

Through these data analyses, we distinguished a large circular structure with a diameter of 35 km surrounding the Shishimuta caldera. This structure appeared also in solution clouds obtained by the Tensor Euler deconvolution. However, we cannot confidently judge what this structure represents using only the gravity gradient tensor. More detailed surveys and studies are required to further discuss this issue.

Acknowledgements

This work was supported partially by JSPS (Japan Society for the Promotion of Science) KAKENHI Grant Number 15K14274. The author is grateful to the agency. The author is also most grateful to Agust Gudmundsson for very useful comments that have considerably improved the manuscript. In addition, the author is most grateful to Karoly Nemeth and Dajana Pemac for their editorial advices and cooperation.

Author details

Shigekazu Kusumoto

Address all correspondence to: kusu@sci.u-toyama.ac.jp

Graduate School of Science and Technology for Research, University of Toyama, Toyama, Japan

References

[1] Smith R L, Bailey R A. Resurgent calderas. Geological Society of America Memoirs 1968; 116: 613–662.

[2] Druitt T H, Sparks R S. On the formation of calderas during ignimbrite eruptions. Nature 1984; 310: 679–681.

[3] Lipman P W. Subsidence of ash-flow calderas: relation to caldera size and magma-chamber geometry. Bulletin of Volcanology 1997; 59: 198–218.

[4] Geshi N, Shimano T, Chiba T, Nakada S. Caldera collapse during the 2000 eruption of Miyakejima Volcano, Japan. Bulletin of Volcanology 2002; 64: 55–68. doi:10.1007/s00445-001-0184-z.

[5] Gudmundsson, A. Magma-chamber geometry, fluid transport, local stress and rock behavior during collapse caldera formation. In: Gottsmann J, Marti J, editors. Caldera

volcanism – analysis, modelling and response. Amsterdam: Elsevier; 2008. p. 313–349. doi:10.1016/S1871-644X(07)00008-3.

[6] Komuro, H. Experiments on caldron formation: a polygonal cauldron and ring fractures. Journal of Volcanology and Geothermal Research 1987; 31: 139–149.

[7] Marti J, Ablay G J, Redshaw L T, Sparks R S J. Experimental studies of collapse calderas. Journal of the Geological Society, London 1994; 151: 919–929.

[8] Acocella V, Cifelli F, Funiciello R. Analogue models of collapse calderas and resurgent domes. Journal of Volcanology and Geothermal Research 2000; 104: 81–96.

[9] Roche O, Druitt T H, Merle O. Experimental study of caldera formation. Journal of Geophysical Research 2000; 105: 395–416.

[10] Walter T R, Troll V R. Formation of caldera periphery faults: an experimental study. Bulletin of Volcanology 2001; 63: 191–203.

[11] Troll V R, Walter T R, Schmincke H U. Cycle caldera collapse: piston or piecemeal subsidence ? Field and experimental evidence. Geology 2002; 30: 135–138.

[12] Ruch J, Acocella V, Geshi N, Nobile A, Corbi F. Kinematic analysis of vertical collapse on volcanoes using experimental models time series. Journal of Geophysical Research 2012; 117: B07301. doi:10.1029/2012JB009229.

[13] Gudmundsson A. Formation and development of normal fault calderas and the initiation of large explosive eruptions. Bulletin of Volcanology 1998; 60: 160–170.

[14] Roche O, Druitt T H. Onset of caldera collapse during ignimbrite eruptions. Earth and Planetary Science Letters 2001; 191: 191–202.

[15] Folch A, Marti J. Geometrical and mechanical constraints on the formation of ring-fault calderas. Earth and Planetary Science Letters 2004; 221: 215–225.

[16] Hardy S. Structural evolution of calderas: insights from two-dimensional discrete element simulations. Geology 2008; 36: 927–930. doi:10.1130/G25133A.1.

[17] Holohan E P, Schôpfer M P J, Walsh J J. Mechanical and geometric controls on the structural evolution of pit crater and caldera subsidence. Journal of Geophysical Research 2011; 116: B07202. doi:10.1029/2010JB008032.

[18] Kusumoto S, Takemura K. Numerical simulation of caldera formation due to collapse of a magma chamber. Geophysical Research Letters 2003; 30: 2278, doi10.1029/2003GL018380.

[19] Kusumoto S, Takemura K. Caldera geometry determined by the depth of the magma chamber. Earth Planets and Space 2005; 57: e17–e20.

[20] Kusumoto S, Gudmundsson A. Magma-chamber volume changes associated with ring-fault initiation using a finite-sphere model: application to the Aira caldera, Japan. Tectonophysics 2009; 471: 58–66. doi:10.1016/jtecto.2008.09.001.

[21] Browning J, Gudmundsson A. Caldera faults capture and deflect inclined sheets: an alternative mechanism of ring dike formation. Bulletin of Volcanology 2015; 77: 1–13. doi:10.1007/s00445-014-0889-4.

[22] Barnes G, Barraud J. Imaging geologic surfaces by inverting gravity gradient data with depth horizons. Geophysics 2012; 77: G1–G11.

[23] Uieda L, Barbosa V C F, Robust 3D gravity gradient inversion by planting anomalous densities. Geophysics 2012; 77: G55–G66.

[24] Lu W, Qian J. A local level-set method for 3D inversion of gravity-gradient data. Geophysics 2015; 80: G35–G51.

[25] Martinetz C, Li Y, Krahenbuhl R, Braga M A. 3D inversion of airborne gravity gradiometry data in mineral exploration: a case study in the Quadrilatero Ferrifero, Brazil. Geophysics 2013; 78: B1–B11.

[26] Mickus K L, Hinojosa J H. The complete gravity gradient tensor derived from the vertical component of gravity: a Fourier transform technique. Journal of Applied Geophysics 2001; 46: 159–174.

[27] Torge W. Gravimetry. Berlin: Walter de Gruyter; 1989. 465 p.

[28] Hofmann-wellenhof B, Moritz H. Physical Geodesy. Berlin: Springer; 2005. 403 p.

[29] Lee J B. Falcon gravity gradiometer technology. Exploration Geophysics 2001; 32: 247–250.

[30] Barnes G, Lumley J. Processing gravity gradient data. Geophysics 2011; 76: I33–I47.

[31] Dransfield M H, Christensen A N. Performance of airborne gravity gradiometers. The Leading Edge 2013; 32: 908–922. doi:10.1190/tle32080908.1.

[32] Blakely R J. Potential theory in gravity and magnetic applications. Cambridge: Cambridge University Press; 1996. 441 p.

[33] Nabighian M N. The analytic signal of two-dimensional magnetic bodies with polygonal cross-section: its properties and use for automated anomaly interpretation. Geophysics 1972; 37: 507–517.

[34] Cordell L, McCafferty A E. A terracing operator for physical property mapping with potential field data. Geophysics 1989; 54: 621–634.

[35] Cooper G R J. The removal of unwanted edge contours from gravity datasets. Exploration Geophysics 2012; 44: 42–47.

[36] Blakely R, Simpson R W. Approximating edges of source bodies from magnetic or gravity anomalies. Geophysics 1986; 51: 1494–1498.

[37] Shichi R, Yamamoto A, Kimura A, Aoki H. Gravimetric evidences for active faults around Mt. Ontake, central Japan: specifically for the hidden faulting of the 1984

Western Nagano Prefecture Earthquake. Journal of Physics of the Earth 1992; 40: 459–478.

[38] Kudo T, Kono Y. Relationship between distributions of shallow earthquakes and gradient of gravity anomaly field in southwest Japan. Zishin 2 1999; 52: 341–350 (in Japanese with English abstract).

[39] Yamamoto A. Gravity anomaly atlas of the Ishikari Plain and its vicinity, Hokkaido, Japan. Geophysical Bulletin of Hokkaido 2003; 66: 33–62 (in Japanese with English abstract).

[40] Elkins T A. The second derivative method of gravity interpretation. Geophysics 1951; 16: 29–50.

[41] Tsuboi C, Kato M. The first and second vertical derivatives of gravity. Journal of Physics of the Earth 1952; 1: 95–96.

[42] Bott M H P. A simple criterion for interpreting negative gravity anomalies. Geophysics 1962; 27: 376–381.

[43] ten Brink U S, Ben-Avarham Z, Bell R E, Hassouneh M, Coleman D F, Andreasen F, Tibor G, Coakley, B. Structure of the Dead Sea pull-apart basin from gravity analyses. Journal of Geophysical Research 1993; 98: 21877–21894.

[44] Miller H G, Singh V. Potential field tilt – a new concept for location of potential field sources. Journal of Applied Geophysics 1994; 32: 213–217.

[45] Cooper G R J, Cowan D R. Enhancing potential field data using filters based on the local phase. Computers and Geosciences 2006; 32: 1585–1591.

[46] Ma G. Edge detection of potential field data using improved local phase filter. Exploration Geophysics 2013; 44: 36–41.

[47] Wijns C, Perez C, Kowalezyk P. Theta map: edge detection in magnetic data. Geophysics 2005; 70: L39–L43.

[48] Li L, Huang D, Han L, Ma G. Optimized detection filters in the interpretation of potential field data. Exploration Geophysics 2014; 45: 171–176. doi:10.1071/EG13059.

[49] Ferreira F J F, de Souza J, de B e S Bongiolo A, de Castro L G. Enhancement of the total horizontal gradient of magnetic anomalies using the tilt angle. Geophysics 2013; 78: J33–J41.

[50] Zhang X, Yu P, Tang R, Xiang Y, Zhao C-J. Edge enhancement of potential field data using an enhanced tilt angle. Exploration Geophysics 2014; 46: 276–283. doi:10.1071/EG13104.

[51] Kusumoto S. Semi-automatic interpretation methods for extracting structural boundaries using gravity gradient tensors. Butsuri-Tansa 2016; 69: 53–64 (in Japanese with English abstract).

[52] Perdersen L B, Rasmussen T M. The gradient tensor of potential field anomalies: some implications on data collection and data processing of maps. Geophysics 1990; 55: 1558–1566.

[53] Beiki M, Pedersen L B. Eigenvector analysis of gravity gradient tensor to locate geologic bodies. Geophysics 2010; 75, I37–I49.

[54] Cevallos C, Kovac P, Lowe S J. Application of curvatures to airborne gravity gradient data in oil exploration. Geophysics 2013; 78: G81–G88.

[55] Cevallos C. Automatic generation of 3D geophysical models using curvatures derived from airborne gravity gradient data. Geophysics 2014; 79: G49–G58.

[56] Koenderink J J, van Doorn A J. Surface shape and curvature scales. Image and Vision Computing 1992; 10: 557–564.

[57] Robert A. Curvature attributes and their application to 3D interpreted horizons. First Break 2001; 19: 85–99.

[58] Beiki M, Analytic signals of gravity gradient tensor and their application to estimate source location. Geophysics 2010; 75: I59–I74.

[59] Sertcelik I, Kafadar O. Application of edge detection to potential field data using eigenvalue analysis of structure tensor. Journal of Applied Geophysics 2012; 84: 86–94.

[60] Zhou W, Du X, Li J. The limitation of curvature gravity gradient tensor for edge detection and a method for overcoming it. Journal of Applied Geophysics 2013; 98: 237–242.

[61] Orç B, Sertçelik I, Kafadar Ö, Selim H H. Structural interpretation of the Erzurum Basin, eastern Turkey, using curvature gravity gradient tensor and gravity inversion of basement relief. Journal of Applied Geophysics 2013; 88: 105–113.

[62] Yuan Y, Huang D, Yu Q, Li P. Edge detection of potential field data with improved structure tensor methods. Journal of Applied Geophysics 2014; 108: 35–42.

[63] Li X. Curvature of a geometric surface and curvature of gravity and magnetic anomalies. Geophysics 2015; 80: G15–G26.

[64] Thompson D T. EULDPH – a new technique for making computer assisted depth estimates from magnetic data. Geophysics 1982; 47: 31–37.

[65] Barongo J O. Euler's differential equation and the identification of the magnetic point-pole and point-dipole sources. Geophysics 1984; 49: 1549–1553.

[66] Reid A B, Allsop J M, Granser H, Millett A J, Somerton I W. Magnetic interpretation in three dimensions using Euler deconvolution. Geophysics 1990; 55: 80–91.

[67] Marson I, Klingele E E. Advantages of using the vertical gradient of gravity for 3-D interpretation. Geophysics 1993; 58: 1588–1595.

[68] Zhang C, Mushayandebvu M F, Reid A B, Fairhead J D, Odegrad M E. Euler deconvolution of gravity tensor gradient data. Geophysics 2000; 65: 512–520.

[69] Beiki M. TSVD analysis of Euler deconvolution to improve estimating magnetic source parameters: an example from the Asele area, Sweden. Journal of Applied Geophysics 2013; 90: 82–91.

[70] Kusumoto S. Estimation of dip angle of fault or structural boundary by eigenvectors of gravity gradient tensors. Butsuri-Tansa 2015; 68: 277–287 (in Japanese with English abstract).

[71] Komazawa M. Gravity grid database of Japan. ver. 2, Digital Geoscience Map P-2 [CD-ROM]. Tsukuba: Geological Survey of Japan; 2004.

[72] Research Group for Active Faults. The Active Faults in Japan: Sheet Maps and Inventories. Rev. ed. Tokyo: University of Tokyo Press; 1991. 437 p (in Japanese with English abstract).

[73] Kamata H. Volcanic and structural history of the Hohi volcanic zone, central Kyushu, Japan. Bulletin of Volcanology 1989; 51: 315–332.

[74] Komazawa M, Kamata H. The basement structure of the Hohi geothermal area obtained by gravimetric analysis in central-north Kyushu, Japan. Reports, Geological Survey of Japan 1985; 264: 305–333 (in Japanese).

[75] Kusumoto S, Fukuda Y, Takemoto S, Yusa Y. Three-dimensional subsurface structure in the eastern part of the Beppu-Shimabara Graben, Kyushu, Japan, as revealed by Gravimetric Data. Journal of the Geodetic Society of Japan 1996; 42: 167–181.

[76] Tsuboi C, Jitsukawa A, Tajima H. Gravity survey along the lines of precise levels throughout Japan by means of a Worden gravimeter. Bulletin of the Earthquake Research Institute, University of Tokyo 1956; Supplementary Volume IV, Part 8: 476–552.

[77] Itoh Y, Takemura K, Kamata H. History of basin formation and tectonic evolution at the termination of a large transcurrent fault system: deformation mode of central Kyushu, Japan. Tectonophysics 1998; 284: 135–150.

[78] Kusumoto S, Takemura K, Fukuda Y, Takemoto S. Restoration of the depression structure at the eastern part of central Kyushu, Japan, by means of the dislocation modeling. Tectonophysics 1999; 302: 287–296.

[79] Okada Y. Surface deformation due to shear and tensile faults in a half-space. Bulletin of Seismological Society of America 1985; 75: 1135–1154.

[80] Kusumoto S, Fukuda Y, Takemura K. A distinction technique between volcanic and tectonic depression structures based on the restoration modeling of gravity anomaly: a case study of the Hohi Volcanic Zone, central Kyushu, Japan. Journal of Volcanology and Geothermal Research 1999; 90: 183–189.

[81] Kamata H. Shishimuta caldera, the buried source of the Yabakei pyroclastic flow in the Hohi volcanic zone, Japan. Bulletin of Volcanology 1989; 51: 41–50.

[82] Kamata H, Danhara T, Yamashita T, Hoshizumi H, Hayashida A, Takemura K. Correlation of the Azuki Volcanic Ash of the Osaka Group and the Ku6C Volcanic Ash of the Kazusa Group to the Imaichi pyroclastic flow deposit in central Kyushu, Japan – a co-ignimbrite ash erupted from Shishimuta caldera. The Journal of the Geological Society of Japan 1994; 100: 848–866.

[83] Aramaki S. Hydrothermal determination of temperature and water pressure on the magma of Aira caldera, Japan. American Mineralogist 1971; 56: 1760–1768.

[84] Watanabe, K., 2010, Aso volcanoes, In: Sano, H. editor. Regional Geology of Japan, 8. Kyushu and Okinawa. Tokyo: Asakura; 2010. p. 267–271 (in Japanese).

[85] Kubotera A, Tajima H, Sumitomo N, Doi H, Izutsuya S. Gravity surveys on Aso and Kuju volcanic region, Kyushu district, Japan. Bulletin of the Earthquake Research Institute, University of Tokyo 1969; 47: 215–225.

[86] Yokoyama I. Volcanic caldera and meteorite craters with the special relation to their gravity anomalies. Journal of the Faculty of Science, Hokkaido University Ser. 7 1963; 2: 37–47.

[87] Komazawa M. Gravimetric analysis of Aso volcanoes and its interpretation, Journal of the Geodetic Society of Japan 1995; 41: 17–45.

[88] Rodrigues R S, de Castro D L, dos Reis J A Jr. Characterization of the Potiguar rift structure based on Euler deconvolution. Revista Brasileira de Geofisica 2014; 32: 109–121.

[89] Itoh Y, Kusumoto S, Takemura K. Evolutionary process of the Beppu Bay in central Kyushu, Japan: a quantitative study of basin-forming process under the control of plate convergence modes. Earth, Planets and Space 2014; 66: 74. doi:10.1186/1880-5981-66-74.

Permissions

All chapters in this book were first published in DSCLPC, by InTech Open; hereby published with permission under the Creative Commons Attribution License or equivalent. Every chapter published in this book has been scrutinized by our experts. Their significance has been extensively debated. The topics covered herein carry significant findings which will fuel the growth of the discipline. They may even be implemented as practical applications or may be referred to as a beginning point for another development.

The contributors of this book come from diverse backgrounds, making this book a truly international effort. This book will bring forth new frontiers with its revolutionizing research information and detailed analysis of the nascent developments around the world.

We would like to thank all the contributing authors for lending their expertise to make the book truly unique. They have played a crucial role in the development of this book. Without their invaluable contributions this book wouldn't have been possible. They have made vital efforts to compile up to date information on the varied aspects of this subject to make this book a valuable addition to the collection of many professionals and students.

This book was conceptualized with the vision of imparting up-to-date information and advanced data in this field. To ensure the same, a matchless editorial board was set up. Every individual on the board went through rigorous rounds of assessment to prove their worth. After which they invested a large part of their time researching and compiling the most relevant data for our readers.

The editorial board has been involved in producing this book since its inception. They have spent rigorous hours researching and exploring the diverse topics which have resulted in the successful publishing of this book. They have passed on their knowledge of decades through this book. To expedite this challenging task, the publisher supported the team at every step. A small team of assistant editors was also appointed to further simplify the editing procedure and attain best results for the readers.

Apart from the editorial board, the designing team has also invested a significant amount of their time in understanding the subject and creating the most relevant covers. They scrutinized every image to scout for the most suitable representation of the subject and create an appropriate cover for the book.

The publishing team has been an ardent support to the editorial, designing and production team. Their endless efforts to recruit the best for this project, has resulted in the accomplishment of this book. They are a veteran in the field of academics and their pool of knowledge is as vast as their experience in printing. Their expertise and guidance has proved useful at every step. Their uncompromising quality standards have made this book an exceptional effort. Their encouragement from time to time has been an inspiration for everyone.

The publisher and the editorial board hope that this book will prove to be a valuable piece of knowledge for researchers, students, practitioners and scholars across the globe.

List of Contributors

Aslıhan Uzel
Department of Orthodontics, Faculty of Dentistry, Cukurova University, Adana, Turkey

Aram J. Keteyian and Yuji Mishina
Department of Biologic and Materials Science, School of Dentistry, University of Michigan, Ann Arbor, MI, USA

Letizia Perillo and Fabrizia d'Apuzzo
Multidisciplinary Department of Medical-Surgical and Dental Specialties, Second University of Naples, Naples, Italy

Sara Eslami and Abdolreza Jamilian
Department of Orthodontics, Cranio Maxillofacial Research Center, Tehran Dental Branch, Islamic Azad University, Tehran, Iran

Alyssa Brzenski
University of California San Diego, San Diego, CA, USA

Ofelia Ham-Mancilla and Silvia Peña-Olvera
Instituto Nacional de Pediatría, Ciudad de México

Amanda Gosman
UC San Diego School of Medicine, University of California San Diego, San Diego, CA, USA

Alicia Sigler
Clínica Ambulatoria Shriners, Tijuana, Baja California, México

Enio Moura
Service of Medical Genetics, Faculty of Veterinary Medicine, School of Life Sciences, Pontifícia Universidade Católica do Paraná (PUCPR), Curitiba, Brazil

Cláudia Turra Pimpão
Department of Animal Science, School of Life Sciences, Pontifícia Universidade Católica do Paraná (PUCPR), Curitiba, Brazil

Mairaj Ahmed
Cleft/Craniofacial Center, Icahn School of Medicine at Mount Sinai, New York City, NY, USA

Yunfeng Xue
University of Texas McGovern Medical School, Houston, TX, USA

Ayisha Ayub
Cleft Hospital, Gujrat, Pakistan

Mustafa Chopan, Lohrasb Sayadi and Donald R. Laub
University of Vermont College of Medicine, Burlington, Vermont, USA

Nikolay P. Serdev
New Bulgarian University, Sofia, Medical Centre "Aesthetic Surgery and Aesthetic Medicine," Sofia, Bulgaria

An-Suey Shiao
Department of Otolaryngology-Head and Neck Surgery, Taipei Veterans General Hospital, Taipei, Taiwan, ROC Department of Otolaryngology, National Yang-Ming University, School of Medicine, Taipei, Taiwan, ROC

Chin-Lung Kuo
Department of Otolaryngology-Head and Neck Surgery, Taipei Veterans General Hospital, Taipei, Taiwan, ROC Department of Otolaryngology, National Yang-Ming University, School of Medicine, Taipei, Taiwan, ROC Institute of Brain Science, National Yang-Ming University, Taipei, Taiwan, ROC Department of Otolaryngology, Taoyuan Armed Forces General Hospital, Taoyuan, Taiwan, ROC

Mairaj K. Ahmed
Cleft/Craniofacial Center, Icahn School of Medicine at Mount Sinai, NY, NY, USA

Anthony H. Bui
Icahn School of Medicine at Mount Sinai, NY, NY, USA

Emanuela Taioli
Institute for Translational Epidemiology, Icahn School of Medicine at Mount Sinai, NY, NY, USA

Norifumi Nakamura and Masahiro Tezuka
Department of Oral and Maxillofacial Surgery, Field of Maxillofacial Rehabilitation, Kagoshima University Graduate School of Medical and Dental Sciences, Kagoshima, Japan

Shigekazu Kusumoto
Graduate School of Science and Technology for Research, University of Toyama, Toyama, Japan

Index

www.ingramcontent.com/pod-product-compliance
Lightning Source LLC
LaVergne TN
LVHW060539210926
848485LV00005B/1225